T0314067

Carpal Ligament Injuries and Instability

FESSH Instructional Course Book 2023

Fernando Corella, PhD
Associate Professor
Department of Surgery
Complutense University of Madrid;
Hand Surgeon
Wrist and Hand Unit
Traumatology Service
University Hospital Quirónsalud Madrid
Madrid, Spain

Carlos Heras-Palou, MD, FRCS (Tr & Orth)
Consultant Hand and Wrist Surgeon
Pulvertaft Hand Centre
Royal Derby Hospital
Derby, UK

Riccardo Luchetti, MD
Private Practice Hand Surgeon
Rimini Hand Surgery and Rehabilitation Center
Rimini, Italy

550 illustrations

Thieme
Stuttgart • New York • Delhi • Rio de Janeiro

Library of Congress Cataloging-in-Publication Data is available from the publisher.

Georg Thieme Verlag KG
Rüdigerstrasse 14, 70469 Stuttgart, Germany
+49 [0]711 8931 421, customerservice@thieme.de

Cover design: © Thieme
Cover image source: © Thieme/Massimiliano Crespi
Typesetting by TNQ Technologies, India

Printed in Germany by Beltz Grafische Betriebe   5 4 3 2 1

DOI: 10.1055/b000000804

ISBN: 978-3-13-245189-6

Also available as an e-book:
eISBN (PDF): 978-3-13-245190-2
eISBN (epub): 978-3-13-245191-9

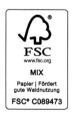

Contents

Contents

Section II: Assessment of the Wrist

Contents

Section IV: Lunotriquetral Injury and Instability

Contents

Section VI: Other Injuries

Videos

Video 22.5: The graft is out of the lunate, and we pull the graft to have a tight reconstruction. (Copyright Jan Ragnar Haugstvedt.)

Video 22.6: From the midcarpal joint we can view the LT interval while pulling the graft to see if the LT joint has been reduced and stabilized. (Copyright Jan Ragnar Haugstvedt.)

Video 22.7: This video shows an animation of the arthroscopic assisted LT lig procedure. It starts with harvesting one half of the ECU tendon. Then a guidewire is drilled through the lunate and when the position is good a 2.8 mm hole is drilled. A guide is placed in the hole in lunate, the guide is used to drill a second hole through the triquetrum. The tendon graft is then pulled through the bones using a tendon shuttle and we perform fixation of the graft using interference screws. Outside the capsule, the graft is then brought back to triquetrum where then tendon graft is sutured back to the ECU tendon. The reconstruction is finalized by reconstructing the DRC ligament. (Copyright Jan Ragnar Haugstvedt.)

Video 22.8: In a patient with coalition, we don't expect any motion across the LT interval. This video displays synovitis and motion in the joint that should have been stable. We find these changes to be signa of instability after a trauma. The patient complains of pain and in these special, seldom cases, we perform arthrodesis. (Copyright Jan Ragnar Haugstvedt.)

Video 22.9: After having resected the dorsal part of the LT joint, grafted bone into the resected part of the joint and have performed osteosynthesis to stabilize the joint, we check the stability from the midcarpal joint. (Copyright Jan Ragnar Haugstvedt.)

Video 26.1: Arthroscopically assisted reduction and fixation in an axial carpal dislocation. (Courtesy Dr. Fernando Corella and Dr. Montserrat Ocampos.)

Preface

Despite incredible advances in the field of wrist surgery, the assessment and management of wrist dysfunctions remain demanding tasks. History taking and clinical examination are still essential for diagnosis, confirmed and staged by imaging including radiographs, computed tomography scans, and magnetic resonance imaging, with or without contrast. Wrist arthroscopy has a well-established role in diagnosis and staging of wrist conditions, and an expanding role in therapeutic procedures.

The fast pace of growth of our knowledge of the precise anatomy and function of the wrist creates new and better treatments for our patients. Our understanding of proprioception is changing the options in conservative management of many wrist disorders and can prevent unnecessary surgery. The rehabilitation for our patients is developing and improving, with more and better protocols that are becoming evidence based.

Understanding detailed anatomy of the wrist allows us to have a better grasp of the mechanics of the wrist and stimulates the imagination of surgeons to improve some existing techniques and describe some new ones. In our careers, we have seen the standard treatment for most wrist conditions change several times; this will continue. Our clinical practice must keep up to date with advancements.

Wrist surgery is still a confusing field for surgeons and therapists, even more so for trainees trying to make sense of the myriad of treatments available. There are three reasons for this: first, the anatomy and mechanics are complicated; second, the semantics we use are misleading; and third, the dearth of published solid clinical outcomes and lack of high quality prospective clinical studies.

In this book we have tried to throw some light on the basic sciences as well as the management of wrist conditions, and for that we have brought together an amazing group of experts from all over the world who have shared their vast experience and knowledge. We are extremely grateful to all of them.

As the field of wrist surgery evolves, some treatments become obsolete and others turn into the standard of care. With this book we have tried to provide an update on ligament injuries of the wrist and the assessment and management of wrist instability. As a community of surgeons, it is important that we continue learning, improving, and innovating. We still have a lot to discover; everything is there to be done and everything is possible.

Fernando Corella, PhD
Carlos Heras-Palou, MD, FRCS (Tr & Orth)
Riccardo Luchetti, MD

Contributors

Cristóbal Martínez Andrade, MD
Hand and Upper Limb Unit
Hospital Quirónsalud Valencia
Valencia, Spain

Andrea Atzei, MD
Pro-Mano, Hand Surgery and Rehabilitation
Treviso, Italy

Vicente Carratalá Baixauli, MD
Hand and Upper Limb Unit
Hospital Quirónsalud Valencia
Valencia, Spain

Jean-Baptiste de Villeneuve Bargemon, MD
Hand and Limb Reconstructive Surgery
AP-HM Hospital de la Timone
Marseille, France

Eva-Maria Baur, MD
Practice
Department for Plastic and Hand Surgery Murnau
Penzberg, Germany

Marion Burnier, MD
Wrist Surgery Unit
Department of Orthopaedics
Claude-Bernard Lyon 1 University
Herriot Hospital
Lyon, France

Luis Cerezal, MD, PhD
Diagnóstico Médico Cantabria (DMC)
Santander, Spain

Jonathan P. Compson, MBBS, BSc, FRCS (Orth)
Consultant Orthopaedic Surgeon
Orthopaedic Department
King's College Hospital
London, UK

Fernando Corella, PhD
Associate Professor
Department of Surgery
Complutense University of Madrid;
Hand Surgeon
Wrist and Hand Unit
Traumatology Service, University Hospital
  Quirónsalud Madrid
Madrid, Spain

Pedro J. Delgado, MD
Head of Orthopaedic Surgery and
  Traumatology Department
Head of Hand Surgery and Microsurgery Unit
Hospital Universitario HM Montepríncipe
Hospital Universitario HM Nuevo Belén;
Associate Professor of Orthopaedics
Universidad San Pablo CEU College of Medicine
Madrid, Spain

Lauren E. Dittman, MD
Resident
Department of Orthopaedic Surgery
Mayo Clinic
Rochester, Minnesota, USA

Liron Duraku, MD
Fellow
The Peripheral Nerve Injury Service
University Hospitals Birmingham NHS
  Foundation Trust
Birmingham, UK;
Plastic, Reconstructive and Hand
  Surgery Department
Amsterdam University Medical Center
Amsterdam, The Netherlands

Mireia Esplugas, MD
Institut Kaplan
Barcelona, Spain

Francisco J. Lucas García, MD
Hand and Upper Limb Unit
Hospital Quirónsalud Valencia
Valencia, Spain

Marc Garcia-Elias, MD, PhD
Institut Kaplan
Barcelona, Spain

Max Haerle, MD, PhD
Professor
Director of Hand and Plastic Surgery Department
Orthopädische Klinik Markgröningen
Markgröningen, Germany

Elisabet Hagert, MD, PhD
Aspetar Orthopedic and Sports Medicine Hospital
Doha, Qatar;
Department of Clinical Science and Education
Karolinska Institutet
Stockholm, Sweden

Jan Ragnar Haugstvedt, MD, PhD
Senior Consultant
Østfold Hospital Trust
Moss, Norway
Oslo Hand Center
Oslo, Norway

**Mike Hayton, Bsc (Hons), MBChB, FRCS
  (Trauma and Orth), FFSEM (UK)**
Consultant Orthopaedic Hand Surgeon
Wrightington Hospital
Lancashire, UK

Carlos Heras-Palou, MD, FRCS (Tr & Orth)
Consultant Hand and Wrist Surgeon
Pulvertaft Hand Centre
Royal Derby Hospital
Derby, UK

Guillaume Herzberg, MD, PhD
Professor of Orthopaedic Surgery
Lyon Claude Bernard University
Herriot Hospital
Lyon, France

**Pak Cheong Ho, MBBS, FRCS (Edinburgh),
  FHKAM (Orthopaedic Surgery), FHKCOS**
Chief of Service
Department of Orthopaedic & Traumatology
Prince of Wales Hospital
Chinese University of Hong Kong
Hong Kong SAR

**Jeffrey Justin Siu Cheong Koo, MBBS (HK), FHKCOS,
  FHKAM (Orthopaedic Surgery), FRCSEd (Orth),
  MHSM (New South Wales), MScSMHS (CUHK)**
Associate Consultant (Orthopaedics Traumatology)
Department of Orthopaedics & Traumatology
Alice Ho Miu Ling Nethersole Hospital
Tai Po, Hong Kong

Hermann Krimmer, MD, PhD
Professor
Hand Center
Ravensburg, Germany

Florian Lampert, PD, MD
Senior Consultant
Orthopädische Klinik Markgröningen
Markgröningen, Germany

Martin Langer, MD
Professor
Department of Traumatology and Hand Surgery
University Clinic Münster
Münster, Germany

Eva Guisasola Lerma, MD
Hand and Upper Limb Unit
Hospital Quirónsalud Valencia
Valencia, Spain

Tommy R. Lindau, MD, PhD (Hand Surgery)
Professor
Consultant Hand Surgeon
Pulvertaft Hand Centre
Derby, UK;
Past President, European Wrist Arthroscopy
  Society (EWAS)

Bo Liu, MD
Department of Hand Surgery
Beijing Jishuitan Hospital
Peking University
Beijing, China

Alex Lluch, MD
Institut Kaplan;
Hand & Wrist Unit, Orthopaedics Department
Vall d'Hebron University Hospital
Barcelona, Spain

Manuel Llusa-Perez, MD, PhD
Full Professor
Department of Human Anatomy, Faculty of Medicine
University of Barcelona;
Orthopaedic Surgeon
Department of Orthopaedic Surgery
Hospital Vall d'Hebron
Barcelona, Spain

Riccardo Luchetti, MD
Private Practice Hand Surgeon
Rimini Hand Surgery and Rehabilitation Center
Rimini, Italy

Lyliane Ly, MD
Department of Orthopedic Surgery of the
    Upper Limb–SOS mains
Edouard Herriot Hospital
Lyon, France

Lorenzo Merlini, MD
International Wrist Center
Institut de la Main
Paris, France

Jane Messina, MD, PhD
ASST Gaetano Pini-CTO Orthopaedic Institute
Milan, Italy

Sara Montanari, MD
Rimini Hand Surgery and Rehabilitation Center
Rimini, Italy

M. Rosa Morro-Marti, MD, PhD
Associate Professor
Department of Human Anatomy, Faculty of Medicine
University of Barcelona;
Orthopaedic Surgeon
Department of Orthopaedic Surgery
Hospital Vall d'Hebron
Barcelona, Spain

Toshiyasu Nakamura, MD, PhD
Professor
Department of Orthopaedic Surgery
School of Medicine
International University of Health and Welfare
Tokyo, Japan

Frank Nienstedt, MD
Center for Surgery St. Anna
Merano, Italy

Montserrat Ocampos, PhD
Department of Orthopedics and Trauma
Hospital Universitario Infanta Leonor
Madrid, Spain

Thomas Pillukat, MD, PhD
Clinic for Hand Surgery
Rhön Klinikum AG
Bad Neustadt an der Saale, Germany

Pietro Randelli, MD
Professor of Trauma and Orthopaedic Surgery
Università degli Studi di Milano;
Direttore Scientiffico
Instituto Orthopedico Gaetano Pini
Milan University
Milan, Italy

Susanne Rein, MD, PhD, MBA
Department of Plastic and Hand Surgery, Burn Unit
Hospital Sankt Georg
Leipzig, Germany;
Martin-Luther-University Halle-Wittenberg
Halle, Germany

István Zoltán Rigó, MD, PhD
Østfold Hospital Trust
Moss, Norway
Oslo Hand Center
Oslo, Norway

David Ring, MD
Professor
Dell Medical School
The University of Texas at Austin
Austin, Texas, USA

Marco J.P.F. Ritt, MD
Professor
Plastic, Reconstructive and Hand
    Surgery Department
Amsterdam University Medical Center
Amsterdam, The Netherlands

Diogo Roriz, MD
JCC Diagnostic Imaging
Viana do Castelo, Portugal

Weston Ryan, MD
Orthopaedic Surgery Resident
Department of Orthopaedics
University of California, Davis School of Medicine
Sacramento, California

Guillem Salva-Coll, MD, PhD
Hand Surgery Unit, Orthopaedics Department
Hospital Universitari Son Espases;
IBACMA Hand Surgery Institute
Palma de Mallorca, Spain

Ana Scott-Tennent, MD
Upper Limb Unit, Trauma & Orthopedics Department
Arnau de Vilanova University Hospital
Lleida, Spain

Alexander Y. Shin, MD
Orthopedic Surgery
Mayo Clinic
Rochester, Minnesota, USA

Robert M. Szabo, MD, MPH
Distinguished Professor of Orthopaedics and
   Plastic Surgery
Department of Orthopaedics
University of California, Davis School of Medicine
Sacramento, California

Teun Teunis, MD
Assistant Professor
Department of Plastic Surgery
University Pittsburgh Medical Center
Pittsburgh, Pennsylvania, USA

Jörg van Schoonhoven, MD
Professor and Senior Consultant
Clinic for Hand Surgery
Rhön Klinikum AG
Bad Neustadt an der Saale, Germany

Rupert Wharton, BM, BSc, FRCS (Tr and Orth),
   Dip Hand Surg (Br and Eur)
Locum Consultant Trauma and
   Orthopaedic Surgeon
Kingston Hospital NHS Foundation Trust
Kingston, UK

Feiran Wu, MD
Birmingham Hand Centre
Queen Elizabeth Hospital
University Hospitals Birmingham
Birmingham, UK

Ezequiel Zaidenberg, MD
Consultant Hand and Wrist Surgeon
Sanatorio Otamendi
Buenos Aires, Argentina

Frantzeska Zampeli, MD, PhD
Hand-Upper Limb-Microsurgery Department
General Hospital "KAT"
Athens, Greece;
Aspetar Orthopaedic and Sports Medicine Hospital
Doha, Qatar

Eduardo R. Zancolli III, MD
Professor in Hand Surgery
Argentine Association for Hand Surgery
   Specialists' Career
Buenos Aires, Argentina;
Past President, Southamerican Federation for
   Surgery of the Hand
Past President, Argentine Association for
   Surgery of the Hand
President, 13th Triennial Congress of the IFSSH 2016

Section I

Anatomy and Biomechanics

1 Anatomy and Histology of Wrist Ligaments

Elisabet Hagert, Frantzeska Zampeli, and Susanne Rein

Abstract

A thorough appreciation of the anatomy and histology of wrist ligaments is the foundation to understand wrist biomechanics and the effects of trauma on wrist function. Wrist ligaments are divided into extra- and intracapsular ligaments, as well as extrinsic, connecting the forearm and the carpus, or intrinsic, connecting bones within the carpus, ligaments. The extrinsic ligaments of the wrist are: the volar radiocarpal, the volar ulnocarpal, and the dorsal radiocarpal ligaments. The intrinsic ligaments consist of the volar and dorsal midcarpal ligaments and the proximal and distal intercarpal ligaments. Ligaments generally have three main functions: (1) to provide passive mechanical stability to joints, thus guiding joints through their normal range of motion when tensile or compressive loads are applied; (2) viscoelasticity, which helps in preserving joint homeostasis; and (3) sensory function, where ligaments are recognized as sensory organs, capable of monitoring and supplying afferent kinesthetic and proprioceptive information. The principal function of a ligament is reflected in its histology, through varied contents of collagen and elastic fibers, as well as presence or absence of innervation. This chapter provides a review of wrist ligament anatomy and histology, with accompanying imaging of all wrist ligaments and microscopic imaging of different histology types.

Keywords: anatomy, carpus, histology, ligaments, wrist

1.1 Wrist Ligaments: Overview of Anatomy and Histology

1.1.1 Anatomy Overview

Wrist ligaments can be described according to their relation with the joint capsule. Three *extracapsular* ligaments are located outside the wrist capsule: (1) the transverse carpal ligament, (2) the pisohamate, and (3) the pisometacarpal ligaments. The majority of wrist ligaments are *intracapsular* or *intra-articular*. Intra-articular ligaments, those found entirely within the joint cavity, are distinguished from the intracapsular ligaments, ligaments composing, in part, the joint capsule, by the degree of coverage by a thin layer of synovial tissue, called synovial stratum. Intra-articular ligaments are covered entirely by synovial stratum, whereas intracapsular ligaments have the synovial stratum only on their deep or joint surface. Depending on which articulations are being linked, these ligaments have been classified as *extrinsic* or *intrinsic*.

Extrinsic ligaments originate from the distal epiphyses of forearm bones and insert on the carpal bones, while *intrinsic ligaments* have their origin and insertion on carpal bones, either of different (midcarpal ligaments) or the same row (intercarpal or interossei ligaments). Different histology of these ligaments accounts for different elastic properties and modes of failure. Extrinsic ligaments mainly insert on bones, are longer, more elastic, and less resistant to tension traction, i.e., lower yield strength, as compared to most intrinsic ligaments, and sustain more midsubstance ruptures rather than avulsions. On the contrary, intrinsic ligaments insert mostly on cartilage and are more frequently avulsed than ruptured. Interossei ligaments show similar failure pattern and are the shortest and stiffest of all ligament types[1,3] (▶ Fig. 1.1).

1.1.2 Histology Overview

The morphology of connective tissue components reflects their biomechanical functions, and histology may thus offer insight into their biomechanical functions and significance in wrist stability. In addition, knowledge of ligament structure is important for the reconstruction of injured ligaments in order to choose a similar substitute graft.[4]

Ligaments generally have three main functions: (1) to provide passive mechanical stability to joints, thus guiding joints through their normal range of motion when tensile or compressive loads are applied; (2) viscoelasticity, which helps in preserving joint homeostasis, which means that intraligamentous tension decreases if constant ligamentous deformation is applied and *"creep"* occurs as a result of elongation under a constant or cyclically repetitive load; and (3) sensory function, where ligaments are recognized as sensory organs, capable of monitoring and supplying afferent kinesthetic and proprioceptive data.[5,6,7,8]

The surface of ligaments is often covered up to the periosteum by a well-vascularized and innervated layer, the epiligament or epifascicular region (▶ Fig. 1.2a).[6,9,10] The arrangement of the collagen fibers reveals interlaced connective tissue types on the one hand and parallel-fibered tight connective tissue types on the other. In densely packed, interlaced, connective tissues, the collagen fibers run as tightly interwoven, parallel, and slightly wavy bundles. The course of the ligamentous collagen fibers is examined through polarized microscopy, which enables to distinguish between parallel and interlacing collagen fiber course (▶ Fig. 1.3b, h).[6,11,12] If the collagen fibers are arranged crosswise/interlaced or spirally with alternating sense of rotation, i.e., in scissors lattice order, the ribbon adapts to the changing shape of its content according to a stocking by changing the mesh lattice angle. Under the polarizing microscope, collagen fibers appear

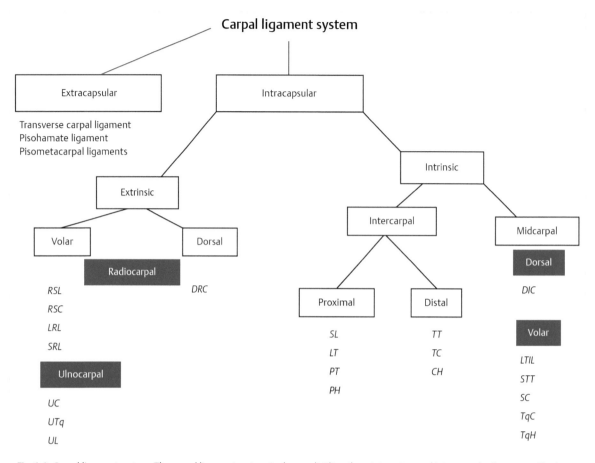

Fig. 1.1 Carpal ligament system. The carpal ligament system is shown, dividing them into extra- and intracapsular ligaments. The latter are subdivided into extrinsic and intrinsic ligaments. CH, capitate-hamate ligament; DIC, dorsal intercarpal ligament; DRC, dorsal radiocarpal ligament; LRL, long radiolunate ligament; LT, lunotriquetral; LTIL, lunotriquetral interosseous ligament; PH, pisotriquetral; PT, pisohamate; RSC, radioscaphocapitate; RSL, radioscapholunate; SC, scaphocapitate; SL, scapholunate; SRL, short radiolunate ligament; STT, scapho-trapezial-trapezoidal ligament; TC, trapezocapitate ligament; TqC, triquetrocapitate ligament; TqH, triquetrohamate ligament; TT, trapezial-trapezoidal ligament; UC, ulnocapitate ligament; UL, ulnolunate ligament; UTq, ulnotriquetral ligament.

anisotropic, are positively uniaxially birefringent, and therefore light up in the diagonal between crossed polars (▶ Fig. 1.3b).[6,12,13]

Depending on the ligament type, loose interstitial connective tissue runs through the collagenous bundles. This tissue can contain nerves, vessels, and even immunocompetent cells, and thus it serves as a water reservoir and displacement layer. Therefore it is important for defense and regeneration processes.[6]

Furthermore, an undulating collagen fiber course indicates that a ligament can be lengthened without injuring it while applying tension.[14] Collagen fibers can be stretched by about 5% and, due to their slightly wavelike arrangement in the connective tissue, can be lengthened by about 3%.[15] The undulating collagen fiber course is generated by the molecular structure of the collagen fibers, which can withstand a tensile force of about 6 kg/mm^2 cross-section. If a stronger tension is applied,

it leads to irreversible elongation by 10% and ultimately to the rupture of the ligament.[15,16]

Crimps in ligaments are composed of parallel, densely packed, collagen fibrils that suddenly change direction in the region of the top angle of each crimp forming 3D special local arrays described as fibrillar crimps. The fibrillar crimps are thought to be the microscopic structure responsible for the mechanical functions of crimps in absorbing/transmitting loads and recoiling of collagen fibers in tendons and ligaments.[17] Crimping makes collagen fibers highly extensible under low tension, protecting them from tearing.[18] The angle of collagen crimping defines its properties for resisting tensile forces and viscoelasticity.[19,20] Therefore, the crimping of collagen fibers of the joint capsule or ligaments plays a crucial role in viscoelasticity of the joints. ▶ Table 1.1 gives a clear overview of the structural collagenous composition in wrist ligaments.

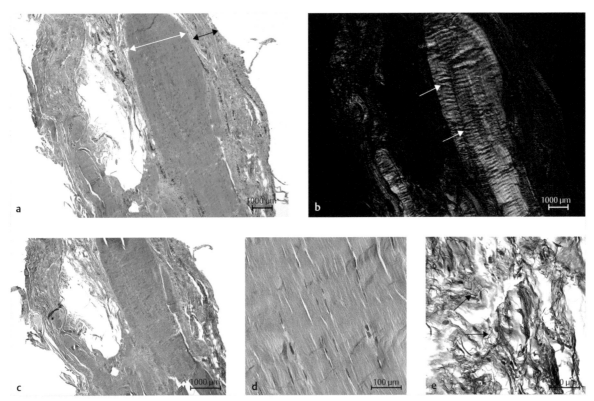

Fig. 1.2 Densely packed parallel collagen bundles. The densely packed parallel collagen fiber structure of an ulnocarpal ligament is shown in the hematoxylin-eosin staining (**a,b**) in the transmission (**a**) and polarization mode (**b**). The epifascicular region (*black two-sided arrow in* **a**), which contains nerves and blood vessels, is clearly distinguishable from the fascicular region (*white two-sided arrow in* **a**). The wavelike structure (*white arrows in* **b**) enables distension during tensile loads. This feature, as well as the absence of interstitial septa and elastic fibers in the fascicular region, indicates resistance to high tensile forces. Elastic fibers are analyzed in the Elastica van Gieson staining (**c–e**). No elastic fibers are visible in the overview magnification (**c**). Elastic fibers are seen in the epifascicular region in the high-power field analysis (**e**, *arrows*). In contrast, there are no elastic fibers in the fascicular region (**d**). Scale bar: 1000 μm (**a–c**), 100 μm (**d,e**). Original magnification: 40 × (**a–c**), 400 × (**d,e**).

The distribution of elastic fibers in the tissue reflects its function.[21] The variability of elastic fiber densities implicates the different adaptability of structures against strain.[22] Elastic fibers lie as accompanying structures of the collagen fibers in the interstitial connective tissue and usually have a netlike structure. The elastic fiber arrangement contributes to the tissue architecture and allows passive contraction to the retraction to the original size after mechanical stress exposure.[5] Elastic fibers serve to rearrange collagen after stretching a ligament or skin.[5,23]

By applying a tensile force of approximately 20 kg/cm^2 cross-section, the reversibly highly stretchable elastic fiber networks can be lengthened up to 150%.[15]

The distribution of elastic fibers depends on the age and the mechanical stress of the respective ligament.[24,25]

The amount of elastic fibers in the fascicular collagenous tissue and its surrounding loose epifascicular connective tissue can be analyzed with the Elastica van Gieson staining. The quantity of elastic fibers is classified as many, few, or none. Many fibers lie in thick bundles and are visible with an overview magnification of 40 × under the microscope. Thin, single fibers are only detectable in the high-power field (400 ×), which are classified as "few elastic fibers." Ligaments with no elastic fibers appear neither in the 40 × nor in the 400 × magnification (▸ Fig. 1.2d, ▸ Fig. 1.3e, f, i, j).[11,13,26] Nearly no elastic fibers are found in the fascicular region of carpal ligaments (DIC, dSL, dLT, CH, TC, STT, TT, UC, UTq, RSC, LRL, SRL, TqC, TqH, vLT, vSL, LTIL). In addition, elastic fibers are observed only occasionally in the epifascicular region of carpal ligaments (DRC, CH, STT, UC, RSC, SRL, TqH, vSL, LTIL). This indicates that the carpal ligaments have low stretching capacity but high resistance against tensile forces.

1.2 Extrinsic Ligaments

1.2.1 Anatomy

Extrinsic ligaments consist of three groups: (1) the volar radiocarpal ligaments, (2) the volar ulnocarpal ligaments, and (3) the dorsal radiocarpal ligament.

I

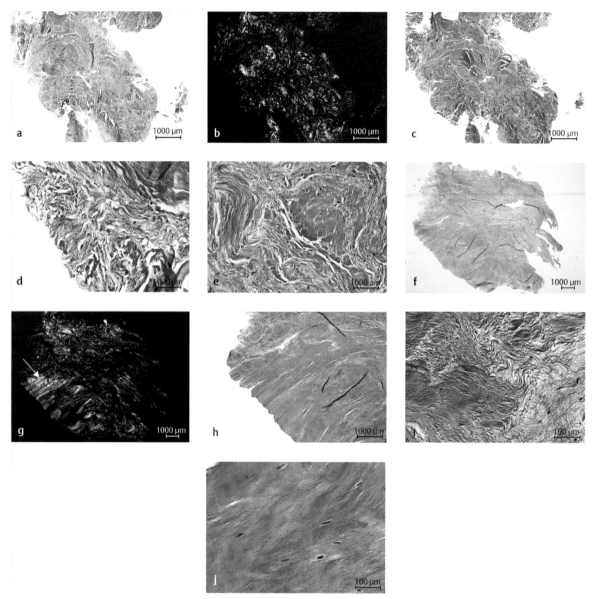

Fig. 1.3 Structural topography of the lunotriquetral ligament. A comparative histological analysis of the collagenous fiber arrangement of the dorsal **(a–e)** and volar **(f–j)** lunotriquetral ligament (dLT, vLT) is shown in the hematoxylin-eosin staining **(a,b,f,g)** in transmission **(a,f)** and polarization mode **(b,g)**. While the vLT has a densely packed parallel structure **(f,g)**, the dLT has a densely packed interlaced structure **(a,b)**, reflecting the high range of movement occurring in the triquetrum during wrist motion. The densely packed parallel collagenous structure of the vLT (*arrow* in **g**) indicates mainly unidirectional tensile forces. No elastic fibers are seen in the overview magnification **(c,h)** or in the high-power field **(d,e,i,j)**. Absence of elastic fibers in both vLT/dLT indicates high resistance and less elasticity, pointing out the important mechanical function of the lunotriquetral ligament. Scale bar: 1000 μm **(a,b,c,f,g,h)**, 100 μm **(d,e,i,j)**. Original magnification: 20 × **(f,g)**, 40 × **(a,b,c,h)**, 400 × **(d,e,i,j)**.

1.2.2 Volar Radiocarpal Ligaments

The volar radiocarpal ligaments originate from the volar rim of the distal radius and include, radially to ulnarly, the radioscaphocapitate (RSC), long and short radiolunate ligaments (LRL and SRL). The radioscapholunate (RSL) ligament of Testut-Kuentz that lies between LRL and SRL is a bundle of loose connective tissue including nutrient vessels to the volar corner of the proximal pole of the scaphoid, rather than a true ligament (▶ Fig. 1.4, ▶ Fig. 1.5).

The RSC has a broad origin that extends from the tip of radial styloid to the middle of scaphoid fossa. It courses distally and obliquely and its fibers display multiple attachments: onto the proximal part of distal scaphoid pole, to the waist of scaphoid, onto the palmar cortex of capitate body, and finally passing around the distal lunate

Table 1.1 Wrist ligaments assigned to the morphological types of collagen ligaments structure

Features	Ligament composition			
	Densely packed		Mixed tight and loose	
	Parallel	Interlaced	Parallel	Interlaced
Course of collagen fiber bundles	Tightly packed, unidirectional, and parallel	Tightly packed, multidirectional	Loosely packed, parallel	Loosely packed, multidirectional, interrupted by loose connective tissue
Loose connective tissue	In thin septa at the ligamentous insertion	Mainly not	Between collagen fiber bundles throughout the structure	Between collagen fiber bundles throughout the structure
Wrist ligaments	DIC, DRC, dSL, CH, TC, TT, UC, RSC, LRL, SRL, vLT, LTIL	dLT, STT, UTq, UL, vSL	TqC, TqH	–

Abbreviations: CH, capitate-hamate ligament; DIC, dorsal intercarpal ligament; DRC, dorsal radiocarpal ligament; dLT, lunotriquetral ligament, dorsal part; dSL, scapholunate ligament, dorsal part; LRL, long radiolunate ligament; LTIL, lunotriquetral interosseous ligament; RSC, radioscaphocapitate; SRL, short radiolunate ligament; STT, scapho-trapezial-trapezoidal ligament; TC, trapezocapitate ligament; TqC, triquetrocapitate ligament; TqH, triquetrohamate ligament; TT, trapezial-trapezoidal ligament; UC, ulnocapitate ligament; UL, ulnolunate ligament; UTq, ulnotriquetral ligament; vLT, lunotriquetral ligament, volar part; vSL, scapholunate ligament, volar part.

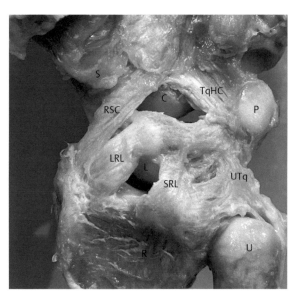

Fig. 1.4 View of the volar extrinsic and volar triquetral ligaments of the wrist. The extrinsic ligaments are the radio-scapho-capitate (RSC), the long radiolunate (LRL), and the short radiolunate (SRL) ligaments. The volar triquetral ligaments include the ulnotriquetral (UTq) and triquetro-hamate-capitate (TqHC) ligaments. C, capitate; L, lunate; P, pisotriquetral articular surface; R, radius; S, scaphoid; U, ulna.

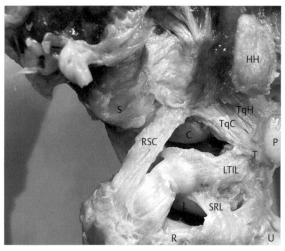

Fig. 1.5 Radiovolar view of the volar wrist ligaments. C, capitate; HH, hook of hamate; L, lunate; LRL, long radiolunate; LTIL, lunotriquetral interosseous ligament; P, pisotriquetral articular surface; R, radius; RSC, radioscaphocapitate; S, scaphoid; SRL, short radiolunate; T, triquetrum; TqC, triquetrocapitate; TqH, triquetrohamate; U, ulna.

to merge with fibers from the ulnocapitate, triquetrocapitate, and palmar scaphotriquetral ligaments to form the arcuate ligament. With its course around the palmar concavity of the scaphoid, the RSC forms a sling over which the scaphoid rotates (▶ Fig. 1.6).

The LRL is an intracapsular ligament that originates from the volar rim of the remaining aspect of the scaphoid fossa, courses obliquely anteriorly to the proximal pole of the scaphoid, and inserts on the radial volar surface of the lunate. The diverging RSC and LRL ligaments

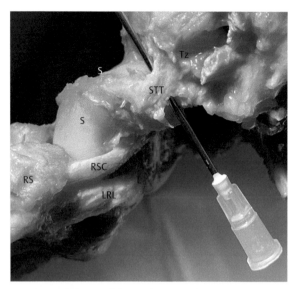

Fig. 1.6 Radial view of the scapho-trapezial-trapezoidal (STT) ligament, in particular the scaphoid-trapezium ligament. Note how the radioscaphocapitate (RSC) ligament curves around the volar scaphoid. L, lunate; LRL, long radiolunate ligament; RS, radius styloid; S, scaphoid; Tz, trapezium.

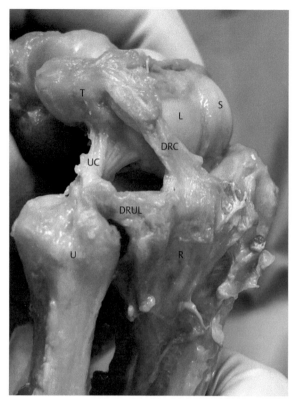

Fig. 1.7 A dorsoulnar view of the ulnocarpal joint, illustrating the relationship between the ulnocarpal ligaments and the dorsal radiocarpal (DRC) ligaments. DRUL, dorsal radioulnar ligament; L, lunate; R, radius; S, scaphoid; T, triquetrum; U, ulna.

are separated by the "interligamentous sulcus," the so-called space of Poirier, a weak zone of the joint capsule with clinical importance in perilunate dislocations.

The RSL lacks true mechanical and histological characteristics of a ligament. It carries small caliber vessels and nerves and travels with a dorsally oriented course, piercing the volar radiocarpal capsule to insert on the interosseous scapholunate ligament.

The most ulnarly located of the volar radiocarpal ligaments, the SRL, originates from the volar rim of the lunate fossa region of the distal radius and has a longitudinal orientation to its insertion on the radial half of the volar lunate. The LRL and SRL form a strong connection of the lunate to the distal radius.

1.2.3 Volar Ulnocarpal Ligaments

There are three volar ulnocarpal ligaments that span the ulnocarpal space palmarly and ulnarly: one superficial (ulnocapitate, UC) and two deep (ulnotriquetral, UTq; ulnolunate, UL) (▶ Fig. 1.4, ▶ Fig. 1.7).

The UC ligament originates from the fovea of the ulnar head. It courses distally and attaches to the volar region of the lunotriquetral interosseous ligament (LTIL); few fibers attach to the capitate body after blending with fibers of the triquetro-hamate-capitate (TqHC) ligament, while the majority of fibers converge with the fibers of the RSC forming the "arcuate" ligament. The UC serves as an ulnar anchor for the wrist.

The UL and UTq ligaments originate from the volar radioulnar ligament and they form the volar and ulnar part of the ulnocarpal joint capsule. The UL attaches along the ulnar part of the proximal lunate just ulnarly to SRL attachment. Due to the indirect origin of the UL and UTq, the forearm rotation does not affect the tightness of these ligaments. The UTq originates from the volar radioulnar ligament. It has a longitudinal orientation and attaches to the proximal and ulnar aspects of the triquetrum. The pisotriquetral orifice divides the UTq in medial and lateral bands, while a second perforation, the prestyloid recess has also been described. It forms as a part of the triangular fibrocartilage complex and acts as a dynamic stabilizer of both the wrist and the distal radioulnar joint (DRUJ) along with the extensor carpi ulnaris tendon system.

1.2.4 Dorsal Radiocarpal Ligament

The dorsal radiocarpal ligament (DRC), also called the dorsal radiotriquetral ligament, has a wide origin from the dorsal rim of the radius extending from the Lister's tubercle to the sigmoid notch. Its width is reduced as it courses obliquely distally and ulnarly, offering some attachment to the dorsal lunate and finally inserting on the dorsal ridge of the triquetrum. At this final insertion

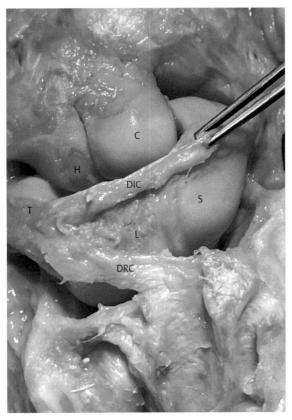

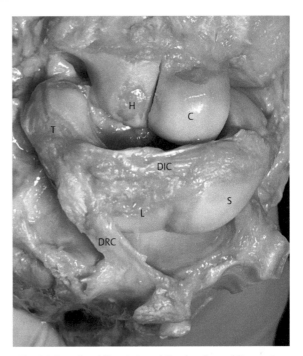

Fig. 1.9 Dorsal and flexed view of the dorsal carpal ligaments, illustrating the tension in the dorsal radiocarpal (DRC) ligament and the transverse expansion of the dorsal intercarpal (DIC). C, capitate; L, lunate; H, hamate; S, scaphoid; T, triquetrum.

Fig. 1.8 Dorsal carpal ligaments: the dorsal radiocarpal (DRC) and dorsal intercarpal (DIC) ligaments. C, capitate; H, hamate; L, lunate; S, scaphoid; T, triquetrum.

it merges with fibers from the dorsal intercarpal ligament (DIC). The DRC reinforces the dorsal LTIL and constrains ulnar translocation of the carpus and ulnocarpal supination (▶ Fig. 1.8, ▶ Fig. 1.9, ▶ Fig. 1.10).

1.3 Intrinsic Ligaments

1.3.1 Anatomy

Intrinsic ligaments may be either midcarpal that connect the bones across the midcarpal joint, or intercarpal (referred by some authors as interosseous[2]) that connect the bones within the same carpal row (either proximal or distal).

1.3.2 Midcarpal Ligaments

The midcarpal joint is crossed by four volar and one dorsal ligament.

Volar Midcarpal Ligaments

The four volar midcarpal ligaments are intracapsular and connect scaphoid and triquetrum with the distal row:

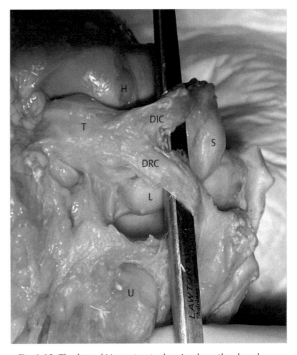

Fig. 1.10 The lateral V-construct, showing how the dorsal radiocarpal (DRC) and dorsal intercarpal (DIC) ligaments insert onto the triquetrum (T) and span across the wrist to provide stability to both the dorsal radiocarpal and midcarpal joints. H, hamate; L, lunate; S, scaphoid; U, ulna.

scaphotrapeziotrapezoid (STT), scaphocapitate (SC), triquetrocapitate (TqC), and triquetrohamate (TqH). The TqC and TqH ligaments form almost mirror images of the STT and SC ligaments. Interestingly, the lunate does not have a connection to the distal carpal row itself.

The STT ligament complex includes four components: the radiopalmar scapho-trapezial ligament (rpSTL), the palmar scapho-trapezial-trapezoidal capsule (pSTTC), the dorsal scapho-trapezial-trapezoidal capsule (dSTTC), and the SC ligament. The rpSTL has been described as the main stabilizer of the STT joint[27] (▶ Fig. 1.6).

The SC originates from the distal pole of the scaphoid at the ulnar half of its volar cortex, courses obliquely, and inserts on the proximal and radial half of volar aspect of capitate body. The SC has the same orientation as the RSC ligament, and this explains the common false impression that the latter inserts on the capitate body.

The TqC and TqH ligaments are important structures for the midcarpal joint stability. The TqC originates from the distal and radial corner of the triquetrum and inserts on the ulnar cortex of the capitate body. The TqH lies just ulnarly to the TqC, originates from the distal volar cortex of the triquetrum, and attaches on the volar cortex of the hamate body. The TqCH complex is also known as the ulnar arm of the arcuate ligament.

Dorsal Midcarpal Ligament

Dorsally the midcarpal joint is coursed by one of the bands of the DIC. Ulnarly it originates from the dorsal tubercle of the triquetrum and courses radially along the dorsal edges of the proximal row bones, distal to the dorsal scaphotriquetral ligament, separated in two bands: the proximal band attaches to the dorsal ridge and radial surface of the distal pole of the scaphoid and the distal band attaches to the dorsal cortex of trapezium and trapezoid.

1.3.3 Intercarpal Ligaments

Proximal intercarpal ligaments include the scapholunate (SL), the lunotriquetral (LT), and the pisotriquetral (PT) and pisohamate (PH) ligaments. Distal intercarpal ligaments include trapeziotrapezoid (TT), trapezocapitate (TC), capitohamate (CH) ligaments (▶ Fig. 1.11).

Proximal Intercarpal Ligaments

The SL joint is stabilized by the three regions of the respective ligament: the volar and dorsal SL (vSL and dSL, respectively) and the proximal fibrocartilaginous membrane that connects them. The dSL is the thickest part and has the greatest yield strength, followed by the thinner vSL and the proximal membrane. The dSL connects the dorsal–distal corners of the scaphoid and lunate bones. It lies deep to the dorsal capsule from which it is clearly differentiated. Its fibers are slightly obliquely

oriented and has significant contribution in maintaining scaphoid stability. The vSL is thinner and can be differentiated from the overlying LRL. Its fibers are more obliquely oriented allowing substantial flexion and extension of the scaphoid relative to the lunate. The proximal fibrocartilaginous membrane follows the proximal arc of scaphoid and lunate, separating the radiocarpal and midcarpal joint spaces. It is composed of fibrocartilage, with no collagen orientation, blood vessels, or nerves[28] (▶ Fig. 1.11, ▶ Fig. 1.12).

Similar to the SL, the LT joint is stabilized by the three parts of LT ligament: the volar, and dorsal that connect the respective surfaces of the two bones, and the proximal fibrocartilaginous membrane that covers the dorsal, proximal, and volar aspects of the LT joint leaving the distal aspect open to the midcarpal joint. Contrary to the SL joint, the volar component (vLT ligament) is thicker and stronger than the dorsal LT (dLT) ligament followed again by the weakest proximal membrane. The vLT is composed of transversely oriented collagen fibers that interdigitate with fibers of the UC. The dLT courses transversely the LT joint and is clearly separated from the DRC. The proximal membrane is composed of fibrocartilage, but lacks collagen orientation, blood vessels, and nerves and prevents communication between the radiocarpal and midcarpal joint spaces (▶ Fig. 1.11, ▶ Fig. 1.12).

Both vLT and dLT are under greater tension throughout the range of motion compared to SL ligaments. The most distal fibers of both vLT and dLT blend with the respective distal fibers of the vSL and dSL, forming the palmar and

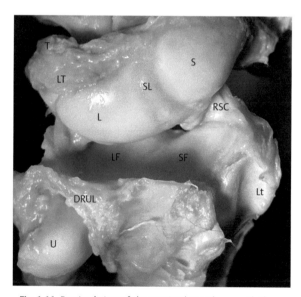

Fig. 1.11 Proximal view of the proximal carpal row, with the interosseous ligaments—the scapholunate (SL) and lunotriquetral (LT) ligaments. DRUL, dorsal radioulnar ligament; L, lunate; LF, lunate fossa; Lt, Lister's tubercle; RSC, radioscaphocapitate; S, scaphoid; SF, scaphoid fossa; T, triquetrum; U, ulna.

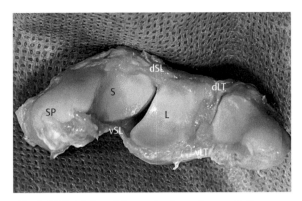

Fig. 1.12 Distal view of the proximal carpal row, with the interosseous ligaments—the dorsal and volar scapholunate (dSL, vSL) and dorsal and volar lunotriquetral (dLT, vLT) ligaments. L, lunate; S, scaphoid; SP, distal scaphoid pole; T, triquetrum.

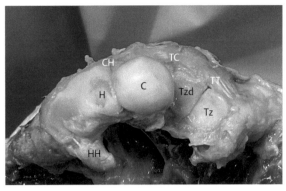

Fig. 1.13 Proximal view of the distal carpal row, with the stout interosseous ligaments—the trapezotrapezoid (TT), trapezoid-capitate (TC), and capitohamate (CH) ligaments. C, capitate; H, hamate; HH, hook of hamate; Tz, trapezium; Tzd, trapezoid.

dorsal scaphotriquetral ligament. The dorsal scaphotriquetral ligament forms a labral extension into the dorsal midcarpal joint and along with the DIC contributes to the stability of the lunocapitate joint.

The PT ligament is a U-shape ligament that covers the radial, distal, and ulnar aspects of the pisotriquetral joint with its radial part being reinforced by fibers of the UC. The proximal part of the pisotriquetral joint, however, is open and communicates with the radiocarpal joint through the pisotriquetral orifice in the UTq. The PH extends from the palmar surface of the pisiform to the hook of the hamate and is formed from the flexor carpi ulnaris tendon.

Distal Intercarpal Ligaments

The stout transverse intercarpal ligaments, i.e., TT, TC, CH strongly connect the bones of the distal carpal row. Each of these ligaments consists of a transversely oriented dorsal and volar component. In the trapezocapitate and capitohamate joints, the respective ligaments attach only onto the body of the capitate crossing only the distal half of the joint because of the proximal extensions of the pole of the hamate and the head and neck of the capitate. For these two latter joints, an intra-articular component exists in addition to the dorsal and palmar components (▶ Fig. 1.13).

Acknowledgment

We wish to express our sincere gratitude to Dr. Theodorakys Fermin, Mr. Ahmad Al Mojaber, and the Surgical Skills Lab of Aspetar Orthopedic and Sports Medicine Hospital, Doha, Qatar for invaluable assistance with anatomical dissections and imaging. Furthermore, we thank Christian Retschke and Rami Al Meklef (both Leipzig, Germany) for logistic support.

References

[1] Berger RA. The ligaments of the wrist. A current overview of anatomy with considerations of their potential functions. Hand Clin. 1997; 13(1):63–82

[2] Berger RA. The anatomy of the ligaments of the wrist and distal radioulnar joints. Clin Orthop Relat Res. 2001(383):32–40

[3] Garcia-Elias M, Lluch AL. Wrist instabilities, misalignments, and dislocations: wrist anatomy. In: Wolfe SW, ed. Green's operative hand surgery, 7th ed. Elsevier; 2017:419–423

[4] Hariri S, Safran MR. Ulnar collateral ligament injury in the overhead athlete. Clin Sports Med. 2010; 29(4):619–644

[5] Frank CB. Ligament structure, physiology and function. J Musculoskelet Neuronal Interact. 2004; 4(2):199–201

[6] Rein S, Hagert E, Schneiders W, Fieguth A, Zwipp H. Histological analysis of the structural composition of ankle ligaments. Foot Ankle Int. 2015a; 36(2):211–224

[7] Rein S, Semisch M, Garcia-Elias M, Lluch A, Zwipp H, Hagert E. Immunohistochemical mapping of sensory nerve endings in the human triangular fibrocartilage complex. Clin Orthop Relat Res. 2015b; 473(10):3245–3253

[8] Solomonow M. Sensory-motor control of ligaments and associated neuromuscular disorders. J Electromyogr Kinesiol. 2006; 16(6):549–567

[9] Chowdhury P, Matyas JR, Frank CB. The "epiligament" of the rabbit medial collateral ligament: a quantitative morphological study. Connect Tissue Res. 1991; 27(1):33–50

[10] Hagert E, Garcia-Elias M, Forsgren S, Ljung BO. Immunohistochemical analysis of wrist ligament innervation in relation to their structural composition. J Hand Surg Am. 2007; 32(1):30–36

[11] Rein S, Kremer T, Houschyar KS, Siemers F, Philipps H. Structural topography of the interosseous membrane of the human forearm. Ann Anat. 2020; 231:151547

[12] Semisch M, Hagert E, Garcia-Elias M, Lluch A, Rein S. Histological assessment of the triangular fibrocartilage complex. J Hand Surg Eur Vol. 2016; 41(5):527–533

[13] Lühmann P, Kremer T, Siemers F, Rein S. Comparative histomorphological analysis of elbow ligaments and capsule. Clin Anat. 2022; 35(8):1070–1084

[14] Amiel D, Chu C, Lee J. Effect of loading on metabolism and repair of tendons and ligaments. In: Funk FJ, Hunter LY, eds. Repetitive motion disorders of the upper extremity. Rosemont: Am Acad Orthop Surg; 1995:217–230

[15] Leonhardt H. Histologie, Zytologie und Mikroanatomie des Menschen. In: Taschenlehrbuch der gesamten Anatomie. Stuttgart, New York: Thieme; 1990

[16] Solomonow M. Ligaments: a source of work-related musculoskeletal disorders. J Electromyogr Kinesiol. 2004; 14(1):49–60

[17] Franchi M, Ottani V, Stagni R, Ruggeri A. Tendon and ligament fibrillar crimps give rise to left-handed helices of collagen fibrils in both planar and helical crimps. J Anat. 2010; 216(3):301–309

[18] Shah JS, Jayson MIV, Hampson WGJ. Low tension studies of collagen fibres from ligaments of the human spine. Ann Rheum Dis. 1977; 36 (2):139–145

[19] Ault HK, Hoffman AH. A composite micromechanical model for connective tissues: Part I–Theory. J Biomech Eng. 1992; 114(1):137–141

[20] Xiao S, Shao Y, Li B, Feng XQ. A micromechanical model of tendon and ligament with crimped fibers. J Mech Behav Biomed Mater. 2020; 112:104086

[21] Kielty CM. Elastic fibres in health and disease. Expert Rev Mol Med. 2006; 8(19):1–23

[22] Baldwin AK, Simpson A, Steer R, Cain SA, Kielty CM. Elastic fibres in health and disease. Expert Rev Mol Med. 2013; 15:e8

[23] Oxlund H, Manschot J, Viidik A. The role of elastin in the mechanical properties of skin. J Biomech. 1988; 21(3):213–218

[24] Barros EMKP, Rodrigues CJ, Rodrigues NR, Oliveira RP, Barros TEP, Rodrigues AJ, Jr. Aging of the elastic and collagen fibers in the human cervical interspinous ligaments. Spine J. 2002; 2(1):57–62

[25] Fullmer HM. A comparative histochemical study of elastic, pre-elastic and oxytalan connective tissue fibers. J Histochem Cytochem. 1960; 8:290–295

[26] Rein S, Zwipp H. Ausprägung der elastischen Fasern in menschlichen Sprunggelenksbändern. Fuss Sprunggelenk. 2016; 14:14–22

[27] Higashigaito K, Pfirrmann CWA, Koch S, et al. Ligaments of the scapho-trapezial-trapezoidal joint: MR anatomy in asymptomatic and symptomatic individuals. Skeletal Radiol. 2022; 51(3):637–647

[28] Berger RA. The gross and histologic anatomy of the scapholunate interosseous ligament. J Hand Surg Am. 1996; 21(2):170–178

2 Biomechanics of the Wrist

Jonathan P. Compson

Abstract

Carpal mechanics has been an area of great interest and controversy for many years but for nonacademic wrist surgeons it is a difficult subject to understand. This view on the subject has been written from the perspective of a surgeon who had to try and extrapolate what was known about biomechanics in the past to useful knowledge for treating acute injuries and their complications rather than treating chronic nontraumatic instabilities. The emphasis is therefore on the functional anatomy and the mechanics of injury causation and treatment. It arose as with other surgeons over a hundred years from a particular interest in fractures of the scaphoid, their fracture patterns, and how they and the carpus collapse in nonunion.

Keywords: wrist, carpal mechanics theory, anatomy, scaphoid fractures, hydromechanics

2.1 Introduction

The anatomy of the eight carpal bones and their soft tissue connections is complex and when united into a single compound joint, the wrist, their combined relationship and function becomes even more complex. How they work together is not yet fully understood, and though this is absolutely fascinating for a few surgeons especially those treating nontraumatic instabilities, for many surgeons it is daunting and confusing. However, for diagnosis and treatment, most wrist surgeons particularly those treating acute trauma require a knowledge of the complex 3D anatomy, both bony and ligamentous, in order to restore normal anatomy and then hopefully function. With this a working knowledge of mechanics is all that is needed as long as one isn't drawn into the minutiae and often arguments and confusing language which dominates the subject. However, a deeper understanding of the mechanics is needed when treating posttraumatic complications due to secondary malalignment and especially for multidirectional instabilities secondary to hyperlaxity and congenital abnormalities.

It is difficult to describe in words alone how things move, particularly about a wrist that has a complex 3D anatomy. However, the advent of the 3D computerized tomography (CT) (▶ Fig. 2.1a, b) has been probably the most important advance for describing, understanding, and treating carpal pathology since wrist arthroscopy was developed.[1,2] By using it to understand and visualize the underlying 3D anatomy it is easy to extrapolate it to the surface anatomy which before such imaging was difficult.[3,4] A good knowledge of surface anatomy is essential not only for diagnosis but also to feel how the normal carpus moves, for instance, the scaphoid flexing and extending on radial and ulnar deviation. In future carpal mechanics will be taught with the aid of moving 3D images, both of bone and eventually with soft tissue additions to the model. Unfortunately, many descriptions of carpal mechanics are still based on fairly unrealistic views of 3D soft tissue anatomy. At the moment the best way to learn is still by dissecting cadaveric hands, observing open carpal surgery and wrist arthroscopy despite the limited views, and radiologically screening one's own patients.

2.2 Functions of the Wrist

The wrist has two main functions. The first with the rest of the upper limb is to place the hand and digits in space to improve dexterity. However, its main function is probably to produce a stable platform for the hand to optimize grip strength in any position.[5] Its ability to maintain stability in many directions and to control the amount of stability at different levels in the joint is probably why the wrist is so complex rather than just a simple ball-and-socket joint.[6]

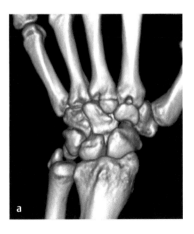
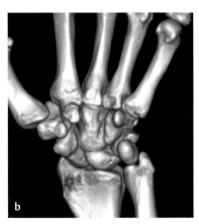

Fig. 2.1 Dorsal **(a)** and palmar **(b)** 3D computed tomography (CT) views of left wrist.

However, as well as bone shape and ligaments, tendons are also important for multipositional grip strength and for stabilizing other joints particularly when the wrist is moving.[8] They not only allow controlled movement and positioning but can also act as dynamic ligaments akin to the rotator cuff in the shoulder. Despite many surgeons' determination to maintain a moving joint, a stable pain-free wrist in the right position, for instance when it is splinted or arthrodesed, may produce a better functioning joint than one with movement and pain.[7]

2.2.1 Optimum Position for Finger Function/Arthrodesis

In a splint maximal grip strength without significantly compromising grip endurance is at 30 degrees of extension.[8] This has significant clinical implications both for splinting and wrist position in arthrodesis. However, for the latter the use of an orthosis, which reduces grip strength in any position, may have some experimental bias. Historically some authors suggest fusing the wrist in extension,[9,10] but others with 10- to 15-degree extension and slight ulnar deviation.[11] Some studies suggest that certain activities are better with wrists in neutral.[12] However clinical studies following fusions can also be biased due to associated etiologies. Sometimes concentration should be more on functional position, for instance, in musicians, rather than grip strength in itself. The author's default position is maximum grip position as seen in the other wrist which corresponds to O'Driscoll et al's study in 1992 that optimal grip strength was self-selected but averaged 35 degrees of extension and 7 degrees of ulnar deviation.[13]

The hand and wrist are very adaptable, especially to lack of full extension and flexion. For instance, people with loss of extension, unconsciously push off with their knuckles or fingers. Except for very specialized functions a full range of movement is not important. However as with any joint, pain at the end of movement is often more a problem than the loss itself.

2.2.2 Functional Range of Movement

When treating any joint it is worth knowing the functional range so as not to overtreat and to have realistic goals. There are many studies for the wrist but most of these have the same conclusion that most activities can be achieved with about 60 degrees of extension, 55 degrees of flexion, 40 degrees of ulnar deviation, and 15 degrees of radial deviation.[14] However, some studies actually show far less than this data, for instance, 5 degrees of flexion, 30 degrees of extension, 10 degrees of radial deviation, and 15 degrees of ulnar deviation.[15]

2.2.3 Dart-Throwing Motion

The so-called "dart-throwing" motion of the wrist has become more important over the past few years, especially since 2007 when the IFSSH Committee produced an extensive report.[16] This report defined it as a plane of movement between full radial extension and ulnar flexion with most movement occurring at the midcarpal joint, which is commonly involved in most actions of the wrist. So, maintenance of a functional range of this movement is particularly important though it is hard to measure or visualize.

2.3 Basic Functional Anatomy of the Wrist

2.3.1 Osteology

Description of the Rows

The wrist, a double diarthrodial joint, was classically looked at as two transverse rows of bone fully separated by the midcarpal joint with a separate joint for the pisiform (▶ Fig. 2.1a, b). They are also functionally different, in that the distal row is rigid and the proximal row is flexible.

Distal Row (▶ Fig. 2.2)

The distal row is a transverse, strongly connected row of bones centered around the capitate with a concave volar curve like downturned wings that essentially behaves as a single functional unit. It is based on the body of the capitate which extends more proximally into a ball-shaped end which is close to the center of rotation of the row. Though predominantly T-shaped the ulnar-side angle is filled in by the hamate, giving it a variably flat surface to articulate with the triquetrum. The radial side, however, leaves a space for the mobile scaphoid and a break in the third Gilula's line.[17]

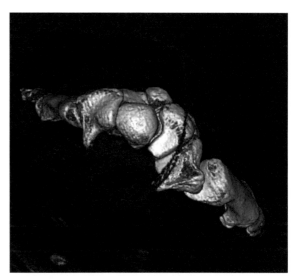

Fig. 2.2 Distal row following removal of proximal row showing the palmar concave curve centered around the capitate.

Proximal Row (▶ Fig. 2.3)

The proximal row is curved but at right angles to the distal row. The long convexity of its proximal face and joints is smooth. The scaphoid points distally into the radial axilla of the T-shaped distal row. The triquetrum also points distally parallel to the wedge-shaped hamate at about 35 degree angle to the transverse axis. Knowing this is useful when making an ulnar midcarpal portal in arthroscopy.

Though the concave distal face of the row looks smooth on X-ray, when viewed from a distal perspective one sees the main feature which is the socket for the capitate head. This is divided in two by the scapholunate joint which varies in shape. The proximal end of the scaphoid is a mirror image of most of the lunate apart from a facet for the hamate.

Tendon Attachments

The tendons which drive movement in the proximal row through the distal row are inserted in optimal positions for movement, especially radial and ulnar deviation and proximal compression away from the center of rotation of the wrist and capitate head.

The Intercalated Segment and the Scaphoid Link

Much has been written about the intercalated bone or segment in wrist mechanics. Initially defined by Landsmeer in 1962[18] its use as a term has been imprecise and produces confusion.[19] However, it can be used in many ways and is in itself not the proximal row or part of it per se. It is a bone or chain of bones which have no tendon attachment and move due to the shape of the adjacent joints or ligament attachments and therefore better used as a description and not a definition.

The scaphoid link first described by Gilford et al[20] again is a term which can be used and defined in several ways but was first used to describe the scaphoid as a strut holding the central column out to length. However, how important it is in controlling the movement of the proximal row is where the controversy lies. It may be better to consider the scaphoid link as the distal half of the bone only. The proximal half is in shape and stability akin to the lunate and its movement is driven by both the head of the capitate through the proximal pole and the distal end pushed into flexion by the trapezium and trapezoid, thus making the scaphoid act as an intercalated segment. Extension of the scaphoid occurs by the distal end being pulled by the distal row through the strong volar scapho-trapezial-trapezoid (STT) and scaphocapitate ligament until it can extend no longer and acting as a strap prevents further ulnar deviation.

The Central Column (▶ Fig. 2.4)

It is worth considering the anatomy of the central column which, as discussed later, is important in the column theory of mechanics. The central column as described by Navarro[21] in 1921 is not a single column of bones which has led to some confusion. Rather than a column it is the T-shaped solid distal row extended proximally through the capitate and lunate (▶ Fig. 2.4). To the ulnar side of this, the angle is filled in by the angle of the hamate. The head of the capitate is part of a centrally located ball-and-socket joint—half of which involves most of the distal surface of the lunate and the other half the proximal half

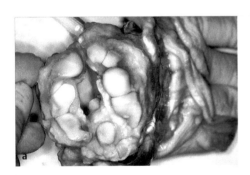
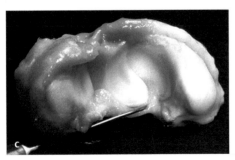
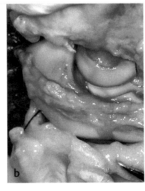
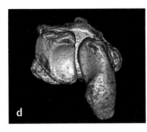

Fig. 2.3 **(a)** Opening up of midcarpal joint in a cadaver right wrist showing the four areas of contact. The ball-and-socket joint, the scaphoid link, the hamate facet on the lunate, and the wide undulating surface of the triquetrohamate joint. **(b)** The "ball" of the scapho-lunate-capitate joint (right wrist). **(c)** The proximal row viewed from the midcarpal joint showing the cup of the scapho-lunate-capitate joint with a lazy S shape of the scapholunate joint, the cups' extension to the side of the scaphoid and prominent hamate facet (right wrist). **(d)** Scapholunate joint visualized distally from 3D computed tomography (CT) showing a straighter scapholunate joint, but still an extension of the cup to the side of the scaphoid.

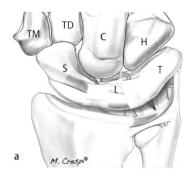
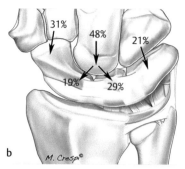

Fig. 2.4 (a,b) The central column. Modified to include proximal half of scaphoid and load distribution in right wrist on compression through the distal row and across the midcarpal joint.

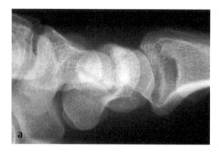
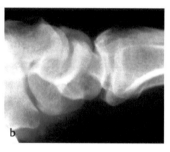

Fig. 2.5 (a) Lateral X-ray of wrist showing five congruous curves. Distal radius, proximal lunate, proximal scaphoid, distal lunate, and proximal capitate. **(b)** Lateral X-ray of wrist with maximum grip. Showing incongruous second and third curves of a scapholunate dissociation whereas all other curves are congruous, but out of line of the longitudinal axis of the radius.

of the scaphoid. The proximal pole of the scaphoid is almost identical in shape to the adjacent lunate (▶ Fig. 2.3c). This column is more complex than the Navarro's model. If one considers both the lunate and proximal pole as part of the central column, then Navarro's column becomes even more inclusive though no less important as a theory to explain carpal mechanics.

Alignment

Looking at the lateral view of the wrist (▶ Fig. 2.5a), it is easy to visualize the central column consisting of five curves in a straight line along the axis of the metacarpals and radius. It is worth considering them in the normal wrist to be like a stack of bowls and when there is compression through the capitate they lock together and the column becomes more stable. In full extension and flexion, the curves remain in position congruent to each other. The ligaments keep the bones in congruency at each joint level by tightening. Either loss of shape (by alignment of the curves) or torn or stretched ligaments results in buckling of the central column.

VISI and DISI (▶ Fig. 2.5a, b)

Ever since Linscheid et al in 1972[22] coined the terms DISI (dorsal-intercalated segment instability) and VISI (volar-intercalated segment instability) for the carpal collapse patterns, there has been a lot of debate about the exact definition. However, though this is an important description of the alignment of the central column in the long axis with the lunate extended in DISI (▶ Fig. 2.5b) and flexed in VISI, it is often variable with load, doesn't relate

to the degree of fixed deformity, and is poor in showing the degree of displacement between all the proximal row bones whereas the congruency of the curves on the lateral film is more useful in treating an individual case. It does however allow one to understand the areas of impingement and probable pain and wear and to assess potential instability and its direction. Precisely defining angles on X-rays appears to engender much controversy[23] with no obvious practical use for individual treatment; therefore, DISI/VISI should probably remain descriptive rather than definitive.

Position in Flexion and Extension

Because most acute injuries to the bones or tendons occur at the extremes of movement or in the wrist on maximal loading, it is worth knowing for any injury the alignment of the carpus during its commonest mechanism of injury and how from that it damages both soft tissue and bone. Hopefully a better understanding of particularly the soft tissue injury will help both with acute treatment and in avoiding secondary mechanical complications. Because of the difficulty in imaging soft tissue injuries, record as much as possible the soft tissue injuries found at surgery, thus looking for consistent injury patterns and extrapolating this back to the mechanics of causation. This has been done for many years in some joints like the ankle but not in the carpus. For instance, though Mayfield et al's explanation of perilunate dislocation[24] covers the intrinsic ligament injuries, it doesn't explain why there is often a Bankart-type capsule and a periosteal lift-off lesion on the dorsum of the radius as well as a capsular lift-off from the lunate.

The Shape and Variability of Individual Bones

To make matters more complex it has been found that there is a significant variation in wrist anatomy which could have significant effects on the mechanics. In 1993[25] Steven Viegas and his team published the results from dissection of 393 wrists. For wrist biomechanics the most significant result is probably the 73% incidence of a separate medial facet on the distal surface of the lunate for the hamate.

2.3.2 Ligaments

Historical Perspective

Historically, functional anatomy has been focused more on bones than the equally important ligaments. However, as with most advances in surgery which require a back-to-basics approach, there was renewed interest in ligament anatomy as a basis to explaining carpal instabilities.[26,27,28,29,30,31] After a great deal of useful work, the impetus tended back toward mechanics and imaging of bone. However, a more kinetic approach as in Sandow's central column theory[32] may help improve understanding of ligament interaction which may be lost by oversimplification. More anatomical investigation is needed. Unfortunately, dividing ligaments into intrinsic and extrinsic puts greater emphasis on the intrinsic structures (ligaments which go from carpal bone to bone) rather than the extrinsic (which go from bones outside the carpus to a carpal bone) and underestimates the combined effect.

It is also difficult to distinguish individual extrinsic ligaments since they run in thick sheets of capsule particularly on the volar side and can be variable as well as indistinguishable. It is easy to make up ligaments to correspond to a theory.

However, despite this and the difficulties of visualizing soft tissue, the positioning of ligaments in extreme positions where they're most likely to be injured has been attempted.[33]

The Capsule and Dorsal Recesses (▶ Fig. 2.6)

The capsule of the wrist joint is a substantial structure which must have significant strengthening and stabilizing effects on the carpus. This is particularly true of the volar capsule which is not only solid but also its individual ligament strands are difficult to distinguish. It is closely adherent to the volar surfaces particularly the central column and also the volar scaphocapitate joint.

The dorsal capsule is much more mobile. The very elaborate V-shaped system appears to allow excellent flexion as the V opens. It is also less adherent to the proximal row than its volar counterpart particularly the lunate and scaphoid which hang from it like a washing line. The

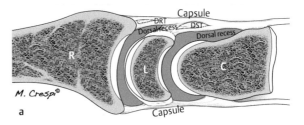

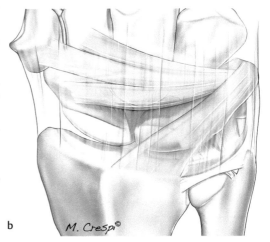

Fig. 2.6 (a,b) A drawing of a sagittal section through the central column of a cadaver wrist showing the different attachments of the capsule dorsal and volar, the dorsal recesses, and position of the "extrinsic ligaments" in the dorsal capsule. The right-hand figure shows direction of the fibers in the dorsal capsule (*pink*) and their attachments to the dorsum of the proximal row (*brown*). C, capitate; L, lunate; DRT, dorsal radiotriquetral ligament; DST, dorsal scaphotriquetral ligament; R, radius.

lunate has a strong dorsal attachment to the capsule as can be seen acutely in a perilunate dislocation when it leaves a large footprint on the undersurface of the capsule. The attachment also lies obliquely producing substantial recesses dorsally over both the capitate and the lunate which also must have some influence on the movement of the proximal row particularly extension and flexion. Interestingly, releasing the dorsal recess over the lunate in a stiff wrist which is stuck down produces flexion but rarely significantly improves extension being probably blocked by thickened capsule.

Tendons

Tendons also act as dynamic ligaments and circumvent the need for collateral ligaments while at the same time can be strongly rigid. Both the first compartment tendons, particularly in the dart thrower's position and the ECU tendon in wrist pronation, act synergistically to control ulnar and radial deviation.

The long extensors and flexors of the digits may also affect wrist mechanics, in that particularly the flexors act as suspension protecting the last degrees of extension both statically and dynamically from damage at the endpoint of carpal bone movement.

2.4 Wrist Stability

The mechanics of wrist stability is probably more clinically important than movement. An arthrodesed wrist in a good pain-free position is more functionally useful than one with pain or in a poor arc of movement, especially flexion. It is also important to understand the mechanics of injury which normally occurs as the stabilizing bone or ligaments fail due to structural damage. The study of loading and function in the wrist has been done by several techniques but with overall similar results.

2.4.1 Trabecular Patterns

The study of trabecular bone orientation and density has long been a way of looking at loading patterns. This is mainly done with X-rays, macroradiology, and now CT scanning. It is of particular interest to the paleoanthropologists who extrapolate hominid hand utilization from fossil bones albeit in limited numbers of specimens.

However, their literature on anatomy, imaging, and hand function is very extensive and, in many ways, more advanced than our own. Even in the late 1980s, there was increased interest in bone functional adaptation resulting from repetitive loading either in compression, tension, and sheer.[34] Many of these studies were done on normal extant hands and wrists due to the paucity of older specimens.

2.4.2 Pressure and Forces Across Wrist

On contracture of the wrist extensors and flexors, a compression force is transferred through the solid distal row and proximally across the midcarpal joint (▶ Fig. 2.7). It is said that when the wrist is in neutral 80% of the force transmitted across the wrist goes radially, 45% through the radiocarpal joint and 35% through the radiolunate joint. The remaining 20% goes through the ulnocarpal joint. Of the load transferred across the midcarpal joint 31% goes through the STT joint, and 48% is transferred through the body and head of the capitate acting as the ball in the ball-and-socket joint of the scapho-lunate-capitate joint. It further transmits forces through both the proximal pole of the scaphoid (19%) and the adjacent part of the lunate (29%) and then into the respective fossae on the radius. The remaining 21% is transferred through the triquetrohamate joint.[35]

This pattern of force transfer assumes that the scaphoid is acting as a rigid strut. However, because of its axis it can act either as an intervening strut passing loads through to its proximal pole or gives way and flexes allowing radial deviation. On the ulnar side, load goes

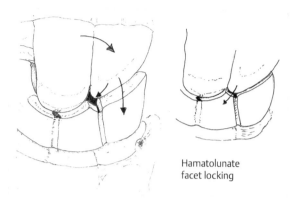

Hamatolunate
facet locking

Fig. 2.7 Hamatolunate facet locking.

through the hamate and its large contact area with the triquetrum and then onto the stretchable trampoline of the triangular fibrocartilage (TFC).

2.4.3 General Aspects and the Importance of Locking

In 1997, Marc Garcia-Elias understood the importance of carpal stability during grip, and demonstrated the complexity of the situation and how several factors affect this. This includes the position of the wrist, the direction of the forces, and the inclination and shape of the articular surfaces of the bones.[36]

2.4.4 Locking of the Midcarpal Joint

The midcarpal joint and the radiocarpal joint appear to stabilize and lock differently as increasing force is transmitted proximally through the wrist by forearm muscle contracture (▶ Fig. 2.4). The midcarpal joint anatomically appears to lock due to varying mechanisms across the joint.

1. Through the head of the capitate. Increasing pressure of the capitate head in the socket of the scapho-lunate-capitate joint appears to act as an interference joint. This mechanism is similar to the locking mechanism described by Marc Garcia-Elias as the "self-stabilizing spring" theory,[37] but the soft tissue spring is produced by the ligaments holding the socket together, the scapholunate ligaments (▶ Fig. 2.3c).
2. Through the hamate and triquetrum. This joint surface has a large surface area which classically was described as a saddle joint. However more recent anatomical studies[38] show a spectrum of variation from a relatively flat oval convex shape to one with an undulating double-faceted surface with presumably different mechanical properties affecting mainly sliding. In both directions, the triangular hamate acts as a unilateral wedge in the distal row on compression.

3. Through the hamate and its facet on the lunate. Three-quarters of people have a facet on the medial side of the lunate which articulates with the hamate.[38] The presence of the facet is variable both in frequency and in its depth. Viegas et al described in 1990[39] two types of lunate. Type 1 lunates which occur in about 25% of dissected cadavers have no real facet but the type 2 lunate have facets ranging from 1 to 6 mm with the commonest size of facet being 2 mm. Also, interestingly about half of type 2 cadaveric lunates were found to have arthritis whereas the type 1 lunates had none. Both the shape of the lunate and the presence of arthritis were difficult to see on predissection X-rays and were not related to ulnar variance or sex.

It is common to find a step-off in the lunotriquetral joint when scoping the midcarpal joint. Though this is probably pathological for the scapholunate joint it appears to be normal or at least common in the lunotriquetral. The prominent triquetrum can be pushed down to the level of the proximal edge of the lunate facet. This mechanism would also occur when the wrist goes into ulnar deviation with increasing grip. The hamate pushes the triquetrum down to joint level and then locks into the facet (► Fig. 2.7).

4. Through the scaphoid. But only probably in certain positions when scaphoid is extended.

2.4.5 Locking Mechanisms in the Radiocarpal Joint

For the radiocarpal joint, a biaxial diarthrodial joint, there is no obvious bony block to movement. On increasing compression, it becomes stiffer due to increasing joint surface friction and resistance. Though the load is spread out, most of the load goes through the radial side rather than the pliant TFC. Increasing pressure over the surface increases resistance and hence motion in both flexion and extension and ulnar and radial deviation. It appears to be able to spread the loads which allows locking in various positions as well as fine control.

2.4.6 Isolated Joints

Carpal mechanical interest over the years has always been more on the wrist as a whole rather than individual joints. However, it may be better to look at individual joints particularly when dealing with traumatic disruption of the mechanics where the injury to both the bone and soft tissue can be limited but occurs often at the extreme ends of functional movement. This may then help better understand the injury patterns and why they occur and how to restore normal anatomy. Also, looking at individual joints may change views on the contribution that joint makes to the overall pattern.

The Radio-Scaphoid-Lunate Joint

The distal end of the radius has two fossae: one for the scaphoid and a second for the lunate. The two surfaces are divided by a central ridge exactly opposite the scapholunate joint. In the normal wrist, loading via the capitate head goes through the lunate more than the scaphoid though the scaphoid fossa is more likely to develop osteoarthritis. However, this doesn't occur without changes in the movement of the scaphoid normally following degeneration or injury of the ligaments producing abnormal movements and it stops being a diarthrodial joint. The normal joint appears to be good at taking extreme loads even on full extension probably due to the increasing contact areas with extension[40] as well as extreme flexion.[41] It is remarkable that the lunate is not involved more often in scapholunate advanced collapse probably because it doesn't rotate and remains with a large contact area in any position of extension or flexion.

However, the compression force of the capitate head which in a normal wrist locks the proximal pole in its fossa may make the unsupported waist of the scaphoid more susceptible to a fracture being at the junction point between a stable proximal end and a distal mobile one.

The Scapho-Trapezial-Trapezoid (STT) Joint (► Fig. 2.8)

This joint is also a gliding joint which occupies the dorsum of the distal half of the 45-degree downturned scaphoid like a tongue. When the distal row extends, it slides the STT over the back of the distal half of the scaphoid to reach the dorsal ridge of the scaphoid (osteology). There is no dorsal ligament but strong volar ones which lift the distal end of the scaphoid. However, at a certain point the proximal pole of the scaphoid cannot extend further and

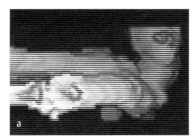
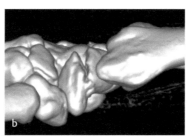

Fig. 2.8 (a) Early 3D computed tomography (CT) showing position of scaphoid on full extension of a cadaver wrist, and trapezium extending to the level of dorsal ridge of scaphoid. **(b)** Displaced acute scaphoid waist fracture with volar comminution.

because of the 45-degree bend on the scaphoid the tubercle lies in the long axis of the radius. This is easily verified by palpating one's own scaphoid tubercle and extending your wrist. Further compressive force through the STT joint in that position through the angulated scaphoid at the weak point of the waist is likely to be the cause of waist fractures, their fracture patterns,[42] their volar comminution (fracture patterns), and lack of associated ligament injuries.

The volar STT ligaments may also need to be secondarily stretched following scapho-lunate dissociation to get delayed DISI deformity.

The Scapho-Luno-Capitate (SLC) Joint (▶ Fig. 2.3)

This joint may be a very underestimated joint in terms of carpal mechanics probably because it is so difficult to visualize. It is a ball-and-socket joint in which the scapholunate joint lies across the center of the cup dividing it in two. Unfortunately, little is known about the mechanics of the cup or even the variability in the shape of each segment which could theoretically change in shape with movement of the capitate head. Also, compressive forces go through the capitate head into both the proximal pole of the scaphoid and the lunate. This may result in strain developing in the scapholunate ligaments which may increase the interference lock of the joint. However, it would also put strain on healing ligament and in tears lead to not only diastasis but also differential rotation of both parts of the cup. Further investigation will be needed but in the interim the author advises the patients not to grip to a level which locks the wrist while the ligaments are healing at the right length until they are strong enough to take the strain at about a month.

2.5 Carpal Movement

Unfortunately, it is still difficult to image abnormalities in carpal stability and movement. A good means of 3D imaging of the moving wrist is still awaited, though for some pathologies such as scapholunate dissociation, wrist cineradiography, which has been used for over 50 years, is accurate.[43] Though complex instabilities are difficult even for experts to diagnose.

2.5.1 Historical Perspective

Most treaties on carpal mechanics contain a long description of the history of carpal mechanical research. Marc Garcia-Elias eloquently describes this as "a long and winding road."[36] The author suggests reading his paper which covers the struggles of wrist surgeons coming to some degree of unified belief, and some of the more accessible original papers from these pioneers. However, it remains complex and until better dynamic imaging

techniques are developed it will remain difficult for most surgeons to visualize being the basis of understanding.

2.5.2 Wrist Movement

At the present time most people agree that the wrist moves through a central column mechanism and that this is driven through the rigid distal row which controls and moves the proximal row. The movement is controlled by both joint surface shape and ligaments. The main center of rotation is in the area of the capitate head though its exact location remains controversial and most people believe the main functional movement is the "Dart Throwers," in which the main movement is at the midcarpal joint.

On radial deviation of the distal row the scaphoid either flexes or slides out of the way[44] allowing the trapezium to move as close as possible to the radial styloid, but eventually it stops at the limits of scaphoid flexion. Sliding is probably stopped by the very strong radiotriquetral ligament.[31] How much the proximal row slides, flexes, or does both may depend on if the wrist is an extension or flexion.

Ulnar deviation is also controlled by the distal row. Instead of flexing like the scaphoid the triquetrum is blocked by the hamate. So, on ulnar deviation the hamate pushes the triquetrum proximally and locks through compression across its large flat interface or into the lunate if it has a facet. Ulnar deviation of the carpus which is normally more than radial deviation appears to be either constrained by the triquetrum on the TFC which has some compliance or from the radial side by the scaphoid unable to extend further and acting as a strap.

2.6 Hydromechanics of the Wrist

Wrist fluid is not often considered to be an important part of wrist mechanics. However, since 1953[45] the mechanical effect of fluid within the wrist joint has been considered and investigated by the rheumatologists as part of their research into the formation of subchondral cysts in osteoarthritis and rheumatoid geodes which are not considered to be cysts but cavities. In an in vivo experiment conducted in 1970 it was noted that the pressure within a distal radial geode in a rheumatoid patient gripping his wrist reached 240 mm Hg.[46] More recently, it was thought osteocyte death followed by hydraulic pressure caused the cavitation in arthritic joints.[47] In 2020 knee surgeons concerned about cyst formation under osteochondral grafts thought this may be in part due to pressure effects.[48] A study done by biochemical engineers in 2022[49] suggested the articular surfaces collapsed due to shear force not to pressure in the medial condyle of the horse. However, the normal resting wrist has minimal or negative pressure in it; any fluid within it results in increasing pressure on gripping which can go well above blood pressure. For the wrist surgeon, it may be the cause of the cystic nonunion found in scaphoid fractures and reducing grip and loading of the hand may be just as important as immobilization for the healing of these fractures.

2.7 Conclusions and Future Developments

Unfortunately, until better imaging and diagnostic techniques are available, treating carpal instabilities is still in the realms of the superspecialist.

However, for most surgeons treating acute trauma, the ability to image bone injuries better is available. However, it is still difficult to extrapolate this to soft tissue injuries and it remains the responsibility of surgeons to collect as much data as possible to improve knowledge of injury patterns. These data are often only available at open surgery for both pure ligament injuries and fracture dislocations. This will help restore normal anatomy, both alignment of the bones and soft tissue healing at the right length, either by conservative treatment or repair depending on the pattern.

A specific injury approach to investigation and research into the mechanical causation of the specific injuries will also help with restoring normal anatomy and hopefully function. In the same way more needs to be known about the way and the time taken for ligaments to heal and how the mechanics of the wrist during recovery may affect this. For instance, Bankart-type injuries due to lifting off of ligaments from bone which are found in certain dislocations may have different mechanical healing mechanics than a midsubstance ligament tear.

A lot still needs to be learnt from both basic science as well as clinical studies before we get to the end of this fascinating "long and winding road."

References

[1] Sandow M. The why, what, how and where of 3D imaging. J Hand Surg Eur Vol. 2014; 39(4):343–345

[2] Bodansky DMS, Sandow MJ, Volk I, Luria S, Verstreken F, Horwitz MD. Insights and trends review: the role of three-dimensional technology in upper extremity surgery. J Hand Surg Eur Vol. 2023; •••: 17531934221150498

[3] Jayasekera N, Akhtar N, Compson JP. Physical examination of the carpal bones by orthopaedic and accident and emergency surgeons. J Hand Surg [Br]. 2005; 30(2):204–206

[4] Srinivas Reddy R, Compson J. Examination of the wrist-surface anatomy of the carpal bones. Curr Orthop. 2005; 19:171–179

[5] Caumes M, Goislard de Monsabert B, Hauraix H, Berton E, Vigouroux L. Complex couplings between joints, muscles and performance: the role of the wrist in grasping. Sci Rep. 2019; 9(1):19357

[6] Kauer JM. Functional anatomy of the wrist. Clin Orthop Relat Res. 1980(149):9–20

[7] Owen DH, Agius PA, Nair A, Perriman DM, Smith PN, Roberts CJ. Factors predictive of patient outcome following total wrist arthrodesis. Bone Joint J. 2016; 98-B(5):647–653

[8] Lee J-A, Sechachalam S. The effect of wrist position on grip endurance and grip strength. J Hand Surg Am. 2016; 41(10):e367–e373

[9] Boyes JH. Bunnell's surgery of the hand. 5th ed. Philadelphia PA: JB Lippincott; 1970:269

[10] Haddad RJ, Jr, Riordan DC. Arthrodesis of the wrist. A surgical technique. J Bone Joint Surg Am. 1967; 49(5):950–954

[11] Hayden RJ, Jebson PJL. Wrist arthrodesis. Hand Clin. 2005; 21(4):631–640

[12] Hinds RM, Melamed E, O'Connell A, Cherry F, Seu M, Capo JT. Assessment of wrist function after simulated total wrist arthrodesis: a compatible a comparison of 6 wrist positions. Hand (N Y). 2016; 11 (4):464–468

[13] O'Driscoll SW, Horii E, Ness R, Cahalan TD, Richards RR, An KN. The relationship between wrist position, grasp size, and grip strength. J Hand Surg Am. 1992; 17(1):169–177

[14] Ryu JY, Cooney WP, III, Askew LJ, An KN, Chao EY. Functional ranges of motion of the wrist joint. J Hand Surg Am. 1991; 16(3):409–419

[15] Palmer AK, Werner FW, Murphy D, Glisson R. Functional wrist motion: a biomechanical study. J Hand Surg Am. 1985; 10(1):39–46

[16] Morimoto H, Apergis EP, Herzberg G, et al. 2007 IFSSH committee report of biomechanics committee: Biomechanics of the so-called dart-throwing motion of the wrist. J Hand Surg Am. 2007; 32A: 1447–1453

[17] Gilula LA. Carpal injuries: analytic approach and case exercises. AJR Am J Roentgenol. 1979; 133(3):503–517

[18] Landsmeer JMF. Power grip and precision handling. Ann Rheum Dis. 1962; 21(2):164–170

[19] Gould HP, Berger RA, Wolfe SW. The origin and meaning of "intercalated segment". J Hand Surg Am. 2015; 40(12):2471–2472

[20] Gilford WW, Bolton RH, Lambrinudi C. the mechanism of the wrist joint with special reference to fractures of the scaphoid. Guys Hosp Rep. 1943; 92:52–59

[21] Navarro A. Luxaciones del carpo. An Fac Med (Lima). 1921; 6:113–141

[22] Linscheid RL, Dobyns JH, Beabout JW, Bryan RS. Traumatic instability of the wrist. Diagnosis, classification, and pathomechanics. J Bone Joint Surg Am. 1972; 54(8):1612–1632

[23] S Braun N, Berger RA, Wolfe SW. Defining DISI and VISI. J Hand Surg Eur Vol. 2021; 46(5):566–568

[24] Mayfield JK. Johnson of P, Kilcoyne RK. Carpal dislocations: pathetic and progressive. perilunar instability. J Hand Surg Am. 1980; 5A: 226–241

[25] Viegas SF, Patterson RM, Hokanson JA, Davis J. Wrist anatomy: incidence, distribution, and correlation of anatomic variations, tears, and arthrosis. J Hand Surg Am. 1993; 18(3):463–475

[26] Taleisnik J. The ligaments of the wrist. J Hand Surg Am. 1976; 1(2): 110–118

[27] Berger RA. The anatomy of the ligaments of the wrist and distal radioulnar joints. Clin Orthop Relat Res. 2001(383):32–40

[28] Berger RA. The gross and histologic anatomy of the scapholunate interosseous ligament. J Hand Surg Am. 1996; 21(2):170–178

[29] Berger RA, Blair WF. The radioscapholunate ligament: a gross and histologic description. Anat Rec. 1984; 210(2):393–405

[30] Berger RA, Landsmeer JMF. The palmar radiocarpal ligaments: a study of adult and fetal human wrist joints. J Hand Surg Am. 1990; 15 (6):847–854

[31] Berger RA, Kauer JMG, Landsmeer JMF. Radioscapholunate ligament: a gross anatomic and histologic study of fetal and adult wrists. J Hand Surg Am. 1991; 16(2):350–355

[32] Sandow MJ, Fisher TJ, Howard CQ, Papas S. Unifying model of carpal mechanics based on computationally derived isometric constraints and rules-based motion - the stable central column theory. J Hand Surg Eur Vol. 2014; 39(4):353–363

[33] Tan J, Chen J, Tang JB. In vivo length changes of wrist ligaments at full wrist extension. J Hand Surg Eur Vol. 2014; 39(4):384–390

[34] Stephens NB, Kivell TL, Pahr DH, Hublin J-J, Skinner MM. Trabecular bone patterning across the human hand. J Hum Evol. 2018; 123:1–23

[35] Berger RA. The anatomy and basic biomechanics of the wrist joint. J Hand Ther. 1996; 9(2):84–93

[36] Garcia-Elias M. Kinetic analysis of carpal stability during grip. Hand Clin. 1997; 13(1):151–158

[37] Garcia-Elias M. Understanding wrist mechanics: a long and winding road. J Wrist Surg. 2013; 2(1):5–12

[38] McLean J, Bain G, Eames M, Fogg Q, Pourgiezis N. An anatomic study of the triquetrum-hamate joint. J Hand Surg Am. 2006; 31(4):601–607

[39] Viegas SF. The lunatohamate articulation of the midcarpal joint. Arthroscopy. 1990; 6(1):5–10

[40] Viegas SF, Wagner K, Patterson R, Peterson P. Medial (hamate) facet of the lunate. J Hand Surg Am. 1990; 15(4):564–571

[41] Chen YR, Wu YF, Tang JB, Giddins G. Contact areas of the scaphoid and lunate with the distal radius in neutral and extension: correlation of falling strategies and distal radial anatomy. J Hand Surg Eur Vol. 2014; 39(4):379–383

[42] Iwasaki N, Genda E, Minami A, Kaneda K, Chao EY. Force transmission through the wrist joint in Kienböck's disease: a two-dimensional theoretical study. J Hand Surg Am. 1998; 23(3):415–424

[43] Compson JP. The anatomy of acute scaphoid fractures: a three-dimensional analysis of patterns. J Bone Joint Surg Br. 1998; 80(2):218–224

[44] Sulkers GSI. Shep NWl, Maas M, van der Horst CMAM, Gosling JC, Strackee SD. The diagnostic accuracy of wrist cine radiography in diagnosing scapho-lunate dissociation. J Hand Surg Eur Vol. 2014; 39:263–271

[45] Eschweiler J, Li J, Quack V, et al. Anatomy, biomechanics, and loads of the wrist joint. Life (Basel). 2022; 12(2):188–205

[46] Craigen MA, Stanley JK. Wrist kinematics. Row, column or both? J Hand Surg [Br]. 1995; 20(2):165–170

[47] Landells JW. The Bone cysts of osteoarthritis. J Bone Joint Surg. 1953; 35B:643–649

[48] Jayson MIB, Rubenstein D, Dixon AS. Intra-articular pressure and rheumatoid geodes (bone 'cysts'). Ann Rheum Dis. 1970; 29(5):496–502

[49] Cox LGE, Lagemaat MW, van Donkelaar CC, et al. The role of pressurized fluid in subchondral bone cyst growth. Bone. 2011; 49(4):762–768

3 Role of Muscles in Wrist Stabilization and Clinical Implications

Mireia Esplugas, Alex Lluch, Guillem Salva-Coll, and Marc Garcia-Elias

Abstract

The wrist needs great mobility, on one side, and to keep normal anatomical relationships throughout the entire range of motion, on the other. We need a mobile wrist to place the hand in the best possible position that allows manipulating all sorts of objects, but we also need to ensure that the joint is able to sustain a considerable amount of force without yielding or suffering injury.

In kinetic terms, a joint is meant to be stable when it is able to sustain physiologic loads without yielding. When the wrist is loaded, capsular ligaments are the first to react. Some ligaments, however, may not resist prolonged tensions; thus, muscles play an important role in protecting them. Muscles play a key role as dynamic carpal stabilizers, and wrist proprioception is what coordinates all the entire process. Ligaments are complex structures containing sensory receptors aimed to provide proprioceptive information to the sensorimotor system to ensure carpal stability. When there is an excessive tension in one or more ligaments, some mechanoreceptors generate a warning message to the central nervous system. Based on this information, the nervous system decides which muscles need to contract and which need to relax to prevent further excessive ligament traction and damage. The wrist ligament-muscular reflexes are the key in this ligament injury protection through muscle activity. For each wrist position, the ligament-muscular reflexes provoke a muscular contraction of the protective muscles or a muscular activity inhibition of the destabilizing muscles.

How could muscles contribute to carpal stability and prevent carpal collapse, if their contraction is likely to compress the carpus? This is the main hypothesis that the authors investigated with many different cadaver biomechanical investigations. They found that wrist muscle activity induces an internal or an external intracarpal rotation relative to the forearm. These different rotations directly modify the carpal bones' positions and, thus, secondarily stabilize or destabilize the different carpal joints.

This chapter summarizes the different muscle-loading effects on the carpal bones alignments and the carpal joints stability in different carpal conditions: (1) interosseous-competent ligaments, (2) scapholunate ligament incompetence, (3) lunotriquetral ligament incompetence, (4) volar midcarpal ligaments deficiency. It also focuses, for the first time, on how the forearm rotation influences the neuromuscular control of the wrist.

Keywords: scapholunate joint muscle control, lunotriquetral joint muscle control, proximal carpal row dyskinesia muscle control, normal wrist muscle control, wrist kinetics, wrist kinematics

3.1 Introduction

From a kinetic point of view, a wrist is considered stable when it can maintain a normal carpal bones relationship, through any range of motion, under any physiological load.[1,2] This wrist stability is achieved by a complex and multifactorial mechanism which relies on four prerequisites: (1) all carpal joints must have normally tilted, reciprocally matching, and smooth articular surfaces, (2) both, capsule and ligaments need to be anatomically intact and properly innervated,[3,4] (3) the sensorimotor system (SMS), a collection of neural structures controlling the mechanisms of neuromuscular control of the joints, must be properly functioning,[5,6,7,8] and (4) the joint neighboring muscles need to be permanently active and ready to effectively neutralize any attempt to destabilize the wrist.[9]

Ligaments are not the only responsible part in joint stability. Even when they are torn, if the SMS and the surrounding muscles are competent, the carpus may still be stable through proprioception and the ligament-muscular reflexes. These allow a joint to receive much greater loads without collapsing than the ones that its proper ligaments can bear. In other words, if the ligaments are the first static stabilization line of the carpus, the muscles that cross the wrist are the second: they are the joint dynamic stabilizers and can stabilize it even when the ligaments are incompetent.

The wrist is a load-bearing joint: any hand activity induces some loading forces across it. These forces carry a predictable kinetical intracarpal alignment modification intended to stabilize the carpus and avoid any carpal collapse.[10] Some neighboring wrist joint muscles contribute to this carpal joints' stability. These muscles actively control the beneficial adaptive carpal alignment in such a way that it does not cross any physiological limit. Other muscles' activity destabilizes the carpal joints: their activity oversizes this adaptive carpal alignment beyond any physiological limit. This is what we call the neuromuscular control of the carpus.

To better understand the accurate stabilizing/destabilizing role of muscles, the authors performed a series of cadaver investigations.[11,12,13,14,15,16,17,18] The purpose of this chapter is to summarize their findings and clarify the role of muscles control in the scapholunate, lunotriquetral, and midcarpal ligaments–deficient wrists. This will become useful in the nonsurgical treatment of the early stages of carpal instabilities or in their pre- or postoperative management programs.

3.2 Interosseous Ligament– Competent Wrist (Normal Wrist)

3.2.1 Kinetic Effect of the Axial Loading on the Carpal Bones Alignment: How Does a Normal Carpus Adapt to the Axial Loading to Avoid Any Collapse?

Kinetics is the branch of physics that deals with the effects of any force applied on a material. Next, we summarize our laboratory findings on how the carpus kinetically adapts to any axial-loading (compression) force (▶ Table 3.1):

- The distal carpal row internally rotates (pronates) around a vertical axis and proximally migrates. This torque movement is transmitted to the proximal carpal row through the midcarpal joint (MCj) ligaments.
- At the proximal carpal row, the scaphoid and the triquetrum (1) slightly volarly translate, (2) ulnarly translate, and (3) reversely rotate around a horizontal axis: the scaphoid flexes and also pronates while the triquetrum extends. The extension moment of the triquetrum counteracts the scaphoid flexion moment, resulting in a stable equilibrium which avoids any carpal collapse under the axial loading.[2,11,12]

Clinical Implications

- Exercises that induce an important axial load through the carpus, such as squeezing a soft object, should be prescribed with caution when the integrity of the interosseous ligaments is uncertain.[2]
- Radiological wrist clenched fist view is sustained by the kinetic effect of an axial-loading force on the carpal bone alignment. Clenched fist radiological view is based on the kinetic effect of an axial load on carpal bony alignment.

Table 3.1 Normal wrist and scapholunate ligament–incompetent wrist

Proximal and distal carpal row bones kinetic adaptation to the axial-loading forces exerted, from distal to proximal, on a wrist kept in neutral position (neutral flexion/extension and neutral radioulnar inclination) when the forearm is in neutral rotation (intracarpal pronation = internal rotation)

Distal carpal row	Intracarpal pronation
Scaphoid bone	Flexion / Intracarpal pronation
Triquetrum bone	Extension

The scaphoid bone and the triquetrum rotate in reverse senses. The scaphoid bone follows the distal carpal row into an internal intracarpal rotation.

3.2.2 Kinetic Effect on the Carpal Bones Alignment of the Isometric Muscle Loading

The most significant experimental findings are summarized in ▶ Table 3.2, ▶ Table 3.3, ▶ Table 3.4, ▶ Table 3.5, ▶ Table 3.6, ▶ Table 3.7, ▶ Table 3.8.

Based on these observations we can conclude that:

- In neutral forearm rotation, the conjoint isometric loading of all the wrist motor tendon muscles induces a distal carpal row intracarpal supination which is totally opposite and, so, it is able to counteract the MCj pronation induced by the forces exerted during the axial loading (▶ Table 3.2).
- In neutral forearm rotation, the forearm muscles can be classified into two categories[11,13] (▶ Table 3.3):
  - The extensor carpi ulnaris (ECU) muscle, whose isometric individual loading rotates the distal carpal row internally: it is the main MCj pronator muscle and its activity aggravates the reactive distal carpal row and the scaphoid and triquetrum bones pronation that are associated to an axial-loading force. The ECU muscle isometric loading destabilizes the scapholunate joint (SLj) space but stabilizes the lunotriquetral joint (LTqj). The ECU is an SLj-unfriendly muscle but an LTqj-friendly muscle (▶ Fig. 3.1).
  - The abductor pollicis longus (APL), extensor carpi radialis longus (ECRL), and extensor carpi radialis brevis (ECRB) muscles, whose isometric individual loading induces a distal carpal row external rotation: they are the MCj supinator muscles. Their kinetic supinating effect counteracts the distal carpal row and scaphoid pronation found during the wrist axial load. Their activity generates an intracarpal scaphoid supination which stabilizes the SLj space. APL, ECRL, and ECRB are the SLj-friendly muscles (▶ Fig. 3.2).
- The APL isometric loading powerfully stabilizes the SLj space in neutral forearm rotation (▶ Table 3.3).
- In forearm pronation, the ECRL and the ECRB turn into great, powerful SLj space-friendly muscles (▶ Table 3.4).

Table 3.2 Normal wrist

Distal carpal row bones kinetic adaptation to the simultaneous isometric loading of the five wrist motor tendons (APL, ECRL, ECU, FCR, FCU) when the wrist is kept in neutral position and the forearm in neutral rotation (intracarpal supination = external rotation)

	Alignment tendency	Muscle load beneficial effect
Distal carpal row	Intracarpal supination	Counteracts the axial-loading effect

The simultaneous isometric loading of the wrist motor muscles stabilizes the carpus when this is axially loaded.

Table 3.3 Normal wrist and scapholunate ligament–incompetent wrist in neutral forearm rotation

Significant results of the proximal and distal carpal row bones kinetic adaptation to the individual isometric loading of the APL, ECRL, ECRB, and ECU muscles when the wrist is kept in neutral position and *the forearm is in neutral rotation* (Supi = external intracarpal rotation; Prona = internal intracarpal rotation; **: Very powerful)

Neutral forearm rotation	APL	ECRL	ECRB	ECRL + ECRB	ECU	ECU + FCU
Distal carpal row	Supi	Supi	Supi	Supi	Prona	Prona
Scaphoid	Supi	Supi	Supi	Supi	Prona	Prona
Triquetrum					Prona	Prona
Stabilizes the SL joint?	Yes**	Yes	Yes	Yes	No	No

In neutral forearm rotation, the isometric APL, ECRL, and ECRB muscles loading stabilizes the SLj. They are the MCj supinator muscles; they are considered the SLj-friendly muscles. In this forearm rotation, the APL stabilizes the joint more powerfully than the other stabilizing muscles.
The individual ECU muscle loading or the simultaneous wrist ulnar inclination muscles loading destabilizes the SLj. The ECU muscle is considered the scapholunate-unfriendly muscle and the FCU muscle loading is not able to counteract this destabilizing role.

Table 3.4 Normal wrist and scapholunate ligament–incompetent wrist in forearm pronation

Most significant results of the proximal and distal carpal row bones kinetic adaptation to the individual isometric loading of the APL, ECRL, ECRB, and ECU muscles when the wrist is kept in neutral position and *the forearm is in pronation* (Supi = external intracarpal rotation; Prona = internal intracarpal rotation; **: Very powerful)

Forearm pronation	APL	ECRL	ECRB	ECRL + ECRB	ECU	ECU + FCU
Distal carpal row	Supi	Supi	Supi	Supi	Prona	Prona
Scaphoid	Supi	Supi	Supi	Supi	Prona	Prona
Triquetrum					Prona	Prona
Stabilizes the SL joint?	Yes	Yes**	Yes**	Yes**	No	No

In forearm pronation, the isometric APL, ECRL, and ECRB muscles loading stabilizes the SLj. They are still the SLj-friendly muscles although, in forearm pronation, the radial extensor wrist muscles (ECRL and ECRB) stabilize the joint more powerfully than the APL muscle does.
The individual ECU muscle loading or the simultaneous wrist ulnar inclination muscles loading destabilizes the SLj.

Table 3.5 Normal wrist and scapholunate ligament–incompetent wrist in forearm supination

Most significant results of the proximal and distal carpal row bones kinetic adaptation to the individual isometric loading of the APL, ECRL, ECRB, and ECU muscles when the wrist is kept in neutral position and *the forearm is in supination* (Supi = external intracarpal rotation; Prona = internal intracarpal rotation; **: Very powerful)

Forearm supination	APL	ECRL	ECRB	ECRL + ECRB	ECU	ECU + FCU
Distal carpal row		Prona	Prona	Prona	Prona	Prona
Scaphoid	Supi	Prona	Prona	Prona	Prona**	Prona
Triquetrum					Prona	Prona
Stabilizes the SL joint?	No	No	No	No	No**	No

In forearm supination, the individual or simultaneous isometric load of any wrist muscle tendon destabilizes the SLj: the scapholunate-friendly muscles become unfriendly muscles and the destabilizing effect of the ECU muscle is maximal.

Table 3.6 Distal radius misalignment: joint surface volarly tilted

Most significant results of the distal carpal row kinetic adaptation to the simultaneous isometric loading of the APL, ECRL, ECB, and ECU muscles when the wrist is ligament-competent and the *distal radius joint surface is 20° volarly tilted* (wrist kept in neutral position with the forearm in neutral rotation)

Distal radius joint surface 20-degree volarly tilted	Alignment tendency	Muscle load–stabilizing effect
Distal carpal row	*Intracarpal pronation*	*No*

When the distal radius joint surface is at least 20-degree volarly tilted, the simultaneous activity of the wrist motor muscles is not able to stabilize the axially loaded carpus. On the contrary, their activity may even destabilize it.

Table 3.8 Distal radius misalignment: joint surface dorsally tilted and shortened

Most significant results of the distal carpal row and scaphoid bone kinetic adaptations to the simultaneous isometric loading of the MCj supinator muscles (APL, ECRL, and ECRB) when the wrist is ligament-competent and *the distal radius joint surface is 20-degree dorsally tilted and 4 mm shortened* (wrist kept in neutral position with the forearm in neutral rotation)

Distal radius joint surface 20-degree dorsally tilted and 4 mm shortened	Alignment tendency	Muscle load–stabilizing effect
Distal carpal row	*Intracarpal pronation*	*No*
Scaphoid bone	*Dorsal translation*	*No*

When the distal radius joint surface is at least 20-degree dorsally tilted, the distal radius is 4 mm shortened, and the scapholunate ligament is competent, the simultaneous wrist motor muscles load induces a dorsal scaphoid bone translation which destabilizes the SLj and the SLj-friendly muscles lose their potential stabilizing role.

Their effect is greater in forearm pronation than in neutral forearm rotation.
- On the contrary (▶ Table 3.5), in forearm supination, the isometric loading MCj supinator muscles induce a contrary intracarpal pronation effect which aggravates the external rotation induced by the axial-loading forces.
- Forearm rotation does not influence the kinetic effect exerted by the ECU muscle even when it is loaded in association with the flexor carpi ulnaris (FCU) (▶ Table 3.5). The ECU muscle loading destabilizes the SLj space and stabilizes the LTqj one, in any forearm rotation, although it becomes much more powerful in forearm supination.

Table 3.7 Distal radius misalignment: joint surface dorsally tilted

Most significant results of the scaphoid bone kinetic adaptation to the simultaneous isometric loading of the APL, ECRL, ECB, and ECU muscles when the wrist is ligament-competent and the *distal radius joint surface is 20-degree dorsally tilted* (wrist kept in neutral position with the forearm in neutral rotation)

Distal radius joint surface 20-degree dorsally tilted	Alignment tendency	Muscle load–stabilizing effect
Scaphoid bone	*Dorsal translation*	*No*

When the distal radius joint surface is at least 20-degree dorsally tilted, the simultaneous wrist motor muscles load induces a dorsal scaphoid bone translation which destabilizes the SLj even when the SLj ligament is competent.

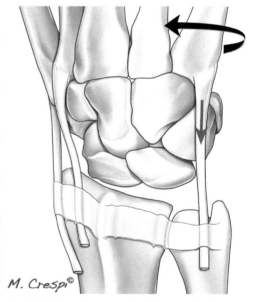

M. Crespi©

Fig. 3.1 ECU muscle contraction induces a distal carpal row internal rotation (intracarpal pronation) relative to the axis of the forearm. This rotation influences both the scapholunate and lunotriquetral joint stability.

- When the articular surface of the radius is at least 20-degree volarly tilted, the beneficial MCj supination carried by the simultaneous loading of all the wrist motor muscles disappears and turns into a negative MCj pronation (▶ Table 3.6). In this situation, muscle loading is not able to counteract the normal intracarpal adaptation to the forces exerted by any axial loading[14]: their protective muscular action against any intracarpal ligament injury secondary to an axial overload is weakened and ligament injuries are facilitated.

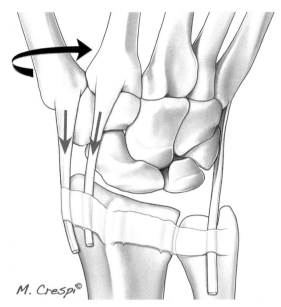

Fig. 3.2 APL and ECRL muscle contraction induce a distal carpal row external rotation (intracarpal supination) relative to the axis of the forearm. This midcarpal joint rotation influences both the scapholunate and the lunotriquetral joint stability.

- When the articular surface of the radius is more than 20-degree dorsally tilted and the wrist motor muscles are conjointly loaded, the scaphoid significantly dorsally translates, even if the SLj ligaments are intact[14] (▶ Table 3.7). So, in this type of distal radius misalignment, even if the scapholunate ligament (SLL) is intact, an early painful radioscaphoid joint degenerative changes may appear.
- When the articular surface of the radius is dorsally tilted and the radius is 4 mm shortened, the SLj-stabilizing effect of the supinator muscles is completely lost[14] (▶ Table 3.8). The scaphoid is dorsally translated and there is no possibility of dynamically stabilizing it. Any superimposed SLL injury associated to this type of distal radius misalignment will hopelessly lead to an early SLAC 1 wrist.

Clinical Implications

- Forearm supination seems to be detrimental to the SLj space stability. Any wrist injury in forearm supination will clearly put at risk the SLL.
- SLj radiographic studies in a true forearm supination clearly better assess the joint space.[15]
- Forearm supination induces some degree of misalignment at the level of the MCj: the SLj space widens and the step increases. Therefore, forearm supination facilitates the arthroscopic evaluation of the SLL-incompetent wrist.
- Forearm rotation is an important factor to consider when planning muscle-strengthening programs to stabilize the wrist.[16,17]

- Forearm pronation protects the SLj space: the scaphoid tends to supinate and the SLj space-friendly muscles are more efficient.
- Casting a wrist sprain patient in 45-degree forearm pronation and carpal supination seems to be the most favorable position for the SLj space and ligaments.
- The ECU contraction always creates an SLj space widening, no matter what rotation the forearm is in. Its activity should be avoided in any pre- or postoperative rehabilitation program after an SLL injury.
- The distal radius joint surface misalignment, even if it is congruent, severely interferes in the muscle control of the carpus and the dynamic scaphoid alignment at the radial scaphoid fossa.
- When an extra-articular distal radius fracture is associated with an SLL injury, the alignment of the radius in the coronal and sagittal planes should be as close to normal as possible, in order to allow and facilitate the efficient dynamic muscular stabilization of the SLj.
- An SLj disconnection may develop osteoarthritic changes (SLAC wrist) faster if it is associated with an extra-articular dorsally tilted distal radius joint surface.
- An SLL reconstruction will easily fail if it lies over a dorsally tilted and shortened malunited distal radius.

3.3 Scapholunate Joint Ligament–Deficient Wrist

3.3.1 Kinetic Effect of the Axial Loading: How Does an SLL-Incompetent Carpus Adapt to the Axial Loading?

As we have previously seen (▶ Table 3.1) when the SLL complex is intact, the axial loading of the wrist induces a slight volar translation of the proximal pole of the scaphoid; nevertheless, the radio scaphoid centroid of pressure still remains in a radial scaphoid fossa area with a good thickness of articular cartilage. On the contrary, when there is a complete SLL injury, the axial loading of the wrist greatly displaces the proximal scaphoid pole toward the dorsal aspect of the radial scaphoid fossa and the centroid of pressure comes where the cartilage is thin and poorly prepared to bear loads.

Clinical Implications

- This finding helps to understand that the SLAC osteoarthritic changes start between the proximal pole of the scaphoid and the dorsal area of the radial scaphoid fossa.
- After performing an SLL reconstruction, the main goal to achieve is not to correct the gap between the scaphoid and the lunate in the coronal plane but to correct: (1) the flexion and intracarpal pronation of the scaphoid and, specially, (2) its dorsoradial translation to prevent the joint degeneration and restore the ability to sustain axial loads.

3.3.2 Muscle Control of the Carpal Bones Alignment When the SLL Is Incompetent[18,19,20]

- The loaded ECU muscle is always incompetent to counteract the SLj alignment induced by an axial load, in any forearm rotation. The truth is that the ECU muscle activity further destabilizes the axially loaded SLj, especially in forearm supination (▶ Table 3.3).
- The coloading of the FCU muscle tendon is not able to counteract the SLj destabilizing effect of the ECU muscle tendon loading (▶ Table 3.3).
- In neutral forearm rotation or forearm pronation (▶ Table 3.3, ▶ Table 3.4), both the ECRL and the ECRB are SLj-stabilizing muscles. Conversely, in forearm supination (▶ Table 3.5), the ECRL and ECRB muscles loading cannot counteract the destabilizing forces exerted on the SLj when the wrist is axially loaded.
- The APL is a good SLj-stabilizing muscle in neutral forearm rotation (▶ Table 3.3).

Clinical Applications

- We may avoid any wrist motor muscle strengthening in forearm supination when we are promoting a conservative treatment of an SLj dysfunction, or when we are conducting a postoperative rehabilitation program: never in forearm supination!
- To dynamically stabilize the SLj, we should promote the APL muscle strengthening in neutral forearm rotation and the wrist radial extensor muscles (ECRL and ECRB) in forearm pronation.
- We should never include the ECU muscle strengthening in the SLj neuromuscular control programs.
- The active co-contraction of the ECU and the FCU muscles in forearm supination maximally destabilizes an SLL-deficient wrist. This maneuver is helpful in order to detect a dynamic SLj dysfunction by radiology.[15]

3.4 Lunotriquetral Joint Ligaments (LTqL) Deficient Wrist

3.4.1 Kinetic Effect of the Axial Loading on the Carpal Bones Alignment: How Does a Deficient LTqL Carpus Adapt to the Axial Loading?

When the LTqL is incompetent, the lunate follows the scaphoid bone position; so, when the wrist is axially loaded, the lunate flexes. On the contrary, the triquetrum, dragged by the triquetrum-hamate helicoidal shape, extends (▶ Table 3.9). This reverse bone rotation undermines the proximal row stability in front of any axial load.

Table 3.9 Lunotriquetral ligament–incompetent wrist: all wrist motor muscles simultaneous loading effect

Proximal and distal carpal row bones kinetic adaptation to the simultaneous five wrist motor muscles isometric loading forces exerted on a lunotriquetral ligament–deficient wrist kept in neutral position when the forearm is in neutral rotation (intracarpal pronation = internal rotation; intracarpal supination= external rotation)

Distal carpal row	*Intracarpal pronation*
Scaphoid and lunate bones	*Flexion/Intracarpal supination*
Triquetrum bone	*Flexion/Intracarpal supination*

Simultaneous loading of all wrist motor tendons always induces a rotation of the entire proximal row into flexion. When the LTqL is incompetent, the ulnar side corner of the wrist overflexes.

Clinical Implications

- The dynamic incompetence of the LTq joint ligaments is difficult to appreciate on a static wrist X-ray as a mild triquetrum extension and a mild lunate flexion are not easy to observe. This is why arthroscopic evaluation of the wrist, with a few amount of axial traction to avoid carpal bones extension, is helpful in this condition.
- The triquetrum extension control directly depends on: (1) the hamate position, (2) the triquetrum-hamate joint surface congruence, (3) the volar triquetrum-hamate ligament, (4) the volar ulno-triquetrum ligament, and (5) the dorsal radio-triquetral ligament competence. It is a constrained carpal bone; its complete collapse is not so common.

3.4.2 Muscle Control of the Carpal Bones Alignment When the LTqj Ligaments Are Incompetent[21,22] (▶ Table 3.10)

- When making a closed fist with an LTq ligament–incompetent wrist in neutral position, the triquetrum rotates into a maximal flexion which is difficult to see on stress X-ray studies.
- On the contrary, the individual isometric loading of the ECU muscle, the MC joint pronator muscle, extends and pronates the triquetrum.

Clinical Implications

- The ECU muscle is the only muscle which tends to realign the LTqj when its ligaments are incompetent: it is the only stabilizing muscle.
- The ECU muscle strengthening and proprioceptive training performed in forearm supination can help to stabilize a ligament-deficient LTqj.

Table 3.10 Lunotriquetral ligament–incompetent wrist: individual wrist motor muscles loading effect

Most significant results of the proximal and distal carpal row bones kinetic adaptation to the individual isometric loading of the APL, ECRL, ECRB, and ECU muscles when the wrist is kept in neutral position and the forearm in neutral rotation (Supi = external intracarpal rotation; Prona = internal intracarpal rotation)

Neutral forearm rotation	APL	ECRL	ECRB	ECRL + ECRB	ECU
Distal carpal row	Supi	Supi	Supi	Supi	*Prona*
Scaphoid	Supi	Supi	Supi	Supi	Prona
Triquetrum	Flexion	Flexion	Flexion	Flexion	Extension/Prona
Stabilizes the LTq joint?	No	No	No	No	**Yes**

The ECU muscle is the only lunotriquetral ligament–deficient dynamic stabilizer: it extends the triquetrum by pronating the distal carpal row and the hamate bone.

Table 3.11 Volar proximal carpal row dysfunction

Most significant results of the proximal and distal carpal row bones kinetic adaptation to the individual isometric loading of the APL, ECRL, ECU, FCR, and FCU muscles when the proximal carpal row is in flexion, the wrist is in neutral inclination, and the forearm is in neutral rotation (Supi = external intracarpal rotation; Prona = internal intracarpal rotation; **: Very powerful)

Wrist in neutral position	APL	ECRL	FCU	FCR	ECU
Controls the proximal carpal row flexion?	No	No	No	No	**Yes**
Avoids "clunking"?	No	No	No	No	**Yes**

When the scapholunate and lunotriquetral interosseous ligaments are competent and the proximal carpal row is flexed in neutral wrist radial-ulnar inclination, the ECU muscle is the only factor able to extend the proximal carpal row and avoid the sudden "clunking" triquetrum-hamate reduction when the wrist gets its maximal ulnar inclination.

3.5 Volar Nondissociative Proximal Carpal Row Dysfunction Secondary to the Midcarpal and Dorsal Radiocarpal Ligaments Incompetence

Until now, we have reviewed the kinetic effect of load (axial or muscular loads) on the proximal carpal row bones alignment when the wrist presents some ligament deficiencies. Now, we will focus on the kinematic effect of the wrist radial/ulnar inclination on the proximal carpal row bones alignment.

3.5.1 Normal Wrist Proximal Carpal Row Kinematics During Wrist Inclinations

When ligaments connecting the proximal and distal carpal rows are competent and the wrist is in radial inclination, the whole first carpal row bones are in flexion. On the contrary, when the wrist is in ulnar inclination, the three proximal carpal bones are in extension. This first carpal row mobility from flexion to extension is smooth, harmonious, and progressive, so, in the midway, the neutral wrist inclination, the three proximal carpal row bones are in a neutral flexion/extension position.

3.5.2 Proximal Carpal Row Kinematics During Wrist Radial/Ulnar Inclination When the Radial MC Ligaments Are Incompetent

In this condition, the whole first carpal row bones still remain flexed in neutral wrist position. Then they, suddenly and abruptly, extend when the wrist gets its maximal ulnar inclination. This abrupt proximal carpal row extension is easily audible with a "clunk" which corresponds to the sudden triquetrum hinging into the helicoidal-shaped triquetrum-hamate joint.[23] This proximal carpal row dyskinesia (abnormal kinematics during wrist mobility) may become symptomatic and clinically unstable.[24,25]

3.5.3 Muscular Control of the Volar Proximal Carpal Row Dyskinesia

- When an abnormal proximal row flexion is created in the lab, the isolated isometric load of the ECU muscle is the only factor that corrects proximal row position while the wrist is in neutral position[26] (▶ Table 3.11).
- In addition, the ECU MCj-pronating effect prevents the sudden and abrupt reduction of the triquetrum-hamate joint.

Clinical Applications

- Proximal carpal row dyskinetic dysfunction was traditionally named as a "midcarpal joint instability." This name should be avoided.
- Proximal carpal row dyskinesia is mostly associated to (1) hyperlaxity (benign or severe), (2) it may also appear after a midcarpal ligaments direct injury, or a (3) wrist neuromuscular control or proprioception impair (after a long wrist immobilization, for instance).
- Conservative treatment is the preferred one. The beneficial effect of the ECU muscle in stabilizing the proximal carpal row should be boosted, especially in symptomatic hyperlax patients and in the pre- and postoperative phases of any MCj ligament repair.
- The orthoses which generate a distal carpal row pronation can be beneficial.

References

[1] Definition of carpal instability. The Anatomy and Biomechanics Committee of the International Federation of Societies for Surgery of the Hand. J Hand Surg Am. 1999; 24:866–867

[2] Garcia-Elias M. Kinetic analysis of carpal stability during grip. Hand Clin. 1997; 13(1):151–158

[3] Hagert E, Forsgren S, Ljung BO. Differences in the presence of mechanoreceptors and nerve structures between wrist ligaments may imply differential roles in wrist stabilization. J Orthop Res. 2005; 23(4):757–763

[4] Hagert E, Garcia-Elias M, Forsgren S, Ljung BO. Immunohistochemical analysis of wrist ligament innervation in relation to their structural composition. J Hand Surg Am. 2007; 32(1):30–36

[5] Hagert E, Lluch A, Rein S. The role of proprioception and neuromuscular stability in carpal instabilities. J Hand Surg Eur Vol. 2016; 41(1):94–101

[6] Lluch A, Salva-Coll G, Esplugas M, Llusá M, Hagert E, Garcia-Elias M. El papel de la propiocepción y el control neuromuscular en las inestabilidades del carpo. Rev Iberoam Cir Mano. 2015; 43(1):70–78

[7] Riemann BL, Lephart SM. The sensorimotor system, part I: the physiologic basis of functional joint stability. J Athl Train. 2002; 37 (1):71–79

[8] Riemann BL, Lephart SM. The sensorimotor system, part II: the role of proprioception in motor control and functional joint stability. J Athl Train. 2002; 37(1):80–84

[9] Hagert E, Persson JK, Werner M, Ljung BO. Evidence of wrist proprioceptive reflexes elicited after stimulation of the scapholunate interosseous ligament. J Hand Surg Am. 2009; 34(4):642–651

[10] Kobayashi M, Garcia-Elias M, Nagy L, et al. Axial loading induces rotation of the proximal carpal row bones around unique screw-displacement axes. J Biomech. 1997; 30(11–12):1165–1167

[11] Salvà-Coll G, Garcia-Elias M, León-López MT, Llusa-Perez M, Rodríguez-Baeza A. Effects of forearm muscles on carpal stability. J Hand Surg Eur Vol. 2011; 36(7):553–559

[12] Salvà Coll G, Garcia-Elias M, Lluch Bergadà Á, León López MM, Llusá Pérez M, Rodríguez Baeza A. Carpal dynamic stability mechanisms. Experimental study. Rev Esp Cir Ortop Traumatol. 2013; 57(2):129–134

[13] Salvà-Coll G, Garcia-Elias M, León-López MM, Llusa-Perez M, Rodríguez-Baeza A. Role of the extensor carpi ulnaris and its sheath on dynamic carpal stability. J Hand Surg Eur Vol. 2012; 37(6):544–548

[14] Fernandez N, Garcia-Elias M, Esplugas M, et al. Influence of post traumatic deformities of the distal radius on muscle control of the carpus. A biomechanical study in cadaver. Federation of European Societies for Surgery of the Hand, FESSH, On(line), Week; 2020

[15] Puig de la Bellacasa I, Salva-Coll G, Esplugas M, Quintas S, Lluch A, Garcia-Elias M. Bilateral ulnar deviation supination stress test to assess dynamic scapholunate instability. J Hand Surg Am. 2022; 47 (7):639–644

[16] Holmes MK, Taylor S, Miller C, Brewster MBS. Early outcomes of "The Birmingham Wrist Instability Programme": a pragmatic intervention for stage one scapholunate instability. Hand Ther. 2017; 22(3):90–100

[17] Lluch A, Esplugas M, Carreño A, et al. ¿Qué hemos aprendido sobre la muñeca en los últimos años? Del laboratorio a la práctica clínica. Cirugía De Mano Y Microcirugía. 2021; 1:50–60

[18] Salvà-Coll G, Garcia-Elias M, Hagert E. Scapholunate instability: proprioception and neuromuscular control. J Wrist Surg. 2013; 2(2): 136–140

[19] León-López MM, García-Elías M, Salvà-Coll G, Llusá-Perez M, Lluch-Bergadà A. Muscular control of scapholunate instability. An experimental study. Rev Esp Cir Ortop Traumatol. 2014; 58(1):11–18

[20] Salva-Coll G, Garcia-Elias M, Lluch-Bergada A, Esplugas M, Llusa-Perez M. Kinetic dysfunction of the wrist with chronic scapholunate dissociation. A cadaver study. Clin Biomech (Bristol, Avon). 2020; 77: 105046

[21] León-Lopez M, Salvà-Coll G, Garcia-Elias M, Lluch-Bergadà A, Llusá-Pérez M. Role of the extensor carpi ulnaris in the stabilization of the lunotriquetral joint. An experimental study. J Hand Ther. 2013; 26: 312–317. Experimental study. Rev Esp Cir Ortop Traumatol 2013;57:129–134

[22] Esplugas M, Garcia-Elias M, Lluch A, Llusá Pérez M. Role of muscles in the stabilization of ligament-deficient wrists. J Hand Ther. 2016; 29 (2):166–174

[23] McLean J, Bain G, Eames M, Fogg Q, Pourgiezis N. An anatomic study of the triquetrum-hamate joint. J Hand Surg Am. 2006; 31(4):601–607

[24] Garcia-Elias M. The non-dissociative clunking wrist: a personal view. J Hand Surg Eur Vol. 2008; 33(6):698–711

[25] Wolfe SW, Garcia-Elias M, Kitay A. Carpal instability nondissociative. J Am Acad Orthop Surg. 2012; 20(9):575–585

[26] Lluch A, Esplugas M, Salvà G, Garcia-Elias M. The role of neuromuscular control in carpal non-dissociative instabilities. Seattle: American Society for Surgery of the Hand Annual Meeting; 2015

4 Ligament Injury and Carpal Instability

Carlos Heras-Palou and Ezequiel Zaidenberg

Abstract

Due to the complexity of the wrist dynamic and static stabilizers, isolated carpal ligament injuries do not cause carpal instability. The terms "ligament injury" of the wrist and "carpal instability" are often used interchangeably, but they are different concepts.

An isolated ligament injury seen on magnetic resonance imaging (MRI) scan, computed tomography (CT) arthrogram, or even wrist arthroscopy is not diagnostic of wrist instability. Ligament injuries without clinical correlation or pain do not constitute a carpal instability and most of them do not require treatment. Furthermore, laxity of the wrist without symptoms should not be understood as a carpal instability and does not require further assessment or treatment. Carpal instabilities are usually caused by failure of several ligament stabilizers leading to a group of dynamic clinical syndromes with defined symptoms and signs that most often require treatment. The diagnosis is based on the clinical history and the examination, and the condition can be further defined and staged with radiographs, fluoroscopy, CT-arthrogram, MRI scan, or wrist arthroscopy.

The decision of management of the unstable wrist must be made based on the clinical findings in the history and examination of every case. Refining and staging the diagnoses are based on imaging and wrist arthroscopy. Clinical assessment must be done before imaging is reviewed to avoid cognitive confirmation bias.

Keywords: carpal instability, wrist instability, wrist ligament injury, management, investigation, assessment of the wrist, wrist injuries

4.1 Introduction

The terms "scapholunate ligament injury" and "scapholunate instability" are often used interchangeably, but they are different concepts.

The wrist is a cardanic joint with a large range of movement and it is able to sustain large compressive and torsional forces (▶ Fig. 4.1). It has been estimated, and then measured, that the force across the wrist is about 10 times the grip force exerted. A young male gripping 50 kg in his hand is applying a force of 500 kg across his radiocarpal joint.[1,2]

A wrist that is not able to keep normal articular alignment when subjected to physiologic deforming forces is said to be unstable.[3] Wrist instability can cause pain, weakness, swelling, inability to perform tasks, and, in the long term, degeneration of the joint surfaces and secondary

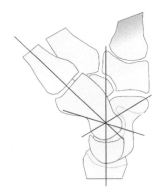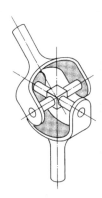

Fig. 4.1 A cardanic (named after G. Cardano, 1501–1576) or universal joint consists of a crosslike piece, opposite ends of which rotate within the forked end of each of the two shafts connected. Your car may have a joint like this to transmit torque to the rear wheels. The wrist has two joints, radiocarpal and midcarpal joints, with their axis at an angle joint by an intercalated segment (scaphoid, lunate, and triquetrum) that allows combined movements at both joints, while sustaining physiological loads without yielding. The intercalated segment moves passively, has no tendon attached to it, controlled only by the ligaments and the shape of the bones.

wrist osteoarthritis. Instability and degeneration can prevent patients from being able to carry out their activities of daily living, their work, and their hobbies, with a significant impact on quality of life.

4.2 Ligament Tears

The carpal ligaments have a very important role to play in providing stability, but they are not the only factor.[4] The stability of the wrist is provided by:
- Smooth and normally orientated joint surfaces.
- An integrated system of intrinsic and extrinsic ligaments.
- A coordinated system of muscles that cross and control the joint.

Wrist arthroscopy and magnetic resonance imaging (MRI) have changed surgeons' practice in the management of ligament injuries of the wrist. As these techniques became popular, surgeons soon realized that there is a low correlation between clinical signs and symptoms and arthroscopic and MRI findings. An early study[5] found no correlation between chondromalacia, synovitis, and ligament tears with mechanism of injury, duration of symptoms, presence of clicking or pain with activity; that is, there was no correlation between ligament changes and carpal instability.

A lot of attention has been given to the intrinsic ligaments, those who link one carpal bone to another, but these ligaments are small and not very strong. The scapholunate ligament has been well studied and the pull-out strength to cause a rupture of the dorsal part of the ligament was measured at 260.3 N or around 26.5 kg.[6] For the palmar component of the lunotriquetral ligament the pull-out strength is 301 N or around 30.6 kg force. The strength of these ligaments does not seem sufficient to control the movement of the bones in the proximal carpal row when they are loaded, and prevent injury, taking into account the huge forces involved.

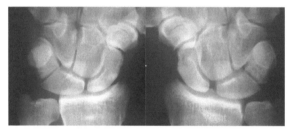

Fig. 4.2 Scapholunate gap in grip view of the right wrist 1 month after injury (clenched fist). (Reproduced from Garcia-Elias M and Mathoulin CL. Articular Injury of the Wrist: FESSH 2014 Instructional Course Book; Copyright © 2014 Thieme. All rights reserved.)

After an injury of the scapholunate ligament, radiographs have a normal appearance; it is only some time later, when the injured extrinsic stretch that malalignment of the bones appear with flexion and pronation of the scaphoid and extension of the lunate (▶ Fig. 4.2 and ▶ Fig. 4.3).

The extrinsic ligaments of the wrist is often described as dorsal and palmar. The dorsal ligaments look like a V, from Lister's tubercle on the dorsum of the radius to the triquetrum and then across to the dorsum of the scaphoid and more distally (▶ Fig. 4.4). The volar ligaments are described like two Vs, a small one from the forearm to the lunate (short and long radiolunate ligaments and ulnolunate ligament) and a bigger V (radioscaphocapitate ligament on one arm and ulnotriquetral, ulnocapitatehamate on the other arm). There is a space in between these two Vs, the space of Poirier, that opens during wrist extension and closes during wrist flexion.

However, it is difficult to deduce the function of these arrangements of the ligaments from their anatomical orientation. A better description has been proposed by Garcia-Elias[7] that explains their function. In this model ligaments work "in teams" to prevent rotational injury and collapse of the wrist. Some of the ligaments form an antipronation sling and some of them form an antisupination sling.

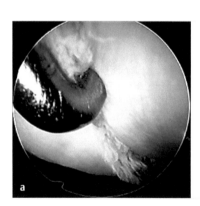
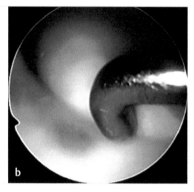

Fig. 4.3 **(a)** Complete fresh rupture of the scapholunate ligament. **(b)** Arthroscopy of the midcarpal joint shows a completely stable scapholunate joint. (Reproduced from Garcia-Elias M and Mathoulin CL. Articular Injury of the Wrist: FESSH 2014 Instructional Course Book; Copyright © 2014 Thieme. All rights reserved.)

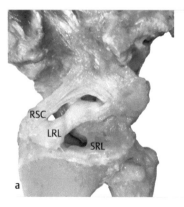
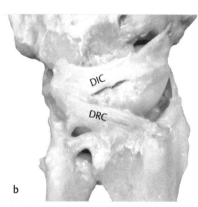

Fig. 4.4 Anatomical dissections showing the extrinsic volar **(a)** and dorsal **(b)** ligaments of the wrist. DIC, dorsalintercarpal ligament; DRC, dorsal radiocarpal ligament; LRL, long radiolunate ligament; RSC, radioscaphocapitate ligament; SRl, short radiolunate ligament.

However, ligaments are not just ropes to keep the bones together, they are part of a complex proprioceptive system that provides muscle control to the wrist to neutralize forces that could injure the joint and allow the hand to operate in space and exert great forces.

Incidental ligament abnormalities seen on MRI or at arthroscopy are common. Many of these "ligament injuries" do not cause symptoms, do not elicit clinical signs, and do not cause long-term damage to the joint. Treating these injuries with surgery is unnecessary as it can be of to both the wrist and the patient.

In the same way, incidental ligaments injuries in cadaveric dissection are found very frequently. One dissection study found scapholunate tears in 35%, lunotriquetral tears in 45%, and triangular fibrocartilage complex (TFCC) tears in 60% of wrists.[8] The reader could think these tears were small and not mechanically significant, but that is not the case. Another study of arthroscopy of cadaveric wrists graded the tears using the Geissler's classification.[9,10] For the tears in the scapholunate ligament they found that 5% were Grade 1, 34% Grade 2, 48% Grade 3, and 1% Grade 4. Similar results were found for the lunotriquetral ligament. With age it seems that ligament tears of the carpal ligaments and the TFFC become the norm rather than the exception. The older the patient the higher the incidence of changes in the ligaments.

The pattern of degeneration caused by scapholunate instability follows a recognized and predictable evolution, involving first the radioscaphoid joint and later the scaphocapitate joint, but the radiolunate joint is spared (▶ Fig. 4.5).

Many of these tears are accompanied by cartilage degeneration in a defined pattern. This pattern corresponds to a scaphoid chondrocalcinosis advanced collapse (SCAC) wrist, where the degeneration is caused by crystal arthropathy (▶ Fig. 4.6). These cases often follow chondrocalcinosis due to calcium pyrophosphate deposition (CCPD), or urate crystals in gout. The radiological image can be confused with a scapholunate advanced collapse (SLAC) pattern but in the SCAC wrist the degeneration seems more generalized, the scaphoid fossa looks excavated, there are more cysts in the carpal bones, and in advanced stages the radiolunate joint is involved. Often crystal deposition in the soft tissues is demonstrated by the radiograph.

In patients with an SCAC wrist, the ligament defects are a degenerative consequence of the process, and are not caused by significant trauma. Trying to repair or reconstruct these ligaments is unnecessary and often futile. Patients often respond very well to conservative treatment when they suffer a flare up of symptoms. A steroid injection and wrist splint for 3 to 4 weeks may be all that is required to return the patient to the PRE-FLAIR status with a reasonably comfortable wrist. Failing that, wrist salvage surgery can be necessary.

4.3 Biomechanical Studies

Several biomechanical studies have carried out experiments with sequential division of the ligaments of the cadaveric wrist to describe and quantify the role of individual ligaments in providing stability. Sectioning the scapholunate ligament does not cause a change in the kinematics of the scaphoid. It has no effect on the range of movement or the center of rotation of the joint (▶ Fig. 4.7).

Further to sectioning the intrinsic ligament, if the dorsal intercarpal ligament is sectioned, kinematic changes

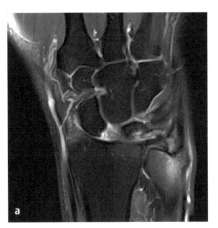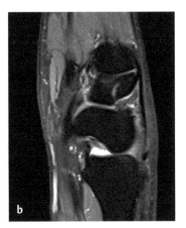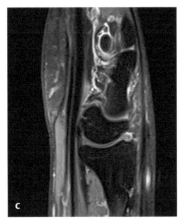

Fig. 4.5 Scapholunate advanced collapse (SLAC). **(a)** Coronal MRI image shows a wrist with a gap between scaphoid and lunate, indicating scapholunate dissociation. **(b)** Sagittal image shows flexion of the scaphoid with dorsal subluxation of the proximal pole over the dorsal edge of the radius. There the area of contact is very small; the scaphoid is clicking in and out with movement. This will cause degeneration of the joint into an SLAC pattern. **(c)** Sagittal image shows the extension of the lunate into a dorsal-intercalated segment instability (DISI). The proximal facet of the lunate is shaped like a section of a sphere. Therefore, in spite of the malalignment, the joint surfaces at the radiolunate joint are congruent and the joint surface in preserved, not involved in the degenerative process. In SLAC wrist, the ligament injury causes instability and this in turn causes degeneration of the joint. It seems reasonable to repair or reconstruct the ligaments.

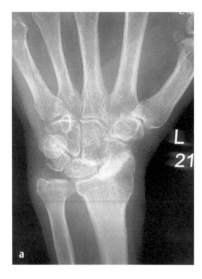

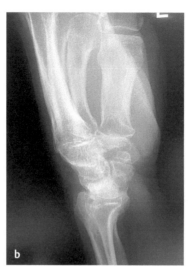

Fig. 4.6 Scaphoid chondrocalcinosis advanced collapse (SCAC). **(a, b)** In the PA view, it can be seen that the scaphoid fossa seems excavated by the scaphoid, there are cysts in several bones. The lateral view shows no joint space at the radiolunate joint, indicating advanced degeneration of this joint. The ligament damage in this joint is the effect of the degeneration, caused by calcium pyrophosphate deposition (CCPD). Repairing or reconstructing the ligament would not change the natural history of the condition.

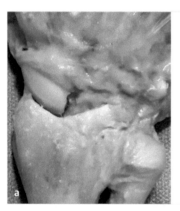

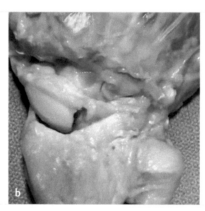

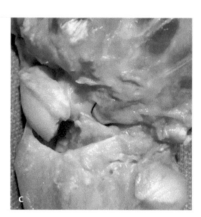

Fig. 4.7 Sequential sectioning of the scapholunate ligament complex. **(a)** Isolated SL ligament section (Including volar, dorsal, and proximal part) showing a minor opening of the SL gap. **(b)** Additional section of the dorsal intercarpal ligament (not including the dorsal scapholunotriquetal ligament). **(c)** Finally, a complete section of the SL and entire dorsal intercarpal ligament showing a complete SL instability.

happen and it can cause scapholunate instability. If the long radiolunate ligament is also sectioned, the instability gets worse.

Wrists with an isolated defect of the scapholunate ligament are unlikely to develop carpal instability, and therefore unlikely to develop degeneration, if the extrinsic ligaments are intact. In the trauma situation, it is easy to assess the intrinsic ligaments with MRI or arthroscopy but it is difficult to assess the extrinsic ligaments. However, it is comparatively easy to take a history of the patient and examine the wrist to decide if there is carpal instability or not, supplemented with fluoroscopy. In the view of the authors the decision to intervene with surgery should be based on the clinical assessment findings, with fluoroscopy, but not based solely on MRI scan or arthroscopy findings.

Arguably, MRI and arthroscopy, to a great extent, are static investigations, while carpal instability is a dynamic problem. These two investigations can guide the choice of

treatment for the patient, but they cannot be the basis of a decision as to whether intervention is required or not. They are not substitute for history taking and clinical examination.

4.4 Carpal Instability

An unstable wrist is the one unable to keep normal articular alignment when bearing physiological load. Normally the wrist moves in a smooth and predictable manner, but with instability the wrist may become malaligned, click, jump from one position to another, and cause pain, swelling, and weakness.

However, many patients with wrist laxity can demonstrate abnormal alignment of the wrist with clicking or clunking but they have no symptoms. In a study published by Wolfe et al[11] assessing the scaphoid shift test, 36% of asymptomatic volunteers had a positive test, recommending fluoroscopy to confirm the test. Is this carpal instability? From a biomechanical point of view, this 36% of healthy volunteers have more movement than normal, but if they do not have any symptoms, this is not clinical instability. They probably compensate very well with good proprioception and muscle control of the wrist. They do not require any investigations or any treatment.

An important clinical question to the patient when examining a wrist and eliciting a click or a clunk is: "do you recognize this click (or clunk or snap)"? The patients can usually distinguish very clearly if that is part of their problem or not. If the patient does not recognize the sensation of the click, it is most likely not relevant, and it is not a sign of clinical wrist instability.

A common example of this situation in clinical practice is the clunk elicited when doing a Litchman's test for nondissociative instability of the proximal carpal row (sometimes called midcarpal instability). It is easy to elicit a clunk while doing the test, but the key to it is to determine if that is the problem bothering the patient or simply an indication of wrist laxity, unrelated to the problem that caused the patient to seek advice.

Carpal instability adaptive is caused by a factor outside the carpus, causing a malalignment of the carpal bones. In general, there is no injury to the ligaments of the wrist. The treatment needs to address the cause of the problem, for example, a malunion of the radius after a fracture, and no surgical intervention to the ligaments is indicated.

The relationship between lunotriquetral ligament injury and lunotriquetral instability is complex.[12] Considering the biomechanics of the lunotriquetral joint it is logical to predict that injury to this ligament will result in a volar intercalated segment instability (VISI), as it has been described many times in articles and books. However, this is extremely rare in clinical practice, in part because traumatic, isolated lunotriquetral injuries are rare; they are often part of a more complex ligament injury. To develop a VISI deformity following trauma, a very significant injury to the extrinsic ligament is required.

Lunotriquetral instability can be degenerative secondary to ulnocarpal abutment, with lunotriquetral ligament and chondral damage to the volar-ulnar corner of the lunate and to the head of the ulna. Although the lunotriquetral ligament is involved, the main treatment is ulnar-shortening osteotomy. This avoids the impaction that is causing the problem, and tightens extrinsic ligaments on the ulnar side of the wrist. This tightens the lunotriquetral joint. Most often no further procedure is required to stabilize this joint.

A patient presenting with pain and clicking or clunking on the ulnar side of the wrist and radiographs showing a VISI malalignment is much more likely to suffer from a nondissociative proximal row instability than a static dissociative lunotriquetral instability. Nondissociative proximal carpal row often presents with no history of trauma, and in many cases is due to congenital reasons. In this case, MRI and arthro-CT scans can be completely normal. A wrist arthroscopy can be completely normal or can show some changes in the extrinsic ligaments. Often the only

remarkable finding during the arthroscopy is that it is technically very easy because the wrist is very spacious.

4.5 Conclusions

The management of patients with wrist conditions demands a systematic approach in order to reach an accurate diagnosis. Clinical history and examination are paramount and help the clinician decide whether this patient needs treatment and what investigations are required. This assessment needs to be done before the imaging and reports are reviewed to avoid confirmation cognitive bias.

Imaging studies and wrist arthroscopy help refine the diagnosis and stage the condition. These findings need to be interpreted with caution due to the incidental findings often seen in wrists, and in conjunction with the clinical findings.

Not all ligament defects cause carpal instability, some do not cause any clinical problem. Not all cases of carpal instability have a demonstrable ligament injury. We need to take a wider view of instability, considering bone geometry, proprioceptive muscle control, and congenital factors, as well as ligament appearance, and assess every case individually. Surgeons need to be wrist surgeons, not just ligament surgeons.

References

[1] Rikli DA, Honigmann P, Babst R, Cristalli A, Morlock MM, Mittlmeier T. Intra-articular pressure measurement in the radioulnocarpal joint using a novel sensor: in vitro and in vivo results. J Hand Surg Am. 2007; 32(1):67–75

[2] Schuind F, Cooney WP, Linscheid RL, An KN, Chao EY. Force and pressure transmission through the normal wrist. A theoretical twodimensional study in the posteroanterior plane. J Biomech. 1995; 28(5):587–601

[3] Garcia-Elias M. Understanding wrist mechanics: a long and winding road. JWrist Surg. 2013;2(1):5–12

[4] Hagert E, Garcia-Elias M, Forsgren S, Ljung BO. Immunohistochemical analysis of wrist ligament innervation in relation to their structural composition. J Hand Surg Am. 2007;32(1):30–36

[5] North ER, Meyer S. Wrist injuries: correlation of clinical and arthroscopic findings. J Hand Surg Am. 1990; 15(6):915–920

[6] Berger RA, Imeada T, Berglund L, An K-N. Constraint and material properties of the subregions of the scapholunate interosseous ligament. J Hand Surg Am. 1999; 24(5):953–962

[7] Garcia-Elias M, Puig de la Bellacasa I, Schouten C. Carpal ligaments: a functional classification. Hand Clin. 2017; 33(3):511–520

[8] Lee DH, Dickson KF, Bradley EL. The incidence of wrist interosseous ligament and triangular fibrocartilage articular disc disruptions: a cadaveric study. J Hand Surg. 2004; 29(4):676–684

[9] Geissler WB, Freeland AE, Savoie FH, McIntyre LW, Whipple TL. Intracarpal soft-tissue lesions associated with an intra-articular fracture of the distal end of the radius. J Bone Joint Surg Am. 1996;78(3):357–365

[10] Rimington TR, Edwards SG, Lynch TS, Pehlivanova MB. Intercarpal ligamentous laxity in cadaveric wrists. J Bone Joint Surg Br. 2010; 92(11):1600–1605

[11] Wolfe SW, Gupta A, Crisco JJ, III. Kinematics of the scaphoid shift test. J Hand Surg Am. 1997; 22(5):801–806

[12] Viegas SF, Patterson RM, Peterson PD, et al. Ulnar-sided perilunate instability: an anatomic and biomechanic study. J Hand Surg Am. 1990; 15(2):268–278

4

5 Surgical Approaches to the Carpus

M. Rosa Morro-Marti and Manuel Llusa-Perez

Abstract

Wrist surgery is characterized by the difficulty in exposing the carpal bones, which require the surgeon to determine the most appropriate technique. In general terms, the anatomical elements that prevent access to the carpus are: on the dorsal side, the extensor tendons of the wrist and fingers, sensory nerves, and dorsal veins; on the volar side, both median and ulnar nerves, the flexor tendons of the wrist and fingers, and the radial and ulnar arteries.

Basically, the wrist can be approached through two surgical approaches: (1) The dorsal approach gives a wide exposure of the radiocarpal and midcarpal joints and is universally used to approach most of the problems of the wrist. (2) The volar approach is rarely used as its exposure to the carpal bones is very limited and it is only recommended when the wrist conditions are limited to the volar side of the wrist. Several variations of these exposures have been described as a better knowledge of the anatomy and biomechanics of the wrist have been widely popularized. In order to minimize injury to vital structures, such as the vascular supply to the carpal bones, or the lesion of important carpal ligaments that would compromise carpal stability, the deeper dissection of these approaches has been modified with fiber-splitting of the ligaments.

Specific approaches have been described to expose a part of the carpus. The structure most often exposed is the scaphoid and can be approached either through a volar or a dorsal approach.

Keywords: carpal bones, approach, exposure, radiocarpal joint, midcarpal joint, scaphoid

5.1 Introduction

General principles of surgical exposures are of utmost importance in the hand and wrist. The relation between superficial and deeper structures is very intimate, so prevention of injury to vital structures and protection of these structures are essential. Preservation of sensory nerves is paramount to prevent painful neuromas. The design of the skin incision must take into account the vascular supply to the skin, the sensory distribution of the superficial nerves of the area, the relationship of deeper structures, and the presence of flexion creases to avoid skin and joint contractures. A precise knowledge of the anatomy of the region is paramount in understanding and applying the surgical approaches of the wrist.[1]

Carpal exposures can be divided into general approaches and specific approaches. General approaches provide a wide exposure to large areas of the wrist and allow for access to pathology that may involve multiple joints or multiple carpal bones. Specific approaches give access to a single bone, such as the scaphoid, or joint for management of a discrete condition, and usually have only one purpose.

5.2 Dorsal Approach

The dorsal carpal exposure is one of the most important general approaches to the carpus, because it gives the surgeon a wider exposure than the palmar approach. There are essentially two dorsal ligaments that are intimate with the dorsal capsule: the dorsal radiotriquetral (radiocarpal) ligament and the dorsal intercarpal (scaphotriquetral) ligament.[2]

5.2.1 Skin and Subcutaneous

The wrist and forearm are placed on a hand table into a neutral rotation position. The incision is centered on the dorsal carpal area in line with the third metacarpal and extended proximally on the distal radius. The length of the incision depends on the surgery performed and the exposure needed. Some authors recommend a curvilinear or zigzag incision; however, we do not particularly recommend it as we have not appreciated an improvement neither of the exposure nor the cosmesis of the wound scar. Furthermore, there is a risk of flap ischemia or necrosis with curvilinear or zigzag incisions, particularly in patients who have poor skin vascularity. Another important consideration of the linear incision is that it will most likely avoid the branches of the cutaneous branch of the radial nerve and the dorsal branch of the ulnar nerve. If distal extension of the incision is needed beyond the base of the third metacarpal, one should be careful with the most ulnar branches of the cutaneous branch of the radial nerve.

Full-thickness flaps containing the skin, subcutaneous tissues, and superficial fascia should be raised together to expose the extensor retinaculum. Besides minimizing the risk of ischemia or necrosis of the skin, this method keeps the cutaneous nerves within the flaps and away from the surgical field. Large longitudinal veins should be preserved, but crossing branches can be divided.

5.2.2 Retinaculum

Starting just ulnar to Lister's tubercle, the course of the extensor pollicis longus (EPL) is identified and the third dorsal compartment opened (▶ Fig. 5.1). The proximal and distal extent of the extensor retinaculum should then be identified and the retinaculum elevated ulnarly by

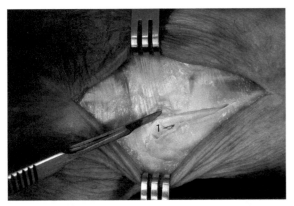

Fig. 5.1 Dorsal approach. Localization of the Lister's tubercle (*star*) and opening of the third extensor compartment where the extensor pollicis longus (1) is identified.

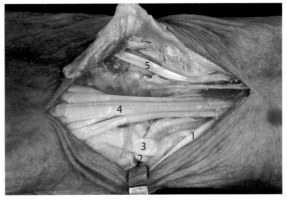

Fig. 5.2 Dorsal approach. Two retinacular flaps are elevated from the third compartment, ulnarward up to the sixth compartment, and radialward up to the first compartment to expose all the extensor tendons of the wrist and fingers. EPL (1), ECRL (2), ECRB (3), ED (4), EDM (5).

dividing the septum between the third and fourth, and fourth and fifth extensor compartments. The fourth compartment can be preserved and a subperiosteal dissection of the compartment performed, but it has been found to add difficulty in the dissection and not improving the functional results.[3]

To gain full exposure of the dorsal carpus, the retinacular flap should be carried ulnarward up to the sixth compartment, opening the fifth extensor compartment (▸ Fig. 5.2). The extensor digiti minimi (EDM) is easier to identify proximally and it facilitates the lifting of the flap without inadvertently sectioning the tendon.

The EPL tendon should be retracted radially with the extensor carpi radialis tendons, and the extensor digitorum (ED), extensor indicis (EI), and EDM tendons should be retracted ulnarly. Once this is done, the floors of the third, fourth, and fifth compartments are exposed, leaving the dorsal wrist capsule and its ligaments exposed. At the radial margin of the fourth compartment lies the posterior interosseous nerve (PIN) with the posterior interosseous artery (▸ Fig. 5.3). Most authors routinely resected the PIN for pain relief as part of the exposure; however, nowadays sometimes it is preserved in order to preserve the proprioception of the wrist and improving the dynamic stability of the wrist.[4]

5.2.3 Capsule

Previous descriptions of capsular incisions included a longitudinal incision that transversely divided the dorsal radiocarpal and intercarpal ligaments; however, a dorsal capsulotomy that preserved the dorsal ligaments was described by Berger and colleagues.[5] In this ligament-sparing capsulotomy, the dorsal intercarpal and radiocarpal ligaments are divided in line with the fibers, and a radial-based capsular flap is created, providing excellent exposure to the entire carpus. Nowadays the so-called

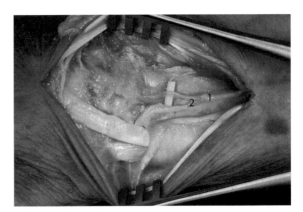

Fig. 5.3 Dorsal approach. Laying on the floor of the fourth compartment, the posterior interosseous nerve (1) and artery (2) can be found entering the dorsal capsule of the wrist.

Berger's capsulotomy is the most used method worldwide. Variations of this approach will allow the surgeon access to the radiocarpal joint, midcarpal joint, ulnocarpal joint, or all of the above.

The landmarks for the ligament-sparing capsulotomy are the dorsal radiocarpal ligament, the dorsal intercarpal ligament, the dorsal tubercle of the triquetrum (where the dorsal intercarpal and dorsal radiocarpal ligaments attach), and the scaphoid.[2] The width of the radiocarpal ligament is estimated and it is sharply divided longitudinally through a fiber-splitting division in the middle of the ligament from the radius to the triquetrum (▸ Fig. 5.4). Care must be taken not to injure the articular cartilage of the carpal bones or the intrinsic ligaments of the carpus. In a similar way, the dorsal intercarpal ligament is sharply divided longitudinally starting in the dorsal tubercle of the triquetrum until its attachment to the scaphoid. It must be performed carefully so that the

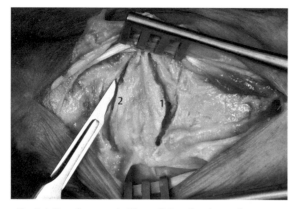

Fig. 5.4 Dorsal approach. Fiber-splitting dorsal capsulotomy through the dorsal radiocarpal (1) and dorsal intercarpal (2) ligaments.

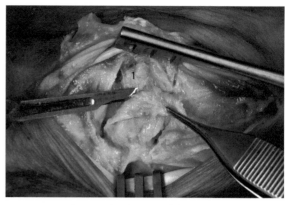

Fig. 5.5 Dorsal approach. Elevation of the capsular flap from the triquetrum (1) and advancing radially and proximally. Note that the scalpel blade is directed dorsally and angulated sufficiently to avoid the dorsal surfaces of the proximal carpal bones and their intrinsic ligaments.

dorsal vascular supply of the scaphoid running in this region is preserved. The capsulotomy is then elevated from the triquetrum and advanced radially and proximally. It is a laborious task as all the capsular attachments to the carpal bones must be cut, preserving the intrinsic (scapholunate and lunotriquetral) ligaments which are intimately related to the capsular flap.[2] When approaching these structures, the scalpel blade must be directed dorsally and angulated sufficiently to dodge the dorsal surfaces of the proximal carpal bones and their intrinsic ligaments (▶ Fig. 5.5). The capsulotomy must be performed until the dorsal edge of the radius is seen. Then, the capsulotomy is completed by radial extension along the distal edge of the radius, leaving a rim of tissue for posterior repair.[5]

5.2.4 Exposure

This capsulotomy will allow exposure of the radiocarpal joint including the distal surface of the radius, proximal scaphoid, lunate, and triquetrum. The midcarpal joint can also be partially exposed including parts of the capitate and hamate (▶ Fig. 5.6).

5.2.5 Modifications

Further radial extension can be achieved by elevating the extensor retinaculum off Lister's tubercle, as a radial retinacular flap exposing the second extensor compartment. This effectively releases the second compartment tendons, allowing greater radial retraction of the extensor carpi radialis brevis (ECRB) and longus (ECRL) for the dorsal capsulotomy to be extended more radially.

Osteotomy of Lister's tubercle is no longer routinely performed although it can be performed if necessary, such as in cases of total wrist fusion where a plate must be placed at the dorsum of the radius.[1]

In order to preserve the PIN, a proximal-based capsular flap can be performed.[4] It is also designed splitting

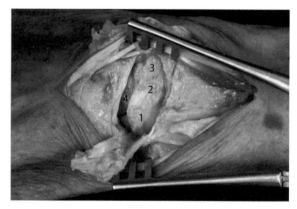

Fig. 5.6 Dorsal approach. Completed capsulotomy with exposure of the radiocarpal joint. The midcarpal joint can also be partially exposed. Scaphoid (1), lunate (2), triquetrum (3), capitate (4).

longitudinally the radiocarpal ligament and the dorsal intercarpal ligament, but instead of detaching the capsule from the distal radius, it should be detached from the scaphoid in their most radial side. It leaves a proximal-based capsular flap containing the PIN which can be rejected proximally.

If exposure of the midcarpal joint is necessary, a distally based capsulotomy can be performed.[1] The landmarks for this are the triquetrum, the scaphoid, and the dorsal intercarpal ligament. The latter is sectioned longitudinally in a fiber-splitting fashion from the triquetrum to the scaphoid. The flap is then elevated from the triquetrum and reflected distally, leaving the capsular attachments to the scaphoid intact. The midcarpal joint will be exposed with the distal articular surfaces of the scaphoid, lunate, and triquetrum, and the proximal surfaces of the trapezium, trapezoid, capitate, and hamate.

Rarely, the entire carpus might need to be exposed. A dorsal pan-carpal capsulotomy can be performed preserving the maximum ligamentous integrity. The proximal edge of the dorsal radiocarpal ligament and the distal edge of the dorsal intercarpal ligament are identified and an incision is made along these borders. The dorsal cortex of the triquetrum is elevated with an osteotome, leaving the common attachments of the dorsal radiocarpal ligament and the dorsal intercarpal ligament intact. This flap is reflected radially until the scaphoid is exposed. The radial origin of the dorsal radiocarpal ligament can be cut but a small rim of tissue should be left on the radius to facilitate posterior repair.

5.2.6 Closure

The radially based dorsal capsular flap is replaced, and the dorsal radiocarpal and dorsal intercarpal ligaments are sutured using absorbable sutures. In order to avoid limitation of wrist flexion, the capsule should not be closed with too much tension placing only a few stitches to hold it in place. The distally based midcarpal capsulotomy can also be similarly repaired to the dorsal intercarpal ligament with sutures.

If a pan-carpal capsulotomy is performed, a stout repair of the radial origin of the dorsal radiocarpal ligament to the rim of the tissue left in the distal radius must be performed, or if there is not enough tissue left, intraosseous sutures anchors should be used. The dorsal triquetral cortex is secured by a small cortical screw, securing the ulnar attachments of the dorsal radiocarpal and dorsal intercarpal ligaments back onto the triquetrum.

Following capsular repair, the extensor tendons are replaced in their original positions except the EPL, and the radial and ulnar retinacular flaps are sutured back together with interrupted absorbable sutures. The EPL is routinely dorsally transposed.

5.3 Volar Approach

The volar carpal exposure is most commonly used to reduce difficult carpal dislocations (perilunate) and for repair or reconstruction of the palmar wrist capsule and the palmar carpal ligaments.[1] Volar approaches are also useful for reduction and fixation of palmar fragments of comminuted distal radius fractures.[3] The volar approach is often used in combination with a dorsal approach in the management of carpal injuries.

The volar side has many extrinsic ligaments which cannot be sectioned, therefore limiting the exposure. These ligaments do not exist in the dorsum of the carpus.[1]

5.3.1 Skin Incision and Subcutaneous Tissue

The carpal tunnel approach has many variations; essentially, they are all an extended carpal tunnel release. The distal part of the incision follows the curve of the thenar muscles to the level of the wrist crease, which is crossed with a zigzag starting in an ulnar direction and going back radially to reach the center of the forearm (▶ Fig. 5.7). The proximal part of the incision is in the middle of the distal wrist and its extension is determined by the surgical needs.

To avoid the palmar cutaneous branch of the median nerve, the incision should be aligned between the long and ring fingers' web space or 5 mm ulnar to the interthenar depression (the deepest point between the thenar and hypothenar eminences).[1] To avoid the palmar cutaneous branch of the ulnar nerve, the palmar incision should not be placed any more ulnar than the proximally extended axis of the ring finger.[1]

The superficial palmar fascia and the antebrachial fascia should then be incised longitudinally.

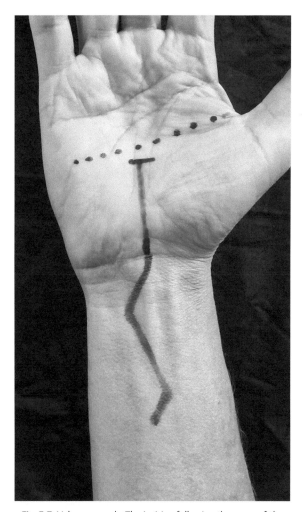

Fig. 5.7 Volar approach. The incision following the curve of the thenar muscles, crossing the wrist crease with a zigzag starting in an ulnar direction and then going radially to reach the center of the forearm.

I

5.3.2 Retinaculum

The median nerve is identified in the distal forearm, radial and deep to the palmaris longus (PL) tendon when present, or ulnar to the flexor carpi radialis (FCR) tendon. Then the flexor retinaculum is identified; it has thick transverse fibers, and it is divided transversally on its ulnar aspect just radial to the hook of the hamate (▶ Fig. 5.8). It can also be divided in a zigzag fashion

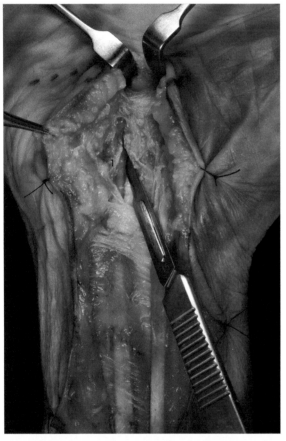

Fig. 5.8 Volar approach. Opening transversely the flexor retinaculum just radial to the hook of the hamate (1) to expose all the flexor tendons of the fingers and the median nerve.

following the contour of the hook of the hamate leaving a small rim of tissue which then facilitates closure of the retinaculum[6] (▶ Fig. 5.9).

The contents of the carpal tunnel (flexor tendons of the fingers, flexor pollicis longus [FPL], and median nerve) can be looped in a Penrose drain and retracted radially or ulnarly to expose the volar wrist capsule and the pronator quadratus (PQ)[1] (▶ Fig. 5.10). It is important to keep in mind that if a proximal extension of the incision is necessary, then the contents of the carpal tunnel should always be retracted radially exclusively to avoid damage to the thenar cutaneous branch of the median nerve (▶ Fig. 5.11).

5.3.3 Capsule

As in the dorsal side, the palmar wrist capsule contains important capsular ligaments. To avoid potential postoperative problems associated with ulnar translation of the carpus, ligament disruption must be avoided. The long radiolunate ligament should be left intact. This ligament tethers the triquetrum to the radius with the palmar lunotriquetral ligament.[1] The space of Poirier which is localized between the long and short volar radiocarpal ligaments[2] is where the capsulotomy should be started using a fiber-splitting approach (▶ Fig. 5.12).

5.3.4 Modifications

If additional exposure is required on the radial side, a subperiosteal elevation of either the radial origin of the radioscaphocapitate ligament or the long radiolunate ligament can be performed following the incision in the space of Poirier. Detaching both ligaments must be avoided as carpal instabilities may appear.[1]

Typically, this approach is used to reduce a perilunate dislocation and repair the space of Poirier in this kind of lesions.

5.3.5 Closure

Usually closure of the space of Poirier is the first step. It is performed using absorbable sutures or with bone anchors when there is not enough tissue to be sutured.

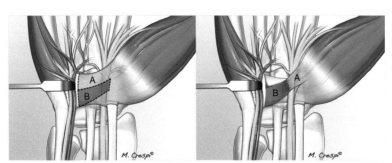

Fig. 5.9 Volar approach. Scheme of the zigzag fashion opening of the flexor retinaculum following the contour of the hook of the hamate described by Lluch.

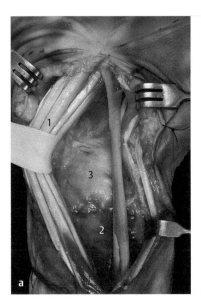
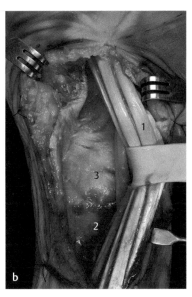

Fig. 5.10 Volar approach. Exposure of the contents of the carpal tunnel (1) which can be looped and retracted ulnarly (a) or radially (b) to expose the pronator quadratus (2) and the volar capsule of the wrist (3).

5

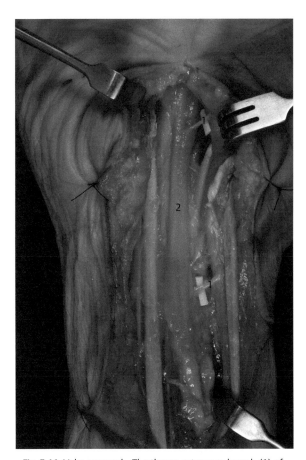

Fig. 5.11 Volar approach. The thenar cutaneous branch (1) of the median nerve (2) is found emerging from the radial side of the nerve in the distal third of the forearm. There can be more than one branch as seen in this figure.

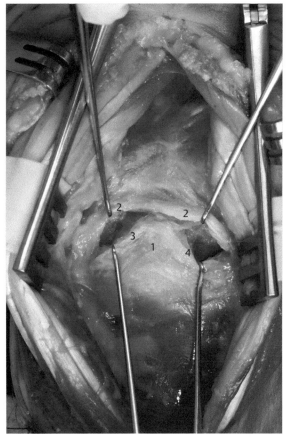

Fig. 5.12 Volar approach. Fiber-splitting palmar capsulotomy starting in the space of Poirier (1) localized between the long (2) and short (3) volar radiocarpal ligaments. The long radio-lunate ligament (4) must be left intact.

Then the contents of the carpal tunnel are put back in place. The flexor retinaculum is usually left open. However, it can be sutured to the rim of the tissue left in the border of the hook of the hamate if it was opened in a zigzag fashion.[6]

5.4 Volar Approach to the Scaphoid

This approach is indicated for the open reduction and fixation of fractures of the waist or distal pole of the scaphoid or treatment of their nonunions.[1] The advantages of this approach are the preservation of the vascularity of the scaphoid by avoiding the dorsal distal blood supply, and an easier ability to correct apex dorsal angulations (humpback deformity) of the scaphoid waist nonunions or malunion. However, one problem is the potential of carpal instability as a result of the division of the radiocarpal ligaments (radioscaphocapitate and long radiolunate ligaments) to access the scaphoid.[7]

5.4.1 Skin Incision and Subcutaneous Tissue

A longitudinal incision over the FCR tendon is performed from the scaphoid tuberosity and followed proximally for 1.5 to 2 cm. The distal part of the incision angles toward the first metacarpal and is in line with it (▸ Fig. 5.13). Care must be taken not to cross the ulnar border of the FCR because the palmar cutaneous branch of the median nerve would be at risk.[2]

5.4.2 Deeper Dissection

In this area, the superficial palmar branch of the radial artery crosses obliquely the volar crease of the wrist from the radial side of the wrist to the center of the hand (see ▸ Fig. 5.13). Sometimes this artery has a great caliber and therefore it must be properly rejected radially in order not to injure it; it can also be ligated if previous to the surgery an Allen test confirms the presence of a superficial palmar arch.

The FCR tendon sheath is then divided longitudinally in line with the skin incision, and the tendon is mobilized as far as the scaphoid tuberosity distally opening the most radial side of the flexor retinaculum. Then the FCR tendon is retracted ulnarward (▸ Fig. 5.14). As long as we are in the tendon sheath of the FCR the palmar cutaneous branch of the median nerve is safe.[1]

Then the deep tendon sheath of the FCR tendon is divided longitudinally, together with the pericapsular fat underlying it. It will reveal the palmar wrist capsule which consists of the radioscaphocapitate and long radiolunate ligaments.

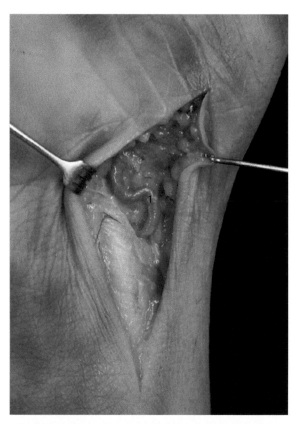

Fig. 5.13 Scaphoid volar approach. Skin incision over the flexor carpi radialis (FCR) tendon and curving toward the first metacarpal in the distal portion. Localization and protection of the superficial palmar branch of the radial artery (1) which crosses obliquely the volar crease of the wrist from the radial side of the wrist to the center of the hand and it can have a great caliber as seen in this figure.

5.4.3 Capsulotomy

The radioscaphocapitate and long radiolunate ligaments are sharply divided, exposing the waist of the scaphoid (▸ Fig. 5.15). This section can originate a carpal instability which can be avoided by dividing longitudinally the radioscaphocapitate ligament in a fiber-splitting fashion and then transversely sectioning each part of this ligament, one in the proximal end and the other in the distal end, opening the ligament in a z-plasty[7] (▸ Fig. 5.16).

5.4.4 Closure

If the radioscaphocapitate and long radiolunate ligaments were sharply divided, they must be repaired stoutly with sutures if one is to avoid potential carpal instability problems.

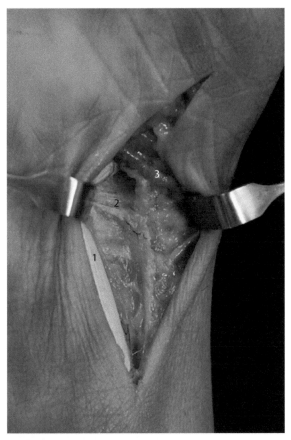

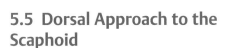

Fig. 5.14 Scaphoid volar approach. Longitudinal division of the flexor carpi radialis (FCR) tendon sheath and opening of the radial side of the flexor retinaculum to allow ulnarward retraction of the FCR tendon (1) to expose the most radial portion of the volar capsule (2). Superficial palmar branch of the radial artery (3).

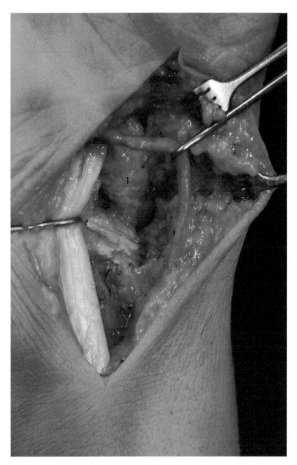

Fig. 5.15 Scaphoid volar approach. Longitudinal section of the radioscaphocapitate and long radiolunate ligaments to expose the waist and distal pole of the scaphoid (1).

5.5 Dorsal Approach to the Scaphoid

The dorsal approach to the scaphoid provides better access to the proximal scaphoid, and is indicated in the fixation of proximal scaphoid fractures or treatment of their nonunions. There is a concern with injury to the vascular supply of the scaphoid[8]; however, recent reports have not shown a significant difference in the union rates when compared with the volar approach.[9]

5.5.1 Skin Incision

It is performed through a transverse or longitudinal incision over the scapholunate interval and radiocarpal joint. The authors prefer a longitudinal incision as it is least likely to injure branches of the superficial radial nerve compared with a transverse incision, although it is less cosmetic (▶ Fig. 5.17).

Skin flaps are elevated and the superficial branch of the radial nerve is identified and protected.

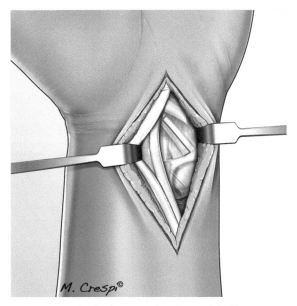

Fig. 5.16 Scaphoid volar approach. Scheme of the fiber-splitting opening of the radioscaphocapitate ligament by opening the ligament in a z-plasty as proposed by Garcia-Elías.

5

I

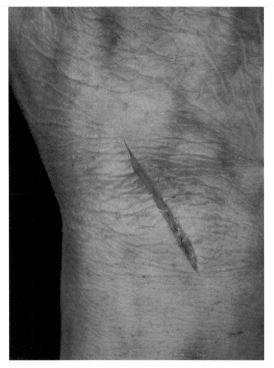

Fig. 5.17 Scaphoid dorsal approach. Longitudinal incision of the skin following the direction of the extensor pollicis longus (EPL) tendon.

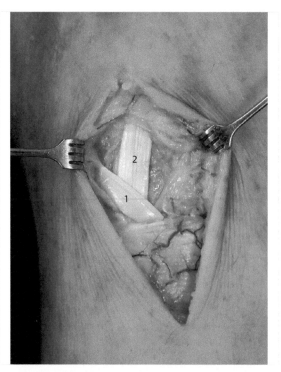

Fig. 5.18 Scaphoid dorsal approach. Opening of the third extensor compartment to expose the extensor pollicis longus (EPL) tendon (1) and retract it radially. ECRB (2).

5.5.2 Retinaculum

The extensor retinaculum over the third dorsal compartment is opened and the EPL tendon is retracted radially (▶ Fig. 5.18). This way the dorsal capsule of the wrist can be exposed.

5.5.3 Capsule

Radial to the insertion of the dorsal radiocarpal ligament, there are no ligamentous structures; only capsule is present.[2] So the capsule can be opened in this region without disruption of any ligamentous structures (▶ Fig. 5.19). If further exposure is necessary, the dorsal radiocarpal ligament can be divided longitudinally and along its fibers, creating a distally based flap.

5.5.4 Exposure

The entire proximal two-thirds of the scaphoid, the radial styloid, and the scaphoid fossa in the distal radius can be exposed.

5.5.5 Closure

The capsule is easily closed with sutures independently of the type of capsulotomy used. The EPL tendon is transposed dorsally to the repaired retinaculum.

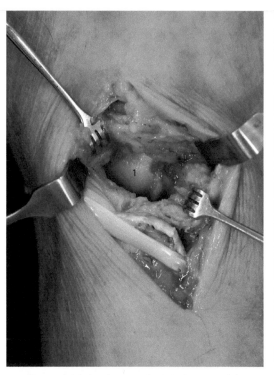

Fig. 5.19 Scaphoid dorsal approach. Capsulotomy radial to the insertion of the dorsal radiocarpal ligament where there are no ligaments, to expose the waist and proximal pole of the scaphoid (1).

References

[1] Tay SC, Shin AY. Surgical approaches to the carpus. Hand Clin. 2006; 22(4):421–434, abstract v

[2] Llusa M, Forcada P, Carrera A, Morro MR, Garcia-Elías M. Atlas of dissection and surgical anatomy of the wrist and hand. 1st ed. Chicago, IL: American Society for Surgery of the Hand; 2022

[3] Hoppenfeld S, deBoer P, Buckley R. Surgical exposures in orthopaedics. The anatomic approach. 4th ed. Philadelphia, PA: Lippincott Williams & Wilkins; 2009

[4] Hagert E, Ferreres A, Garcia-Elias M. Nerve-sparing dorsal and volar approaches to the radiocarpal joint. J Hand Surg Am. 2010; 35(7): 1070–1074

[5] Berger RA, Bishop AT, Bettinger PC. New dorsal capsulotomy for the surgical exposure of the wrist. Ann Plast Surg. 1995; 35(1):54–59

[6] Lluch A. Reconstruction of the flexor retinaculum. In: Luchetti R, Amadio P, eds. Carpal tunnel syndrome. Berlin: Springer; 2007: 226–238

[7] Garcia-Elias M, Vall A, Salo JM, Lluch AL. Carpal alignment after different surgical approaches to the scaphoid: a comparative study. J Hand Surg Am. 1988; 13(4):604–612

[8] Gelberman RH, Menon J. The vascularity of the scaphoid bone. J Hand Surg Am. 1980; 5(5):508–513

[9] Morsey M. Vascular anatomy of the scaphoid and implications in surgery. In: Bhatia DN, Bain GI, Poehling GG, Graves BR, eds. Arthroscopy and endoscopy of the elbow, wrist and hand. Cham: Springer; 2021: 845–853

5

Section II

Assessment of the Wrist

6 Physical Examination of the Wrist

Guillem Salva-Coll

Abstract

Wrist pain is a common reason of consultation. Both complex anatomy and biomechanics of the wrist often make the diagnosis complicated. Deep knowledge of the anatomy and a focused medical history, together with a systematic physical examination, help to dramatically reduce the differential diagnosis of possible injuries of the wrist and plan a correct treatment. However, a final diagnosis may require complementary imaging investigations, such as X-rays, magnetic resonance imaging (MRI), or computed tomography (CT) scan. It is mandatory to emphasize that "complementary" refers to complementing the medical history and physical examination. Therefore, to base the diagnosis on imaging is unfortunately a common error. In this chapter a systematic approach to physical examination focused on carpal instabilities of the wrist is proposed, which includes inspection, palpation, range of motion, and special tests.

Keywords: wrist, clinical examination, physical examination, ligament injuries, provocative maneuvers, carpal instability

6.1 Medical History

A detailed medical past history is one of the most important part of the patient's evaluation. This history can be brief, in cases of a posttraumatic injury, or long, in cases of nontraumatic injuries. This helps us to narrow the differential diagnosis. Next step is to delimit the area where the patient has pain. With this information, possible diagnoses become more apparent. Next, it is interesting to know what the patient can and cannot do, as a consequence of the symptoms. It is also helpful to establish the nature of the pain, as well as how this pain relates to activity or sleep. Finally, all the information regarding the general state of health, involvement of other joints, surgical history, family history, received treatments, and current treatment must be collected. At this point, you should have an approximate idea of the possible pathology and where to focus your efforts to reach the diagnosis.

6.2 Inspection

Visual inspection provides a lot of information when compared to the healthy wrist. It is important to assess the visual appearance and the resting position of the forearm and hand. Scars, skin appearance and color, swelling, and lumps and bumps can be made more obvious by using light in the room to create shadows on the wrist, or by using dark clothing in the background to increase contrast. Loss of normal skin folds suggests inflammation of the underlying area. Wrist position can give us some clues for the diagnosis and should always be recorded. Normal dorsal view of the wrist at rest reveals that the hand is in slight ulnar deviation. If the hand appears radially deviated or straight, then the radius should be relatively shorter than the ulna, for example, as a consequence of a distal radius malunion. The prominence of the distal ulna should also be assessed. It is often described as a prominent ulna head, but it often has nothing to do with the ulna. In many cases, it is the ulnar part of the carpus that is subluxed in supination, giving the impression of a prominent ulnar head. Rheumatic diseases or injuries to the dorsal stabilizers such as triangular fibrocartilage complex (TFCC) are the most common causes of this sign. Other data on nearby joints, such as fingers and elbow, should also be recorded. ▶ Fig. 6.1 shows the relationship between the palmar creases and the bony skeleton of the wrist and hand.

6.3 Palpation

Palpation is one of the most useful tools in the diagnosis of wrist pathology, especially in chronic problems. In acute injuries, due to the involvement of multiple structures, the patient does not usually locate well the area of pain, and instead of marking specific points delimitates an area. Palpation should be started away from the painful area. Painful sites should be located and remembered, and return to that area repeatedly, to check the reproducibility of that pain with the exploration maneuvers. The structures proximal to the radiocarpal joint should first be explored, palpating the dorsal extensor compartments from I to VI, as well as the capsule of the distal radioulnar joint (DRUJ) and the head of the ulna.

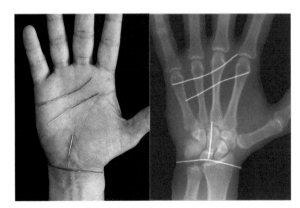

Fig. 6.1 Relationship of the palmar creases and the bony structures of the hand and wrist.

Next, the bones of the proximal row of the carpus should be palpated from the scaphoid tuberosity, the dorsal part of the scaphoid, the scapholunate ligament, the lunate, the lunotriquetral ligament, the triquetrum, to the pisiform in the volar part of the carpus. The more distal structures should then be palpated, although they are rarely the cause of pathology.

It is important to remember that scars around the wrist (surgical or traumatic) can be the source of severe pain if there is an injury such as a neuroma. The diagnosis of this condition will be made by the presence of dysesthesias and a positive Tinel's sign.

6.4 Range of Motion

Wrist mobility has to be measured in flexion/extension, radial/ulnar deviation, and pronation/supination (▶ Fig. 6.2). The average of the maximum normal values of movement of the wrist are as follows[1]: flexion 78 degrees, extension 60 degrees, radial inclination 21 degrees, ulnar inclination 38 degrees, pronation 76 degrees, and supination 82 degrees. When assessing wrist mobility, care must be taken that the patient does not falsely increase the range of motion by combining movements of extension at the end of radial deviation, and flexion at the end of ulnar deviation, or rotation of the entire arm.

For this reason, it has to be performed with the patient seated in front of the examiner, and with the elbow resting on the examination table. In this way, any attempt to compensate for a movement will be instantly detected. Forearm rotation occurs over the entire length of the forearm. Once the end of rotation (pronation or supination) is reached, the patient can further increase this movement with carpal supination. Measurement of forearm rotation should be made at the level of the DRUJ, and not in the palm of the hand (▶ Fig. 6.2c). If the arm is free at the time of the examination and there is a supination deficit, the patient performs an adduction movement to compensate for this mobility deficit in supination, or abducts the arm to compensate for a pronation deficit. It is important to compare the measurements with the contralateral side.

6.5 Specific Tests

6.5.1 Scapholunate Dysfunction

The oblique position of the scaphoid with respect to the longitudinal axis of the radius and the ligamentous connections with the lunate and the distal carpal row play a fundamental role in wrist biomechanics and joint function, maintaining movement and transmitting loads

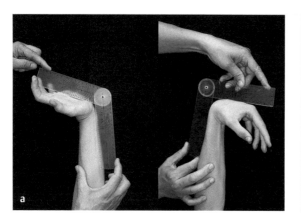
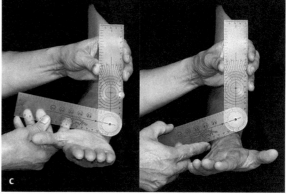
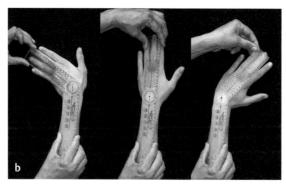

Fig. 6.2 Measurement of the range of motion using a goniometer. **(a)** Flexion/Extension; **(b)** radial/ulnar tilt; **(c)** pronation/supination.

without pain. Most of the injuries of the wrist are caused by a fall on the hand with the wrist in extension, ranging from fractures of the distal radius or scaphoid, to partial or complete tears of the scapholunate ligament. The three most common causes of dorsal scapholunate pain with normal wrist radiographs are (1) occult dorsal carpal synovial cyst, (2) scaphoid impaction on the dorsal edge of the radius, and (3) dynamic or predynamic scapholunate instability.[2]

Scaphoid Shift Test or Watson Test

Passive mobilization of an unstable scapholunate joint helps us in not only determining the presence of abnormal scaphoid subluxation but also reproducing pain. The examiner places the index finger on the dorsal scapholunate area and the thumb on the scaphoid tuberosity (distal pole). The other hand is used to passively move the wrist from ulnar to radial deviation. In ulnar deviation, the scaphoid is extended, a position more aligned with the forearm. In radial deviation, the scaphoid flexes. Pressure on the distal pole of the scaphoid as the wrist moves from ulnar to radial deviation prevents the scaphoid from flexing. If the scapholunate ligament is torn or incompetent, the proximal pole of the scaphoid subluxes dorsally over the dorsal edge of the radius, inducing pain on the dorsoradial aspect of the wrist. When the pressure is released, a typical clunk may occur, indicating automatic reduction of the scaphoid[3] (► Fig. 6.3).

Finger Extension Test

This test is used to assess minor injuries of the scapholunate ligament. The patient is asked to extend the fingers as much as possible against resistance with the wrist flexed (► Fig. 6.4). This maneuver increases the joint reaction force between the capitate and the scapholunate unit, pushing the head of the capitate between the two bones and increasing tension on the scapholunate ligament. In patients with an injury or insufficiency of the

dorsal scapholunate ligament, acute pain is elicited in the scapholunate area, probably due to the presence of synovitis in the radioscaphoid joint. This maneuver is very sensitive but not specific for this pathology.[2,4]

Differential Diagnosis of Radial Wrist Pain

There are many causes of wrist pain, from tendon and joint problems to ligament injuries. The medical history and palpation will help us define the painful area and focus our examination on specific injuries. It is important to explore the contralateral side to detect differences that are often subtle. Specific tests for specific pathologies will help us in the diagnosis.

WHAT Test

De Quervain tenosynovitis is the most common condition involving inflammation of the abductor pollicis longus and extensor pollicis brevis tendons within the first dorsal compartment and it is a very common cause of radial wrist pain. Patients' Wrist Hyperflexion Abduction of the Thumb (WHAT) is the test used for de Quervain's tendinitis, and it is the one with the best sensitivity (0.99) and specificity (0.28), compared to the Finkelstein's and Eichhoff's tests.[5] It is an active test in which the patient is asked to hyperflex the wrist and actively abduct the thumb against resistance. The examiner uses their index finger to counteract this movement, which will reproduce the pain in the first dorsal compartment if the patient has a tendinitis (► Fig. 6.5).

De Quervain's tendinitis should not be confused with intersection syndrome, which is a tendinopathy that affects the radial extensors of the wrist at the point where the muscle bellies of the abductor pollicis longus and extensor pollicis brevis intersect with them. Symptoms may be similar to de Quervain's tenosynovitis, but are more severe with wrist flexion and extension.

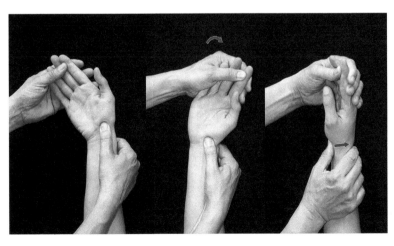

Fig. 6.3 Watson's test to assess scapholunate instability.

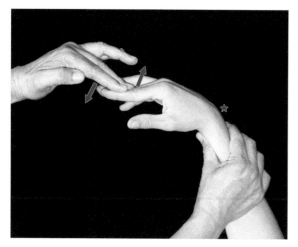

Fig. 6.4 Finger extension test.

Trapeziometacarpal Stress Test

The trapeziometacarpal stress test, known as the Grind test, is used to diagnose trapeziometacarpal joint pathology.[6] This is a biconcave joint, which has little inherent stability; therefore, it is a common area of degenerative pathology. This test is performed by compressing the metacarpal on the trapezium and rotating the metacarpal. It is important to block the movement of the rest of the carpal bones to limit a single zone of movement, in this case the trapeziometacarpal joint. The patient's wrist is placed in ulnar tilt and the examiner grasps the wrist from the ulnar side, delimiting the trapezium between the examiner's index finger and thumb. With the other hand, compression and rotation of the neck of the first metacarpal is applied (▶ Fig. 6.6).

In this same position, the stability/laxity of the trapeziometacarpal joint can be assessed. With the examiner's free hand, the first metacarpal is rotated and pronated to tighten the ligaments, and the base of the metacarpal is grasped between the thumb and index finger. In this position, a lateral force is applied to radially subluxate the base of the metacarpal. This highlights joint laxity, often reproducing painful symptoms at the base of the thumb (▶ Fig. 6.7).

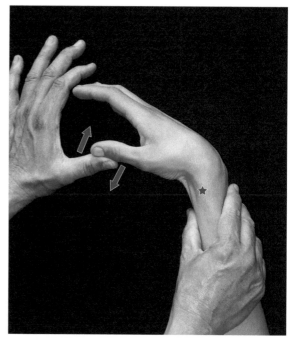

Fig. 6.5 WHAT test for the examination of de Quervain's tendinitis.

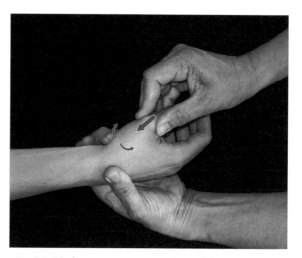

Fig. 6.6 Grind test to assess osteoarthritis of the base of the thumb.

6.5.2 Lunotriquetral Instability

Under axial load the scaphoid tends always to rotate into flexion and pronation owing to its oblique alignment with respect to the longitudinal axis of the forearm, and its unique relationship with the obliquely oriented radioscaphocapitate ligament.[7,9] This tendency to rotate into flexion and pronation is constrained by the tendency of the lunate to extend, due to its palmar wedge-shaped configuration[9] and, as suggested by Weber,[10] because of the helical slope of the triquetrum–hamate joint which tends to extend the triquetrum. Complete lunotriquetral ligament injuries will result in the scaphoid and lunate progressing into flexion, while the triquetrum extends. Partial ligament injuries can be more difficult to diagnose on examination and standard radiographs. The following

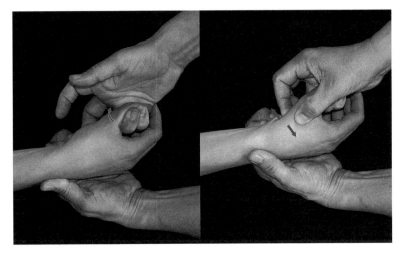

Fig. 6.7 Trapeziometacarpal stress test to assess laxity/instability. It is necessary to place the thumb in pronation to tighten the ligaments, especially the dorsoradial ligaments.

6

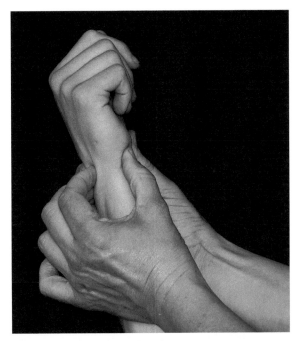

Fig. 6.8 Reagan test.

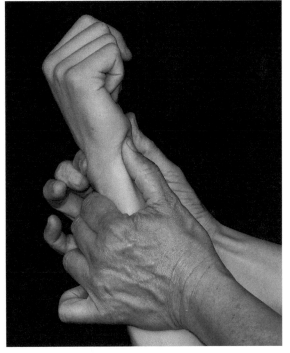

Fig. 6.9 Kleinman test.

specific tests can be used to evaluate lunotriquetral ligament injuries.

Ballottement Test or Reagan Test

This test was described to assess lunotriquetral instability.[11] The lunate is firmly stabilized with one hand, while the triquetrum and pisiform are moved dorsally and palmarly with the other hand. This test is considered positive when the joint can be passively mobilized beyond normal limits, that is, more than the contralateral side (► Fig. 6.8).

Shear Test, Shuck Test, or Kleinman Test

This test applies a palmar to dorsal force on the lunotriquetral ligament, with one hand. To perform the test, the opposite hand to the one being explored is used. The lunotriquetral complex is compressed by performing a digital clamp, in which the index finger compresses the lunate palmarly, while the thumb exerts dorsal force on the pisiform. This test is positive when there is a tear or injury to the lunotriquetral ligament[2] (► Fig. 6.9).

Historically, problems on the ulnar side of the wrist have been described as a mixed bag of pathologies to highlight the diagnostic challenge that this anatomical region represents for many clinicians. Ulnar-sided wrist pain is also commonly referred to as the "low back pain" of hand surgery: a complaint that is pervasive, vague, and frustrating to both patient and physician. Here more than ever, a good medical history and a meticulous physical examination are essential, since there are up to 25 possible pathologies originating in the ulnar side of the wrist. Systematization is very important in order to avoid forgetting specific tests. This will help us to narrow the range of possible diagnoses. The goal of these tests is to reproduce pain or demonstrate instability. These are the most frequently used specific tests in order to diagnose different causes of ulnar wrist pain.

Radioulnar Compression Test

The head of the ulna is compressed against the sigmoid fossa of the radius, while the forearm is passively brought from full pronation to full supination. This maneuver helps to assess the cartilage status of the DRUJ.[12] If this maneuver causes a painful crepitus, osteoarthritis is likely present (▶ Fig. 6.10).

Pisotriquetral Compression Test

Symptomatic osteoarthritis of the pisiform-triquetral joint is a relatively common cause of pain on the ulnar side of the wrist. To perform the test, the pisiform must be compressed against the triquetrum, with slight flexion and ulnar inclination of the wrist, while a rotational movement is applied to the pisiform[12] (▶ Fig. 6.11).

Ulnar Impaction

Pronation places the radius in an oblique position with respect to the ulna. This may cause the radius to be relatively shorter than the ulna in pronation. Soft tissues located at the distal end of the ulna may be compressed against the triquetrum in full pronation. Ulnar impaction is positive when symptoms are reproduced by pronation the forearm, ulnar deviation the wrist while a pressure is applied in a palmar direction to the head of the ulna and dorsal pressure to the pisiform. Therefore, in this test there are three factors that increase the pressure at the TFCC level[12] (▶ Fig. 6.12).

Ulnocarpal Stress Test

This test is used to verify that the pathology is on the ulnar side and to assess the ability of the TFCC to withstand rotational shear forces.[13] The examiner's one hand holds the patient's hand at the level of the metacarpals while the examiner's other hand stabilizes the distal forearm in a vertical position. This test is performed with the wrist in maximum ulnar deviation, the forearm in neutral rotation, and the elbow in 90-degree flexion, an axial load is applied while performing rotational movements in supination and pronation (▶ Fig. 6.13). The test is positive when it reproduces pain, sometimes with an audible click in the area of the ulnar fovea.

Distal Radioulnar Joint Stability Test

This test is performed in various degrees of rotation of the forearm (neutral, full pronation, and full supination)

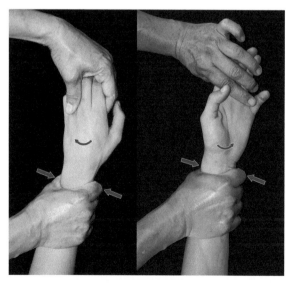

Fig. 6.10 Distal radioulnar compression test.

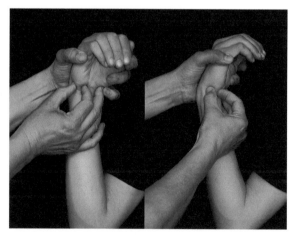

Fig. 6.11 Pisotriquetral compression test.

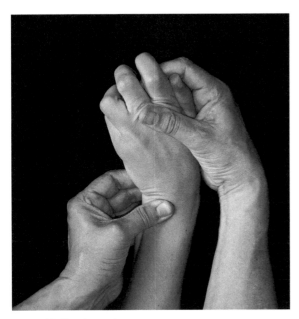

Fig. 6.12 Ulnar impaction test.

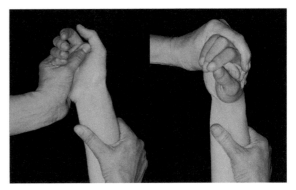

Fig. 6.13 Ulnocarpal stress test or Waiter's test.

with the elbow in 90 degrees of flexion. The distal ulna is stabilized by the examiner's hands 4 cm proximal to the DRUJ to avoid palpation of structures that may be a cause of pain. In neutral forearm rotation, up to 5 mm of translation may be normal. In contrast, in the extreme supination and pronation positions, no translation should be noted, because the TFCC tightens and constricts the DRUJ (▶ Fig. 6.14a). To further assess the integrity of the DRUJ, the wrist is radially deviated using the ulnocarpal component of the TFCC to add stability. In cases in which the tension caused in the ulnocarpal ligaments by the radial inclination does not improve the stability of the joint, it will be highly suggestive of a peripheral tear of the TFCC[14] (▶ Fig. 6.14b).

Piano Key Test

This test is useful to assess the stability of the DRUJ. It is performed with the hand flat and pronated on the examination table. The examiner exerts pressure on the prominent ulnar head, with the goal of reducing the dorsally subluxed ulna (▶ Fig. 6.15). Most of the time, the joint is passively reduced, but returns to the starting position as soon as the pressure is released. A key point that determines the positivity of this test is that there is minimal restriction to volar displacement of the ulna relative to the distal radius.

Axial Compression Test

Although the compression test was initially described to diagnose TFCC tears, it can also be used to diagnose bidirectional or dorsal DRUJ instability. The patient is asked to

get up from a sitting position in a chair, with the help of both hands extended and supported on the armrests of the chair. The test is considered positive when it reproduces pain, or an asymmetric and increased depression of the distal ulna is observed (▶ Fig. 6.16).

Extensor Carpi Ulnaris Synergy Test

In addition to palpating the extensor carpi ulnaris (ECU) tendon along its course at the dorsoulnar margin of the wrist, the ECU synergy test is helpful in assessing ECU tendonitis. This test is performed with the patient's elbow resting on the examination table at 90 degrees of flexion, with the wrist in a neutral position and the fingers extended. The examiner grasps the patient's thumb and index finger with one hand, and palpates the ECU tendon with the other hand and the patient is asked to spread the fingers against resistance (▶ Fig. 6.17). The test is positive if pain is reproduced along the dorsal ulnar aspect of the wrist.[12]

Extensor Carpi Ulnaris Instability Test

ECU instability resulting from disruption or dysfunction of the ECU sheath may be reproduced on physical examination. While the examiner holds the patient's wrist in maximum flexion and ulnar deviation, the patient supinates the wrist against resistance (▶ Fig. 6.18). This test is positive if it produces a visible subluxation of the tendon.[12]

6.5.3 Midcarpal Instability

The term "midcarpal instability" covers a range of conditions characterized by a painful clunk, usually felt in ulnar deviation of the wrist. It has been suggested that the term "instability of the proximal carpal row" would be a more accurate description because the mechanical problem is a carpal instability nondissociative, affecting the radiocarpal or the midcarpal joints or both. The scaphoid, lunate, and triquetrum move like one unit, but not in a predictable,

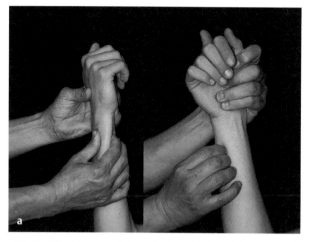
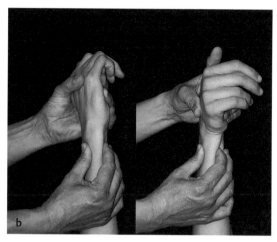

Fig. 6.14 Test to assess distal radioulnar stability. **(a)** Anteroposterior translation to assess in different degrees of pronation and supination. **(b)** Anteroposterior translation in neutral rotation of the forearm and ulnar and radial tilt.

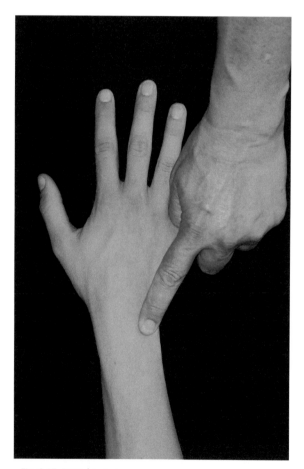

Fig. 6.15 Piano key test.

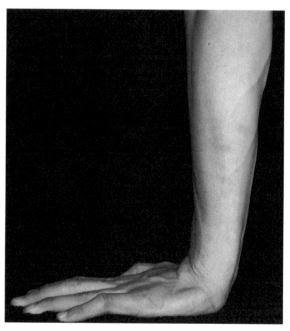

Fig. 6.16 Axial compression test (getting up from a chair).

proximal carpal row remains flexed until terminal ulnar deviation, at which time it is suddenly forced into extension. This sudden extension causes the so-called catch-up clunk felt by the patient and often clearly seen and heard by observers.[15]

Midcarpal Shift Test

smooth manner. In a wrist with palmar midcarpal instability, there is palmar subluxation of the capitate head with the wrist in radial deviation in the midcarpal joint, and the

This test was described by Lichtman et al[16] to determine the degree of laxity of the midcarpal joint. This test consists of subluxing the midcarpal joint in palmar direction,

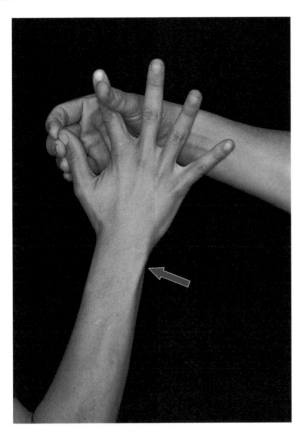

Fig. 6.17 Extensor carpi ulnaris synergy test.

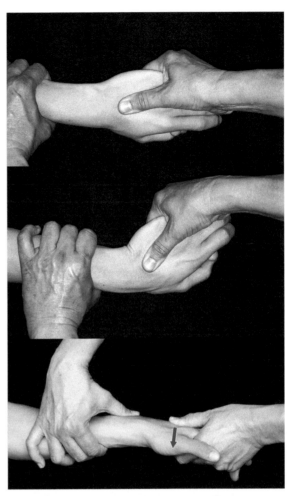

Fig. 6.19 Lichtman test to assess midcarpal laxity.

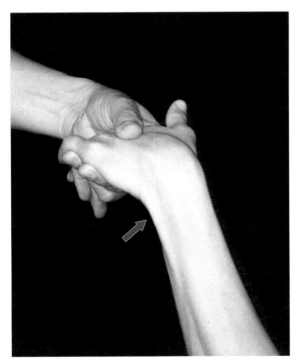

Fig. 6.18 Extensor carpi ulnaris stability test.

while the wrist is ulnarly deviated with the forearm in pronation (▶ Fig. 6.19). Depending on how much force is necessary to maintain the palmar subluxation in ulnar deviation, they are classified into five degrees. Grade 1 is when the distal row cannot be displaced palmarly due to the presence of strong and tight palmar midcarpal ligaments. Grades 2 and 3 are found among normal individuals and represent increasing levels of midcarpal laxity. In those individuals, palmar subluxation can be obtained, but it is reduced when force is stopped. Grade 4 is an abnormal level of laxity in which the midcarpal joint remains subluxed when external force is released. Grade 5 instability is when the patient can actively sublux the joint without assistance. This test evaluates the level of laxity of the palmar midcarpal ligaments. It is important to remember that high degrees of laxity should not be interpreted as pathological unless painful dysfunction is present.

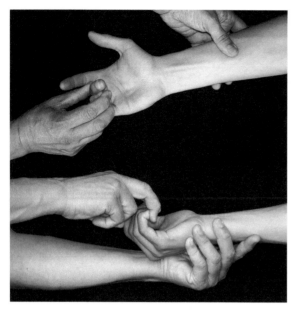

Fig. 6.20 Hook traction test of the hamate.

hook, in an attempt to widen the carpal concavity. If the hook is fractured or unattached, localized pain is likely.

References

[1] Ryu JY, Cooney WP, III, Askew LJ, An KN, Chao EYS. Functional ranges of motion of the wrist joint. J Hand Surg Am. 1991; 16(3):409–419

[2] Kleinman WB. Physical examination of the wrist: useful provocative maneuvers. J Hand Surg Am. 2015; 40(7):1486–1500

[3] Watson HK, Ashmead D, IV, Makhlouf MV. Examination of the scaphoid. J Hand Surg Am. 1988; 13(5):657–660

[4] Garcia-Elias M, Lluch A. Wrist instabilities, misalignments, and dislocations. In: Wolfe SW, Hotchkiss RN, Kozin SH, Pederson WC, Cohen M, eds. Green's operative hand surgery. 7th ed. Elsevier Churchill Livingstone; 2017:418–478

[5] Goubau JF, Goubau L, Van Tongel A, Van Hoonacker P, Kerckhove D, Berghs B. The wrist hyperflexion and abduction of the thumb (WHAT) test: a more specific and sensitive test to diagnose de Quervain tenosynovitis than the Eichhoff's Test. J Hand Surg Eur Vol. 2014; 39(3):286–292

[6] Gelberman RH, Boone S, Osei DA, Cherney S, Calfee RP. Trapeziometacarpal arthritis: a prospective clinical evaluation of the thumb adduction and extension provocative tests. J Hand Surg Am. 2015; 40(7):1285–1291

[7] Garcia-Elias M. Kinetic analysis of carpal stability during grip. Hand Clin. 1997; 13(1):151–158

[8] Garcia-Elias M, Geissler WB. Carpal instability. In: Green DP, Hotchkiss RN, Pederson WC, Wolfe SW, eds. Green's operative hand surgery. 5th ed. Elsevier Churchill Livingstone; 2005:535–604

[9] Kauer JM. Functional anatomy of the wrist. Clin Orthop Relat Res. 1980(149):9–20

[10] Weber ER. Concepts governing the rotational shift of the intercalated segment of the carpus. Orthop Clin North Am. 1984; 15(2):193–207

[11] Reagan DS, Linscheid RL, Dobyns JH. Lunotriquetral sprains. J Hand Surg Am. 1984; 9(4):502–514

[12] Garcia-Elias M. Clinical examination of the ulnar-sided painful wrist. In: Del Piñal F, Mathoulin C, Nakamura T, eds. Arthroscopic management of ulnar pain. Springer-Verlag; 2012:24–44

[13] Nakamura R, Horii E, Imaeda T, Nakao E, Kato H, Watanabe K. The ulnocarpal stress test in the diagnosis of ulnar-sided wrist pain. J Hand Surg Br. 1997; 22(6):719–723

[14] Sanz L. Dias R, Heras-Palou C. A modification of the ballottement test in the assessment of the distal radioulnar joint instability. J Bone Jt Surg Br. 2009; 91 Suppl I:80

[15] Heras-Palou C. Midcarpal instability. In: Slutsky DJ, Osterman AL, eds. Fractures and injuries of the distal radius and carpus. Elsevier; 2009:417–423

[16] Lichtman DM, Schneider JR, Swafford AR, Mack GR. Ulnar midcarpal instability-clinical and laboratory analysis. J Hand Surg Am. 1981; 6 (5):515–523

6.6 Other Specific Tests

6.6.1 Hamate Hook Pull Test

The hamate should be considered not only as the ulnar wall of the carpal tunnel but also as a pulley that increases the mechanical advantage of the little finger flexor tendons. Because the two flexor tendons change direction at the level of the hook of the hamate, contraction of these muscles generates a laterally directed force against the hook. The hamate hook pull test is based on the use of these two tendons to tension the hamate hook. The patient's wrist is placed in slight flexion and ulnar deviation. In this position, the angulation of the tendons around the hook is maximized. The patient is then asked to flex the little finger against resistance (▶ Fig. 6.20). In doing so, tension on the tendon increases, producing a vector directed ulnarly against the

7 Arthroscopic Examination of the Wrist

Fernando Corella, Jane Messina, Montserrat Ocampos, and Pietro Randelli

Abstract

Arthroscopy has revolutionized the practice of wrist surgery. The wide list of indications for wrist arthroscopy is continuously growing. Today it is possible to carry out arthroscopic repair and reconstruction techniques for all kind of carpal instabilities and wrist ligament injuries through a minimal invasive procedure.

Furthermore, as preoperative explorations and image studies still do not have high sensitivity or specificity for ligament injuries, arthroscopy continues to be the gold standard tool for evaluating these kinds of pathologies. After arthroscopic evaluations we can accurately define the stage of each ligament injury, assess its chronicity, and detect associated injuries. Therefore, this tool helps surgeons to obtain a more accurate diagnosis and hence a more accurate method of treatment.

For performing a precise and safe wrist arthroscopy (both for the diagnosis and treatment), it is mandatory to have a deep knowledge of portal placement, of arthroscopic anatomy, and of specific arthroscopic classification and tests for each carpal instability and ligament injury.

The aim of this chapter is to explain the following in detail: (1) the arthroscopic portals and general joint exploration; (2) the specific pathological evaluation and arthroscopic classification of the scapholunate ligament, lunotriquetral ligament, and extrinsic ligaments.

Keywords: Wrist arthroscopy, carpal instabilities, scapholunate ligament, lunotriquetral ligament, extrinsic ligaments

7.1 Introduction

The development of many technological innovations in the field of wrist arthroscopy has made it possible to carry out arthroscopic repair and reconstruction techniques for wrist ligament injuries. For this, it is essential to make a correct diagnosis of these pathologies. The detection rate of scapholunate (SL) or lunotriquetral (LT) ligament tears is up to 55 to 60% for plain magnetic resonance imaging (MRI) compared to arthroscopy,[1] and the accuracy and clinical relevance of MRI for extrinsic ligaments assessment remains undetermined.[2]

For this reason, wrist arthroscopy is the gold standard in diagnosis of wrist ligament injuries, allowing staging of each injury, assessing its chronicity, and detecting associated injuries. This chapter describes the arthroscopic diagnosis of intrinsic and extrinsic ligaments of the wrist and how to assess their injuries.

7.2 Arthroscopic Portals and General Joint Exploration

7.2.1 Radiocarpal Joint (Video 7.1)

Arthroscopic examination of the wrist begins exploring the radiocarpal joint. The arthroscopic portals are named considering their relationship with the extensor tendon compartments.

The two common portals used for the exploration of the radiocarpal joint are the 3/4 and 6 R. The 3/4 portal is firstly performed in a blinded manner and then the 6 R portal under arthroscopic visualization. The radial side is usually examined first and then the ulnar side of the radiocarpal joint.

3/4 Portal

It is located in the space between the extensor pollicis longus (EPL) and the extensor digitorum (ED), 1 cm distal to the Lister's tubercle and in line with the radial edge of the third metacarpal bone.

At the entry point of this portal the proximal view corresponds to the articular surface of the radius and the ridge that separates the scaphoid and lunate fossa. In front of the portal and in the middle of the vision field, the radioscapholunate (RSL) ligament of Testut is observed. If the vision is moved distally, the membranous portion of the SL ligament appears.

Turning the scope to the radial side, the radial styloid and the scaphoid fossa of the radius are observed proximally, the scaphoid distally, and on the volar side, the radioscaphocapitate (RSC) and long radiolunate (LRL) ligaments.

When the scope is moved to the ulnar side, the lunate fossa of the radius and the triangular fibrocartilage complex (TFCC) are observed proximally, the lunate distally, and on the volar side, the short radiolunate (SRL) ligament (covered by synovial membrane) and the ulnocarpal ligaments. Just ulnar to the ulnotriquetral (UT) ligament is the prestyloid recess.

6 R Portal

It is located on the radial side of the extensor carpi ulnaris (ECU) and distal to TFCC. As mentioned before, to avoid any damage to the TFCC, this portal must be carried out under arthroscopic vision.

If the arthroscope is advanced to the radial side and placed under the lunate, the proximal vision corresponds to the lunate fossa. If it is moved more radially, this proximal vision corresponds to the scaphoid fossa. Distally, the proximal pole of the lunate is observed and radially, the membranous portion of the SL ligament and proximal pole of the scaphoid.

On the dorsal side, the dorsal capsule is visualized along with the dorsal radiocarpal (DRC) ligament (that is covered by synovial tissue). If the arthroscope is moved over the dorsal side of the lunate, the dorsal capsuloligamentous scapholunate septum (DCSS)[3] is visualized.

Just at the entry point, moving the scope distally, the proximal pole of the lunate and membranous portion of the LT ligament can be observed.

7.2.2 Midcarpal Joint (Video 7.2)

The arthroscopic examination of the wrist in the midcarpal joint is performed through the ulnar midcarpal (UMC) and radial midcarpal (RMC) portals.

Usually, the UMC portal is performed firstly in a blinded manner and secondly the RMC under arthroscopic visualization.

Ulnar Midcarpal Portal

It is located 1 cm ulnar and 1 cm distal to the 6 R. It is in line with the fourth metacarpal bone.

Unlike the RMC portal (which is located just distal to the SL ligament), the UMC portal is not located above the LT ligament, but above the triquetrum bone. That is why it is safer to establish this portal firstly, in a blinded manner, and then the RMC portal under arthroscopic visualization.

At the entry point, the proximal view corresponds to the surface of the triquetrum and the lunate, separated by the LT joint.

In front of the portal, the triquetrocapitate (TC) ligament (which is the distal and ulnar portion of the arcuate ligament) is observed.

If the arthroscope is advanced to the radial side and located over the distal surface of the lunate, the proximal view corresponds to the articular surface of the lunate and scaphoid as well as the SL joint. The distal view corresponds with the proximal pole of the capitate and hamate.

The dorsal intercarpal (DIC) ligament is found on the dorsal side and the RSC ligament (which is the distal and radial portion of the arcuate ligament) on the volar side, both covered by the synovial tissue.

Radial Midcarpal Portal

It is located 1 cm distal to the 3/4 portal, in line with it and with the radial edge of the third metacarpal bone. As mentioned before, since it is just above the SL ligament, it is preferable to be performed under arthroscopic control.

Proximal to the entry point, the concave surface of the scaphoid and the lunate are observed. The space between them corresponds to the SL joint and the RSC ligament is viewed in front of the portal.

The scaphoid can be followed on the radial side for its entire length, up to the midcarpal joint until scaphotrapeziotrapezoidal (STT) joint is reached.

If the arthroscope is advanced to the ulnar side of the midcarpal joint and located over the distal surface of the lunate, the proximal view corresponds to the articular surface of the lunate and triquetrum and the LT joint. The capitate and hamate are observed distally. The DIC ligament is found on the dorsal side and the TC ligament on the volar side.

7.3 Scapholunate

7.3.1 Generalities and Normal Arthroscopic Anatomy

The exploration of SL ligament and joint should always be done from both the radiocarpal and midcarpal joint. Even though each injury is best evaluated and visualized from a specific portal, it is important to switch portals and explore them from different positions.

Scapholunate Visualization from the Radiocarpal Joint

Many portals can be used to visualize the proximal portion of the SL ligament and joint, but the two common radiocarpal ones are the 3/4 portal and the 6 R portal.

At the entry point of the 3/4 portal, if the scope is turned distally, the membranous portion of the SL ligament and its insertion on the proximal pole of the scaphoid and lunate are observed (▶ Fig. 7.1).

Through the 6 R portal, the membranous portion of the SL ligament is also viewed. On the dorsal side, if the scope is turned distally, a fibrous structure that links the dorsal capsule and the dorsal aspect of the SL ligament, which corresponds to the DCSS,[3] is visualized (▶ Fig. 7.2).

It must be remembered that the normal intact interosseous ligaments are almost invisible even in arthroscopic examination as they are in perfect continuity with the scaphoid and lunate articular surfaces. If there is a significant rupture, the intrinsic ligaments, and particularly the SL ligament, will protrude in the joint (▶ Fig. 7.3).

Scapholunate Visualization from the Midcarpal Joint

Through the UMC portal, the SL joint is viewed proximally (▶ Fig. 7.4). On the dorsal side, the dorsal portion of the SL ligament and the DIC ligament (covered by synovial tissue) can be visualized (▶ Fig. 7.5). On the volar side of the SL joint, the volar portion of the SL ligament can be observed, but it is usually covered by synovial tissue.

Through the RMC portal, the SL joint is observed proximally and in front of the portal, the anterior portion of the scaphoid, the anterior horn of the lunate, the volar

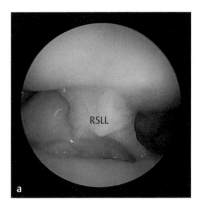
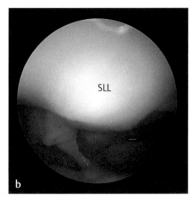

Fig. 7.1 View of the RSLL and SLL through the 3/4 portal. **(a)** RSLL in front of the 3/4 portal. **(b)** Membranous portion of the SLL. RSLL, radioscapholunate ligament; SLL, scapholunate ligament.

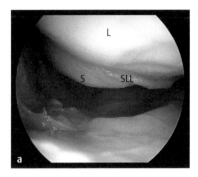
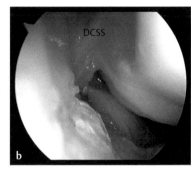

Fig. 7.2 View of the SLL and DCSS through the 6R portal. **(a)** The scaphoid and lunate fossae proximally and the lunate, membranous portion of the SLL and the scaphoid distally are observed. **(b)** View of the DCSS sliding the scope distally and turning it dorsally. SLL, scapholunate ligament; DCSS, dorsal capsuloligamentous scapholunate septum; L, lunate; S, scaphoid.

7

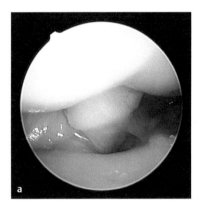
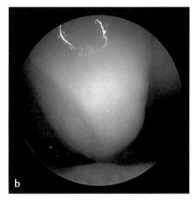

Fig. 7.3 "Baby buttock sign" through the 3/4. **(a)** Normal: regular invisible SL ligament between the scaphoid and lunate. **(b)** Pathological: SL ligament is protruding in the joint.

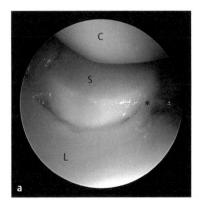
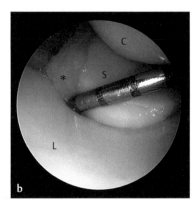

Fig. 7.4 View of the scapholunate (SL) joint through the ulnar midcarpal (UMC) portal. **(a)** The asterisk marks the dorsal portion of the SL ligament. **(b)** The asterisk marks the volar portion of the SL ligament that is masked by synovial membrane. C, capitate; L, lunate; S, scaphoid.

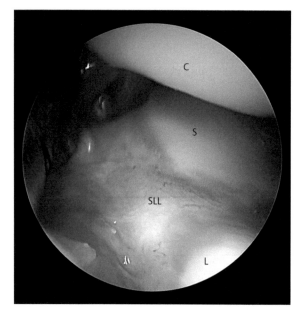

Fig. 7.5 View of the dorsal portion of the scapholunate ligament though the ulnar midcarpal (UMC) portal. C, capitate; L, lunate; S, scaphoid, SLL, scapholunate ligament.

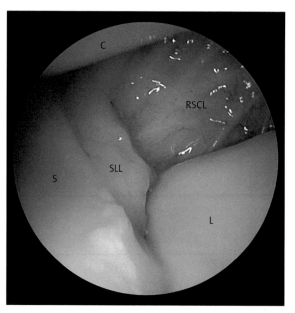

Fig. 7.6 View of the volar portion of the scapholunate ligament through the radial midcarpal (RMC) portal. Just volar to the SLL is the RSC ligament, both of which are covered by synovial membrane. C, capitate; L, lunate; S, scaphoid; RSCL, radio-scaphocapitate ligament; SLL, scapholunate ligament.

portion of SL ligament, and the RSC ligament are also observed (▶ Fig. 7.6).

7.3.2 Arthroscopic Pathological Exploration

The SL pathology is a spectrum of injuries and for understanding and defining them, many issues must be explored. They can be grouped in the 7-items arthroscopic exploration for SL pathology.

Gap Between the Bones

This the most common exploration. The probe enters through the RMC portal and the degree of instability is evaluated considering the passage of the tip and the grade of twisting of the probe. Most of the arthroscopic classifications use this kind of exploration for grading the SL lesion. They will be explained in detail below.

However, it is important to recognize that there is no ligament in the SL joint in the midcarpal joint (different from the radiocarpal joint, where the membranous portion covers the joint). So, when exploring the gap between the bones, we are neither testing nor directly visualizing the SL ligament, but interpreting the state of the ligament evaluating the laxity of the joint.

Acute vs Chronic

Most of the times the suspicion of an acute or chronic injury is easy, considering when the trauma occurred.

However, there can be doubts when evaluating injuries associated to distal radius fractures or carpal bone fractures. In these cases, old and chronic injuries can be found and no specific treatment is needed.

That is why, it is important to look for signs of acute injury, which are a hemorrhagic ligament along with fresh torn stumps. In these acute cases the associated injuries can be treated, but if there are no acute signs, they should be classified as chronic and not be overtreated (▶ Fig. 7.7; **Video 7.3**).

Quality of the Ligament Remnant

A direct visualization of the different three portions of the SL ligament can be performed arthroscopically. However, the most important portion to be evaluated is the dorsal one, as a complete injury with no remnant or a bad quality remnant of the ligament will lead to a reconstruction technique. On the other hand, lesions in continuity, with a ligament of enough quality, could be treated with a reinforcement technique.

To evaluate the SL dorsal portion, the arthroscope is introduced through the UMC portal and turned to visualize the dorsal SL joint and RMC portal. The synovial tissue is removed over the dorsal rim of the scaphoid and lunate, until the transverse fibers of the ligament and their insertion in both bones are observed.

To evaluate the quality and attachments of the dorsal portion of the SL ligament, a "hook test" can be performed.

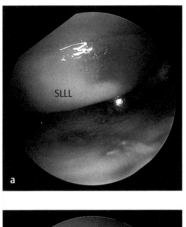 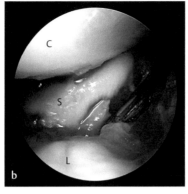

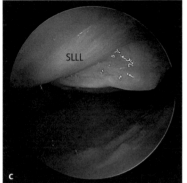 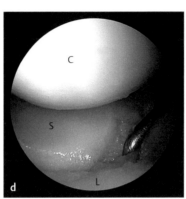

Fig. 7.7 View of the SL ligament through the 6 R (*left*) and ulnar midcarpal (UMC) portals (*right*). **(a,b)** Acute injury of the SL ligament. **(c,d)** Chronic injury of the SL ligament. C, capitate; L, lunate; S, scaphoid; SLL, scapholunate ligament.

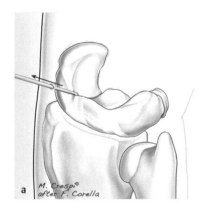 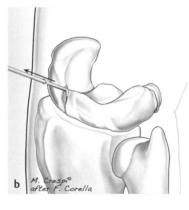

Fig. 7.8 Schematic representation of Hook test of the scapholunate (SL) ligament. **(a)** The SL ligament is competent; the probe does not pass. **(b)** The SL ligament is torn; the probe passes through it.

The probe is introduced in the SL joint, and a dorsal traction is performed, capturing the dorsal portion of the ligament. If there is a competent ligament, the probe is caught in the dorsal SL ligament (positive hook test); if not, there will be no capture (negative hook test) (▶ Fig. 7.8, ▶ Fig. 7.9; **Video 7.4**).

Dorsal Displacement of the Scaphoid

Patients with SL pathologies complain of pain in the dorsal side of the wrist. This may occur due to the dorsal displacement and impingement between the proximal pole of the scaphoid and the dorsal edge of the radius.

This dorsal displacement can be explored with the "arthroscopic scaphoid 3D (dorsal, dynamic, displacement) test."[4] This test can be useful if there are doubts about the mechanical repercussion of an SL tear and could help in the decision making of the kind of treatment.

The test should be performed in both the radiocarpal and midcarpal joints (▶ Fig. 7.10, ▶ Fig. 7.11; **Video 7.5**).

Test in the midcarpal joint: The arthroscope is introduced through the UMC portal and placed over the lunate. Then, traction is released, and the scaphoid is pushed dorsally from the scaphoid tubercle. If there is no SL misfunction, the proximal row moves dorsally together (a negative 3D test). If there is an SL instability, the

7

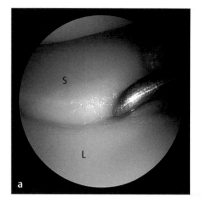 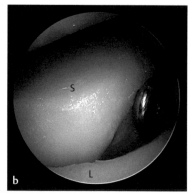

Fig. 7.9 Hook test of the scapholunate ligament. **(a)** Positive hook test. **(b)** Negative hook test. L, lunate; S, scaphoid.

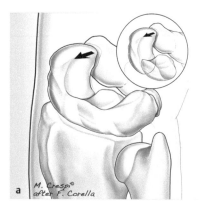 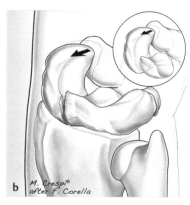

Fig. 7.10 (a,b) Schematic representation of "Arthroscopic Scaphoid 3D test."

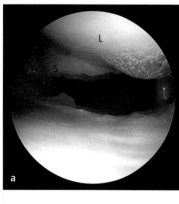 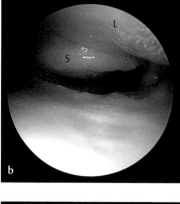

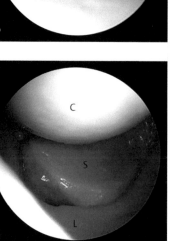

Fig. 7.11 Arthroscopic scaphoid 3D (dorsal, dynamic, displacement) test. **(a,b)** Positive arthroscopic scaphoid 3D test in the radiocarpal joint; the scaphoid is moved dorsally. **(c,d)** Positive arthroscopic scaphoid 3D test in the midcarpal joint; the scaphoid is moved dorsally separately from the lunate. C, capitate; L, lunate; S, scaphoid.

scaphoid moves dorsally while the lunate remains in the same position (a positive 3D test).

Test in the radiocarpal joint: The arthroscope is introduced through the 6 R portal under the lunate. The scaphoid is pushed dorsally again. If there is no SL misfunction, the proximal row moves dorsally together (negative 3D test), but if there is a dysfunction the scaphoid is displaced over the dorsal rim of the radius, while the lunate remains static (positive 3D test).

Reducibility

This is one of the key points when deciding the treatment in SL pathologies. If the scaphoid cannot be easily reduced to its normal position, palliative surgeries are recommended, but if it is reducible, reconstruction techniques can be performed.

Arthroscopically, this reducibility can be checked easily. The arthroscope is introduced through the UMC portal and placed over the lunate while the probe is introduced through the RMC portal. In an easily reducible instability, the scaphoid should be reduced and positioned to the height of the lunate only by pushing with the arthroscopic probe. But if not, the scaphoid cannot be positioned to its normal height in the midcarpal joint (▶ Fig. 7.12, ▶ Fig. 7.13; **Video 7.6**).

Associated Ligament Injuries

Two important ligament structures should be explored when evaluating the SL ligament, as they can be injured along with the SL ligament. They are the DCSS and the LT ligament.

The DCSS is an anatomic structure linking the SL ligament and the dorsal capsule of the wrist. In the past few years the interest in this structure has increased as it is considered an important stabilizer of the SL joint.

With the scope in the 6 R portal, which needs to be oriented posteriorly up, it is possible to identify a detachment of DCSS.[3] The probe from the membranous portion of the SL ligament is moved dorsally around the SL curved articular surfaces up to the extreme dorsal portion. There, if the DCSS is intact, it is not possible to continue as the probe is stopped by the insertion of DCSS to scaphoid and lunate. When DCSS is ruptured, the probe goes up in the midcarpal joint and it is possible to visualize the midcarpal joint from the radiocarpal joint (▶ Fig. 7.14). The specific classification for the DCSS injuries will be explained later.

The concurrence of tears of the SL and LT ligaments is not unusual and can also occur without an apparent perilunate dislocation. Badia and Khanchandani called this combined lesion a "floating lunate."[5] More recently

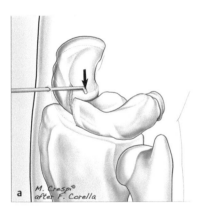
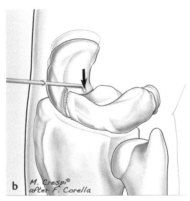

Fig. 7.12 (a,b) Schematic representation of reducibility of the scaphoid in the midcarpal joint.

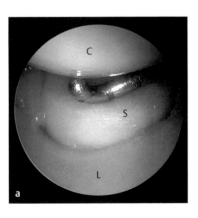
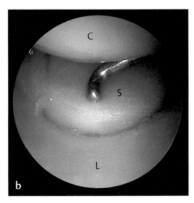

Fig. 7.13 (a,b) Reducibility of the scaphoid in the midcarpal joint. The scaphoid should be easily reduced and positioned to the height of the lunate by pushing with the arthroscopic probe.

Herzberg has described this pathology as perilunate dislocations in which there was no dislocation of the capitate from the lunate on the initial radiographs and called them perilunate injury not dislocated (PLIND).[6]

As the image studies can underestimate this combined injury, it is important to discard the presence of a floating lunate. This can be done with the "Rocking Chair Sign."[7]

With the scope in the UMC portal and over the triquetrum, a vision of the SL joint, lunate bone, and LT joint should be obtained. The probe should enter through the RMC portal. An oscillating movement of the probe is performed, from the posterior to the anterior horn of the lunate and back again. In a normal wrist, without an SL or LT injury, the lunate bone remains static when this oscillating movement is performed. However, if there is a

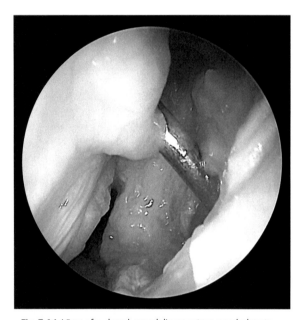

Fig. 7.14 View of a dorsal capsuloligamentous scapholunate septum (DCSS) tear through the 6 R portal.

"floating lunate," the lunate would make a movement that resembles a rocking chair, whereas the scaphoid and lunate would remain static (▶ Fig. 7.15; **Video 7.7**).

Degenerative Changes

As a nonreducible instability precludes the performance of a reconstruction technique, the presence of cartilage damage will lead to indicate palliative procedures.

Watson and Ballet have described this process as the degenerative process of an SL ligament injury and have called it the scapholunate advanced collapse (SLAC) of the wrist.[8]

The three stages of a SLAC wrist can be distinguished in radiographs. In Stage I, there is damage only to the most radial aspect of the radioscaphoid joint. In Stage II, narrowing of the whole radioscaphoid joint occurs, and in Stage III, there is an additional narrowing of the midcarpal joint.

During the decision-making process, defining the exact stage of osteoarthritis plays a central role. The correlation between cartilage lesions, classified by arthroscopy and MRI, is low.[9] Furthermore, MRI in detecting wrist chondral loss, despite a high specificity of 97%, has a low sensitivity of 65%.[10] That is why, the gold standard for assessing the status of the cartilage is wrist arthroscopy.

Four different locations should be explored arthroscopically for cartilage loss to correctly define the stage of the collapse.[11] According to the Outerbridge classification and ICRS classification it is possible to stage cartilage damage (▶ Table 7.1).[11]

Dorsal Aspect of the Radioscaphoid Fossa

This is the location of the first degenerative changes in a SLAC wrist. It is important to notice that although SLAC I and scaphoid nonunion advance collapse (SNAC) I have been published to be similar, with cartilage loss in the radial styloid, the initial degeneration is not similar.[11] In SNAC I the proximal scaphoid is linked to the lunate via

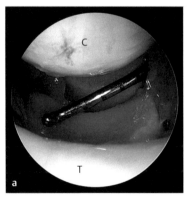 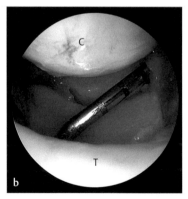 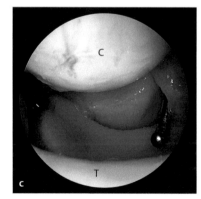

Fig. 7.15 (a–c) The "rocking chair sign." If there is combined injury of the SL and LT ligaments, the lunate performs a "rocking chair"-like motion with the aid of an arthroscopic probe. C, capitate; T, triquetrum.

an intact SL ligament, and the joint space is usually preserved. However, there is an impingement between the distal fragment of the scaphoid and the radial styloid; thus, the initial degeneration occurs at this location.

On the other hand, when there is a complete rupture of the SL, as there is a dorsal displacement of the scaphoid over the dorsal rim of the radius (as explained before), the initial degenerative cartilage loss occurs in the dorsal portion of the radioscaphoid fossa and not in the radial styloid (▶ Fig. 7.16).

This is important because in SLAC I the resection of this area (dorsal portion of the radioscaphoid fossa) could be indicated, while in SNAC I, the resection should correspond to the radial styloid.

Radioscaphoid Fossa

If the degeneration evolves, all radial fossa is affected (▶ Fig. 7.17). The degree of compromise of this fossa is essential to indicate a partial resection of the dorsal rim of the radius or other treatments that involve both the resection of the scaphoid (four corner arthrodesis) or the fusion of the radioscaphoid joint (RSL arthrodesis).

Midcarpal Joint

As the congruence in the midcarpal joint is lost due to the pronation and dorsal subluxation of the scaphoid and because of the dorsal intercalated segment instability (DISI) deformity of the lunate, the next joint to suffer

cartilage loss is the midcarpal joint. The initial degenerative changes should be looked for in the proximal pole of the capitate and in the dorsal aspect of the lunate (▶ Fig. 7.18).

7.3.3 Arthroscopic Classifications

Classifications are useful to understand and stage pathological cases and then to plan surgical treatment. As defined by Garcia Elias (2006)[12,13] the SL lesions are a spectrum of lesions and each of them must be correctly staged before planning a surgical repair.

The first paper which identifies the abnormalities of intrinsic ligaments arthroscopically was published by Dautel in 1993.[14] He developed a simple classification of three stages performed from the midcarpal joint.[15] Lindau also described several SL injuries associated to distal radius fractures and made a classification.[16] Geissler also proposed a classification in four stages of acute SL injuries associated to distal radius fractures, which have been widely used.[17]

Nevertheless, these classifications were described in acute injuries only and did not consider the different parts of the SL ligament involved, the radiological findings, and the ligaments involved in each stage. Therefore, the European Wrist Arthroscopy Society (EWAS) group, now International Wrist Arthroscopy Society (IWAS), has been working on creating a new classification over the past few years to clarify these aspects and has described the EWAS classification[3,18]. This classification was based on a study done on cadaver specimens under fluoroscopic and arthroscopic evaluation in order to correlate the arthroscopic findings to the anatomopathological damage in SL injuries.[3,18] The EWAS classification can be found in ▶ Table 7.2 (**Video 7.8**).[3,18]

The scope is positioned in the UMC portal while the probe is positioned in the RMC portal. A dynamic instability test is performed with a 2-mm probe. In the midcarpal joint, the probe is inserted in the SL joint and twisted. The test must be performed in the anterior part, then in the central part, and finally in the posterior part of SL joint. This way it explores which part of the

Table 7.1 Outerbridge classification

Grade	Outerbridge classification—1961
I	Softening of hyaline cartilage surface
II	Superficial fibrillation and fissuring of small areas
III	Deep fibrillation in the articular surface irrespective of the size
IV	Full-thickness defect down to bone

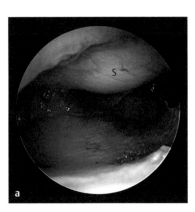
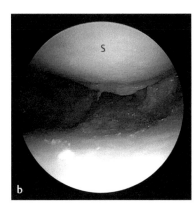

Fig. 7.16 (a,b) View of scapholunate advanced collapse (SLAC) I and scaphoid nonunion advance collapse (SNAC) I wrist through the 6 R portal. **(a)** SLAC I wrist; initial degenerative cartilage loss occurs in dorsal portion of the radial scaphoid fossa. **(b)** SNAC I wrist; initial degenerative cartilage loss occurs in the radial styloid. S, scaphoid.

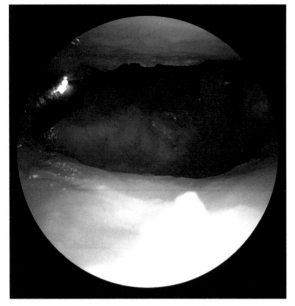

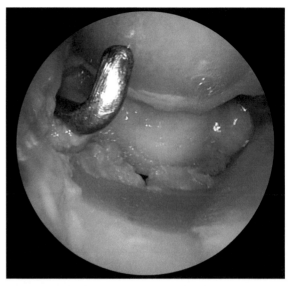

Fig. 7.18 View of scapholunate advanced collapse (SLAC) III wrist through the ulnar midcarpal (UMC) portal. The capitolunate joint is affected. C, capitate; L, lunate.

Fig. 7.17 View of scapholunate advanced collapse (SLAC) II wrist though the 6 R portal. The entire radial fossa is affected. LF, lunate fossa; L, lunate.

Table 7.2 EWAS SL staging

EWAS SL staging A: acute/C: chronic Ligaments involved		Arthroscopic findings RC: radiocarpal MC: midcarpal
I	A only	RC: attenuation of SL ligament, hemorrhage MC: attenuation of SL ligament, hemorrhage No passage of the probe through SL joint
II Tear of central part	A/C	RC: attenuation of SL ligament MC: tip of probe or the whole probe can go through SL space (central part) **Dynamic SL testing neg (no widening of SL space)**
IIIA Tear of anterior part	A/C	RC: thickening of Testut ligament, possible protrusion of SL MC: anterior SL widening at dynamic instability test, possible involvement of extrinsic volar ligaments (LRL, RSC) **Dynamic anterior widening of SL space**
IIIB Tear of dorsal part	A/C	RC: protrusion of SL ligament MC: partial posterior SL widening at dynamic instability test. Possible injury to DCSS, possible involvement of DIC **Dynamic posterior widening of SL space**
IIIC Complete SL tear, DIC, LRL	A/C	RC: protrusion of SL ligament, possible step-off, dynamic gap MC: complete SL widening at dynamic instability test, possible step-off, involvement of extrinsic ligament **Dynamic complete widening of SL space—reducible**
IV Complete SL tear, DIC, DRC, LRL, RSC, SRL	A/C	RC: marked protrusion of SL ligament with gap, possible step-off MC: gap and **passage of the arthroscope** from midcarpal to radiocarpal joint through SL joint, SL dissociation
V Complete SL tear + multiple extrinsic ligament injuries	C	RC: marked protrusion of SL ligament with gap, step-off, incongruency of SL, **drive through sign** MC: gap and **passage of the arthroscope** from midcarpal to radiocarpal joint through SL joint, SL dissociation, **drive through sign** **Radiological signs of instability**, rotatory subluxation of scaphoid

Abbreviations: DCSS, dorsal capsuloligamentous scapholunate septum; DIC, dorsal intercarpal; EWAS, European Wrist Arthroscopy Society; LRL, long radiolunate ligament; MC, midcarpal; RC, radiocarpal; RSC, radioscaphocapitate; SL, scapholunate.

ligament is damaged and whether the extrinsic ligament attachments are still in place or are detached. Afterwards the scope is moved to the RMC portal and a new testing of SL ligament is performed.

In Stage I, there is a hemorrhagic SL ligament.

In Stage II, the tip of the probe can pass through the SL space, but the probe cannot be twisted and there is no widening of the SL space. Stages I and II are stable injuries which can be treated with simple immobilization.

In Stage IIIA, there is widening of SL space in its anterior part. In these cases of anterior widening, there is damage not only to the anterior part of the SL ligament, but also to the LRL, RSC, and SRL ligaments. This damage is not always clearly seen by dorsal portals. Sometimes it is necessary to perform a volar radial portal. In this stage, the Testut ligament can appear thickened and hemorrhagic (pseudothickening of Testut ligament). This is not a real thickening, but an indirect sign of involvement of the volar portion of the SL ligament and the volar attachment of extrinsic ligaments around the SL joint (such as the RSC and the LRL ligaments), which are volar to the Testut ligament.

In Stage IIIB, there is a widening of the posterior part of the joint. This dorsal widening means there is damage to the posterior portion of the SL ligament and the extrinsic ligaments such as the DIC. A detachment of the DCSS can also be seen at this stage.

In Stage IIIC, the tear is complete, and the scaphoid and lunate can be pulled apart by twisting the probe. As there is a widening of the whole space with the probe, the damage is anterior, proximal, and posterior. When the probe is removed, the SL interval is closed spontaneously.

In Stage IV, the widening of the two bones is wider and the arthroscope can go from the midcarpal to the radiocarpal joint. In this stage there are still no radiological abnormalities. Nevertheless, several extrinsic ligaments are involved, such as the DIC, the LRL, and the RSC ligaments.

In Stage V the "drive-through sign" is present which means that when the scope is introduced in the 3/4 portal, it passes directly in the SL space because there is a wider gap (static SL injury). At this stage there are radiological abnormalities (increased SL gap, DISI deformity) and more extensive involvement of extrinsic ligaments (DIC, DRC, STT, LRL, RSC, SRL).[3,18.]

Advanced stages are commonly found in old chronic injuries, as these injuries evolved in several subsequent steps over time.[3,18] However, they can also be present in acute and high-energy traumas, such as perilunate injuries, high-energy distal radius fractures, etc.

7.4 Lunotriquetral

7.4.1 Generalities and Normal Arthroscopic Anatomy

As in the SL evaluation, the exploration of the LT ligament and joint should also be done from both the radiocarpal and midcarpal joints.

Lunotriquetral Visualization from the Radiocarpal Joint

Many portals can be used to visualize the proximal portion of the LT ligament and joint, but the most common one is the 6R portal and sometimes the 6U portal. It is difficult to visualize this proximal portion from radial portals (as the 3/4).

Through the 6R portal, with the arthroscope over the TFCC and moving the vision field distally, the proximal pole of the lunate and membranous portion of the LT ligament can be observed (▶ Fig. 7.19; **Video 7.9**).

The 6U portal, located ulnar with respect to the ECU and over the TFCC, can also be used to visualize the LT ligament. In fact, the visualization of the proximal portion of the LT ligament is as good or even better than from the 6R portal. However, the sensory branch of the ulnar nerve is very close to the portal, so great precaution should be taken when performing it.

Lunotriquetral Visualization from the Midcarpal Joint

The two portals used in the midcarpal joint to test and visualize the LT ligament and joint are the RMC and UMC portals.

Through the UMC portal, the LT joint is viewed proximally. In front of the portal, the anterior portion of the triquetrum, the anterior horn of the lunate, the volar portion of the LT ligament (covered by synovial tissue), and the TC ligament are observed (▶ Fig. 7.20).

Through the RMC portal, the scope is moved to the ulnar side and the LT joint is observed.

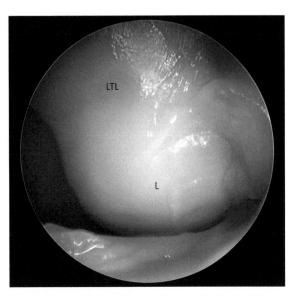

Fig. 7.19 View of the LT ligament through the 6R portal. L, lunate; LTL, lunotriquetral ligament.

It is important to be aware that it could be a crest in the lunate that separates an articular fossa for the capitate and a smaller fossa for the hamate, a finding that Viegas classified as lunate type I (without a crest and concave shape) and type II (with a crest and biconcave shape).[19] If the crest is too close to the LT joint, it could be mistaken as a step-off (▶ Fig. 7.21).

7.4.2 Specific Pathological Evaluation

Although less well established than the SL ligament, the LT ligament may be injured to varying degrees. To understand and define the type of injury, many issues must be explored. They can also be grouped in the 7-items arthroscopic exploration.

Gap Between the Bones

This the most common exploration, but unlike the SL joint assessment, the probe enters the LT joint obliquely through the UMC portal, which makes it more difficult to explore the gap (▶ Fig. 7.22). There is also a classification for the LT ligament considering the twisting of the probe that will be explained later.

Acute vs Chronic

As previously detailed in the SL ligament exploration, the signs of acute injury are a hemorrhagic ligament along with a fresh torn stump. As with the SL ligament, when the LT injuries are assessed in the context of carpal or distal radius fractures, it is important to differentiate

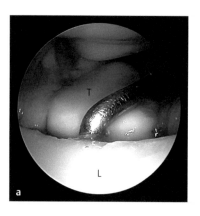

Fig. 7.20 View of the TC ligament through the ulnar midcarpal (UMC) portal. C, capitate; H, hamate; T, triquetrum; TCL, triquetrocapitate ligament.

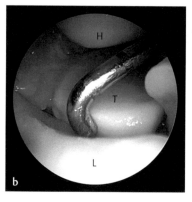

Fig. 7.21 **(a)** Lunate type I without articular facet for the hamate. **(b)** Lunate type II with articular facet for the hamate. L, lunate; H, hamate; T, triquetrum.

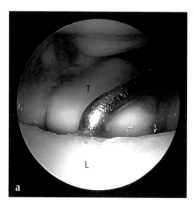
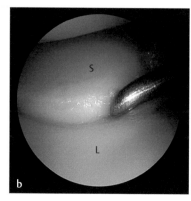

Fig. 7.22 Gap between bones. **(a)** Lunotriquetral (LT) ligament assess; the probe enters the LT joint obliquely through the ulnar midcarpal (UMC) portal. **(b)** Scapholunate (SL) ligament assess; the probe enters in line with LT joint through the radial midcarpal (RMC) portal. L, lunate; S, scaphoid; T, triquetrum.

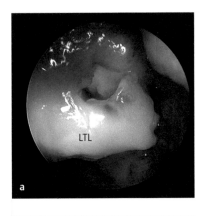
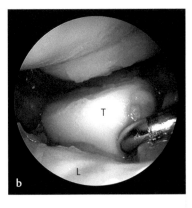
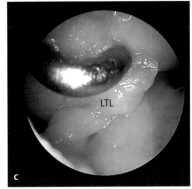
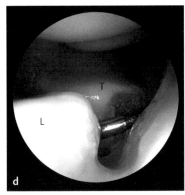

Fig. 7.23 View of the lunotriquetral (LT) ligament through the 6 R (*left*) and radial midcarpal (RMC) portals (*right*). (**a,b**) Acute injury of the LT ligament. (**c,d**) Chronic injury of the LT ligament. L, lunate; T, triquetrum; LTL, lunotriquetral ligament.

between chronic and acute injuries and not to overtreat an old one (▶ Fig. 7.23).

Quality of the Ligament Remnant

Different from the dorsal portion of the SL ligament, the dorsal portion of the LT ligament is not easily seen as it is thinner and more integrated with the dorsal capsule and the DIC ligament. On the volar side of the LT joint, the volar portion of the LT ligament is located, generally covered by synovial tissue. The most important portion to be evaluated is the volar one as it is the strongest portion.

To evaluate the volar portion, the arthroscope is introduced through the UMC portal and the scope is turned volarly to visualize it (▶ Fig. 7.24). The synovial tissue can be removed over the volar LT midcarpal joint, but the debridement is more difficult to perform through the UMC portal without the risk of injuring the lunate or triquetrum cartilage. To avoid this, the synovial tissue could be also debrided through a volar portal.[20,21]

As explained before there can be doubts between the laxity of the joint or a real ligament injury. In these cases, it is useful to explore the LT ligament in the radiocarpal joint through the 6 R portal. In a complete injury the lunate will be completely detached from the triquetrum and there will be an injury of the membranous portion that allows a direct visualization of the LT joint (▶ Fig. 7.25).

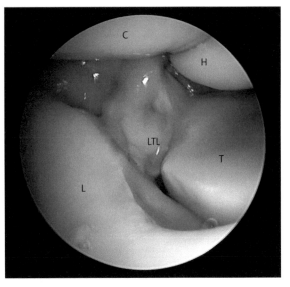

Fig. 7.24 View of the volar portion of the lunotriquetral (LT) ligament that is masked by synovial membrane through the radial midcarpal (RMC) portal. L, lunate; H, hamate; T, triquetrum; LTL, lunotriquetral ligament.

Arthroscopic Ballottement Test

An arthroscopic ballottement test with a direct visualization of the LT joint can be performed.[22] The arthroscope is introduced through the RMC portal and located over the lunate. Then, traction is released, and the triquetrum is pushed dorsally and volarly. If there is no LT instability, the triquetrum will move along with the lunate. If there is an LT injury, the triquetrum will move dorsally and volarly while the lunate remains static (▸ Fig. 7.26; **Video 7.10**).

Reducibility

Arthroscopically, this reducibility can be checked in the same way as in the SL joint. The arthroscope is introduced through the RMC portal and placed over the lunate while the probe is introduced through the UMC portal. The triquetrum is easily reduced if the normal height of the LT joint is reached by pushing it with the probe (▸ Fig. 7.27).

Combined Injuries

As explained before, the concurrence of tears of the SL and LT ligaments can occur.[5,6] So, this combined injury can be explored as explained before with the "rocking chair sign."[7]

It is also important to look for other combined injuries, especially the lesions that appear in an ulnar abutment syndrome. This pathology is not a carpal instability, but it is commonly associated with LT lesions, so it will be explained in the next heading.

Degenerative Changes

The presence of cartilage damage can modify the type of treatment in LT pathology.

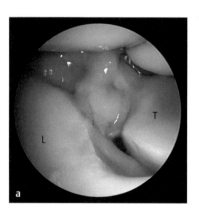

Fig. 7.25 View of a lunotriquetral (LT) ligament injury through the 6R portal. L, lunate; T, triquetrum; LTL, lunotriquetral ligament.

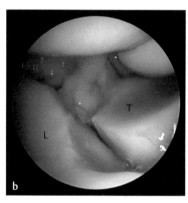

Fig. 7.26 (a,b) Arthroscopic ballottement test of the lunotriquetral (LT) joint. The triquetrum moves dorsally and palmarly separately from the lunate if there is an injury to the LT ligament. L, lunate; T, triquetrum.

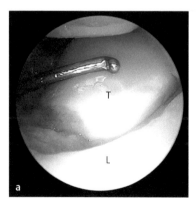
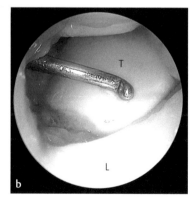

Fig. 7.27 (a,b) Reducibility of the triquetrum in the midcarpal joint. The triquetrum should be easily reduced and positioned to the height of the lunate by pushing with the arthroscopic probe. L, lunate; T, triquetrum.

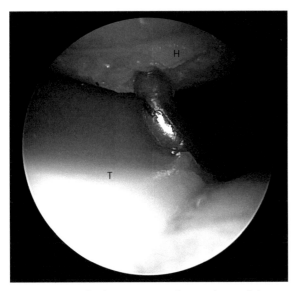

Fig. 7.28 View of a degenerative cartilaginous lesion of the proximal pole of the hamate through the radial midcarpal (RMC) portal. H, hamate; T, triquetrum.

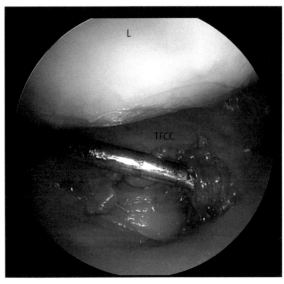

Fig. 7.29 View of a degenerative central lesion of the TFCC through the 3/4 portal. L, lunate; TFCC, triangular fibrocartilage complex.

Similar to the SL injury which can develop in a SLAC wrist, the LT instability can develop in degenerative changes especially in the proximal pole of the hamate. This lesion has been described as HALT (Hamate Arthrosis Lunotriquetral Ligament tear) due to its association with LT injuries and is usually associated to type II lunate.[23] This degenerative changes of the proximal surface of the hamate can be viewed through both RMC and UMC portals (► Fig. 7.28).

The ulnar abutment syndrome, in patients with ulnar positive variance, can develop different lesions that must be considered.[24] One of these lesions is the LT ligament injury. In this situation, a reconstruction of the LT ligament is not the main aspect to assess, but the restoration of the correct length of the ulna.

Four different locations should be explored arthroscopically, as described in the following text.

Triangular Fibrocartilage Complex (TFCC) and Ulnar Head

This is the location of the first degenerative changes in the ulnocarpal abutment syndrome. The TFCC is assessed with the scope through the 3/4 portal and the probe through the 6R portal. Usually, a degenerative central to radial lesion of the TFCC is found (the edges are frayed and not hemorrhagic) (► Fig. 7.29).

Articular Surface of the Lunate and/or Ulnar Head

If the compression evolves, degenerative changes of the distal and radial articular surface of the ulnar head or proximal and ulnar articular surface of the lunate can occur. The degenerative changes of the articular surface of

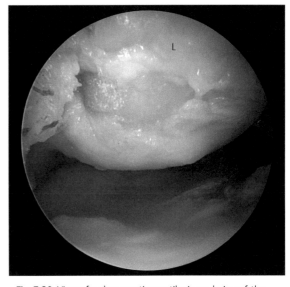

Fig. 7.30 View of a degenerative cartilaginous lesion of the proximal surface of the lunate through the 6R portal. L, lunate.

the ulnar head can be visualized through the 3/4 portal if there is a degenerative perforation of the TFCC.

The degenerative changes of the proximal surface of the lunate are best viewed through the 6R portal, sliding the scope distally (► Fig. 7.30).

LT Ligament

The next injury to appear is a lesion of the LT ligament. As mentioned before this is not a primary carpal instability, but secondary to the ulnar abutment syndrome.

Proximal Hamate

As mentioned previously, degenerative injuries of the proximal pole of the hamate can develop with time after an LT injury.

7.4.3 Arthroscopic Classifications

LT injuries are less frequent compared to SL lesions. Therefore, the classification of SL is commonly used for the LT instabilities as well. Nevertheless, there are some differences in the pathological cases and ligaments involved as the anatomy is different at the LT joint.

First, the volar part of LT ligament is very strong and isolated volar lesions are rare. Moreover, wrist traumas mostly affect the radial side of the wrist as they usually occur with the wrist in extension, ulnar deviation, and intercarpal supination. According to Mayfield the LT ligament is involved only at the very end of a perilunate injury.[25] However, ulnar-sided trauma has been described and can cause LT injuries.[26,27] Finally, chronic injuries are manly caused by ulnocarpal abutment syndrome or repetitive minor trauma. As explained before the most important thing to consider in these cases is restoring the length of the ulna and not the LT injury.

Although the arthroscopic classifications for SL ligament injuries have been commonly used for LT injuries, a specific arthroscopic classification for the LT ligament can be found in ▶ Table 7.3 (**Video 7.11**).

7.5 Extrinsic Ligaments

7.5.1 Generalities and Normal Arthroscopic Anatomy

Some extrinsic ligaments can be easily observed arthroscopically but others cannot since they are lined by a synovial tissue.

Palmar Radiocarpal Ligaments

There are four palmar radiocarpal ligaments: RSC ligament, LRL ligament, RSL ligament, and SRL ligament.[28]

Table 7.3 EWAS LT staging

EWAS LT staging A: Acute/C: Chronic Ligaments involved		Arthroscopic findings RC: radiocarpal MC: midcarpal
I	A only	RC: attenuation of LT ligament, hemorrhage MC: attenuation of LT ligament, hemorrhage No passage of the probe through LT joint
II Tear of central membranous portion	A/C	RC: attenuation of SL ligament MC: tip of probe or the whole probe can go through LT space (central part) **Dynamic LT testing neg (no widening of LT space)**
IIIA Tear of anterior part	A/C	RC: hypermobility and LT malalignment MC: anterior LT widening at dynamic instability test, tear involvement of extrinsic volar ligaments (UL, UT) **Dynamic Anterior widening of LT space**
IIIB Tear of dorsal part	A/C	RC: hypermobility of LT joint MC: partial posterior LT widening at dynamic instability test. Possible injury to DRC, possible involvement of DIC **Dynamic posterior widening of LT space**
IIIC Complete LT tear Involvement of UL, UT, DRC	A/C	RC: Hypermobility and malalignment, dynamic gap MC: complete LT widening at dynamic instability test, possible step off, involvement of extrinsic ligament **Dynamic complete widening of LT space—reducible**
IV Complete	A/C	RC: possible step off MC: gap and **passage of the arthroscope** from midcarpal to radiocarpal joint through LT joint, LT dissociation floating lunate, Rocking chair sign
V Complete SL tear + multiple extrinsic ligament injuries	C	RC: gap, step-off, incongruency of LT MC: gap and **passage of the arthroscope** from midcarpal to radiocarpal joint through LT joint, LT dissociation **Radiological signs of instability**

Abbreviations: DRC, dorsal radiocarpal; EWAS, European Wrist Arthroscopy Society; LRL, long radiolunate ligament; LT, lunotriquetral; MC, midcarpal; RC, radiocarpal; SL, scapholunate; UL, ulnolunate; UT, ulnotriquetral.

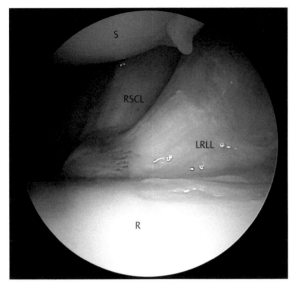

Fig. 7.31 View of the RSC and LRL ligaments through the 3/4 portal. R, radius; RLLL, radiolunate ligament; RSCL, radioscaphocapitate ligament; S, scaphoid.

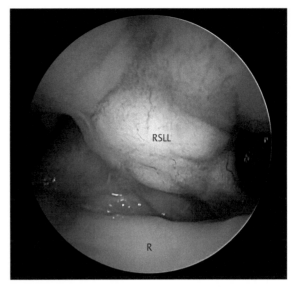

Fig. 7.32 View of the radioscapholunate (RSL) ligament through the 3/4 portal. R, radius.

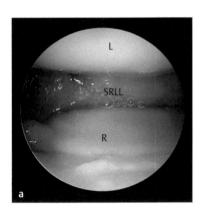
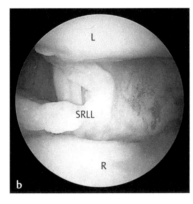

Fig. 7.33 View of the SRL ligament through the 3/4 portal. **(a)** The ligament is masked by synovial membrane. **(b)** View of the ligament when the synovial membrane is partially detached. L, lunate; R, radius; SRLL, short radiolunate ligament.

The RSC and LRL ligaments are well-differentiated structures, so they are easily visualized from all the DRC portals. Nonetheless, the portal commonly used to view the palmar radiocarpal ligaments is the 3/4 portal.

With the scope in the 3/4 portal, the ligaments visualized from radial to ulnar are the RSC, LRL, RSL, and SRL.

RSC Ligament

From the 3/4 portal, the radiocarpal part of this ligament is visualized. It extends from the tip of the styloid process to approximately the middle portion of the radioscaphoid fossa.

LRL Ligament

Just ulnar to the RSC ligament, the LRL ligament is spread over the rest of the scaphoid fossa. There is space between the RSC and LRL ligaments which is named interligamentous sulcus.[28] The LRL ligament slightly overlaps the RSC ligament in its more proximal region[29] (▶ Fig. 7.31).

RSL Ligament

This ligament is not considered a true ligament but a mesocapsule which holds vessels and innervation to the SL ligament and proximal pole of the scaphoid.[28] It is covered by a thick synovial tissue with many capillaries. Its attachment is located at the interfossal ridge of the radius (▶ Fig. 7.32).

SRL Ligament

Ulnar to the RSL ligament, the SRL ligament spans the lunate fossa. This ligament is covered by synovial tissue (▶ Fig. 7.33).

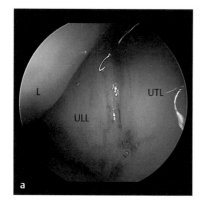
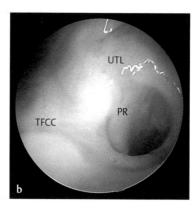

Fig. 7.34 (a,b) View of the ulnocarpal ligaments through the 6 R portal. Just ulnar to the UT ligament prestyloid recess is found. L, lunate; ULL, ulnolunate ligament; UTL, ulnotriquetral ligament; PR: prestyloid recess; TFCC, triangular fibrocartilage complex.

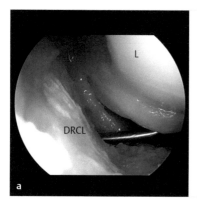
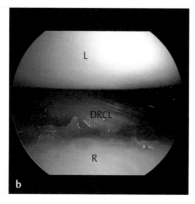

Fig. 7.35 (a) View of the DRC ligament through the 6 R portal after shaving the synovial membrane. **(b)** View of the DRC ligament through the volar central portal. DRCL, dorsal radiocarpal ligament; L, lunate; R, radius.

Ulnocarpal Ligamentous Complex

The ulnocarpal ligamentous complex (UCLC)[30] is made up of the ulnocapitate (UC), ulnolunate (UL), and ulnotriquetral (UT) ligaments. The UC ligament is anterior to the junction of the UL and UT ligaments[28,31] so it is not visualized with the scope. The UL and UT ligaments can be visualized through the 3/4, 4/5, and 6 R portals. They are indistinguishable in their most proximal region and are in continuity with the TFCC. The prestyloid recess is found immediately ulnar to the UT ligament. Through the 6 R portal, both ligaments can be differentiated in their distal region by sliding the scope distally and turning it volarly (▶ Fig. 7.34).

Dorsal Radiocarpal Ligament

The DRC ligament can be partially viewed from the 3/4 and 6 R portals if the synovial membrane that lines over it is removed. The volar central portal[21] is best for fully viewing this ligament which spans from the 3/4 portal to the junction of the TFCC and radius (▶ Fig. 7.35).

Palmar Midcarpal

There are four palmar midcarpal ligaments: STT ligament, scaphocapitate (SC) ligament, triquetrocapitate ligament, and triquetrohamate (TH) ligament.[28] Of these four ligaments, only the TC ligament is visualized from the dorsal midcarpal portals. It spans along the radial

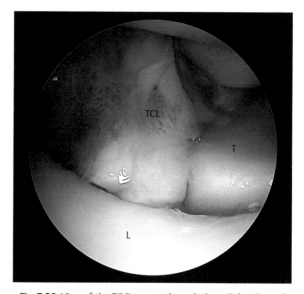

Fig. 7.36 View of the TC ligament through the radial midcarpal (RMC) portal. Sometimes, the TH ligament is observed just ulnar to the TC ligament. L, lunate; T, triquetrum; TCL, triquetrum capitate ligament.

half of triquetrum (▶ Fig. 7.36). The other ligaments are masked by synovial tissue. If the synovial tissue is removed, the ligaments that could be viewed from radial

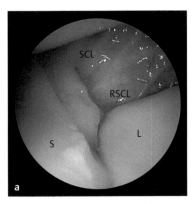 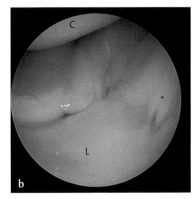 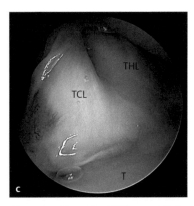

Fig. 7.37 View of the midcarpal (and radiocarpal) palmar ligaments. **(a)** SC ligament and the midcarpal portion of the RSC ligament that are masked by synovial membrane. **(b)** The asterisk sign shows the UC ligament that is covered by synovial membrane. **(c)** Ulnar midcarpal ligaments: TC and TH ligaments. C, capitate; L, lunate; S, scaphoid; RSCL, radioscaphocapitate ligament; SCL, scaphocapitate ligament; T, triquetrum; TCL, triquetrocapitate ligament; THL, triquetrohamate ligament.

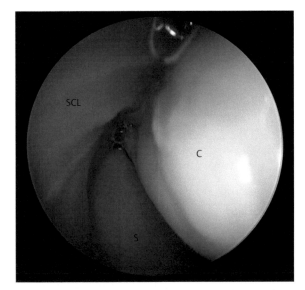 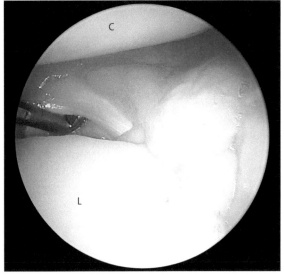

Fig. 7.38 View of the SC ligament through the volar central portal sliding the scope distally and turning it palmarly. C, capitate; S, scaphoid; SCL, scaphocapitate ligament.

Fig. 7.39 View of the Poirier space that is signaled by an arthroscopic probe, through the ulnar midcarpal (UMC) portal. C, capitate; L, lunate.

to ulnar would be the SC ligament and the midcarpal portion of the RSC ligament on the scaphoid, the midcarpal portion of the UC ligament just radial to the RC ligament, and the TH ligament just ulnar to the TC ligament on the triquetrum[28] (▶ Fig. 7.37). The SC ligament can also be viewed through the volar central portal of the midcarpal joint, sliding the scope distally and turning it volarly (▶ Fig. 7.38). Immediately distal to the distal and palmar edge of the lunate is the Poirier space (▶ Fig. 7.39).

Dorsal Intercarpal Ligament

The DIC ligament can be partially viewed from the dorsal midcarpal portals if the synovial tissue that lines it is

removed. The volar central portal[21] is best for fully viewing this ligament which spans from the triquetrum to the scaphoid (▶ Fig. 7.40).

7.5.2 Specific Pathological Evaluation and Arthroscopic Classification

Extrinsic ligament testing can be also performed under arthroscopy with a probe. The laxity of their incompetence can be graded according to Van Overstraeten.[33]

It is not always easy to test these extrinsic ligaments by arthroscopy, as they are covered by synovial tissue (which has to be removed first) and may not be so well defined,

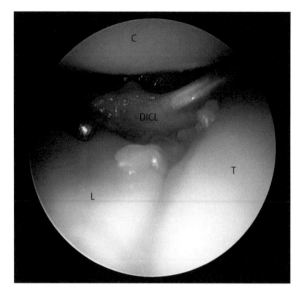

Fig. 7.40 View of the dorsal intercarpal ligament portal through the volar central portal once the synovial membrane is shaved.

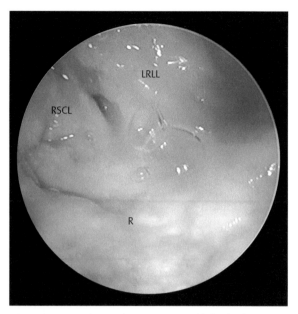

Fig. 7.41 From 3/4 portal we can see an old distal radius fracture with chronic lesion of extrinsic ligaments LRL and RSC; on x-ray there is an initial ulnar translocation of carpus. LRLL, long radiolunate ligament; R, radius; RSCL, radioscaphocapitate ligament.

especially in chronic cases and in patients with degenerative changes. In fact, in chronic cases the definition of the lesion is not so clear as a scar tissue may be present. This scar tissue may be incompetent, and the resistance of the ligament reduced.

The testing is performed hooking each ligament with a probe and pulling it under arthroscopic visualization.

The different degrees of ligament tears or laxity are staged, in which "E" means extrinsic ligament:

E0: normal tension.

E1: slight laxity, fibers elongated < 50%.

E2: moderate laxity, the ligament is elongated > 50% of its fibers.

E3 complete rupture, complete detention of the ligament, or the ligament has disappeared.

With the scope in the 6 R portal and the probe in the 3/4 portal it is possible to test the radiocarpal part of the RSC ligament, the LRL ligament, and the SRL ligament.

With the scope in 3/4 portal and the probe in 4/5 or 6 R portals it is possible to test the UL ligament and the UT ligament.

In order to test the DRC ligament, slide the probe along the proximal surface of the triquetrum and hook the dorsal insertion of this ligament on the triquetrum.

With the scope in RMC portal and the probe in UMC portal it is possible to test the midcarpal portion of the RSC ligament, the TC ligament, and TH ligament.

To test the DIC ligament, rotate the probe dorsally at the distal surface of the proximal pole of scaphoid and pull it outwards. It is possible to withdraw the scope extra-articularly to directly visualize the dorsal edge of the scaphoid where the probe is hooking the DIC for testing.

To test the scaphotrapezial (ST) ligament it is better to place the scope in UMC portal and the probe in RMC portal, in order to hook the ligament on the radial side of the STT joint.

Specific pathological evaluation can be done for instance in ulnar wrist trauma; a TFCC injury can be associated to a tear of UL and UT ligaments. This is a frequent finding in the radiocarpal joint. In the midcarpal joint, damage to TH and TC ligaments can be found associated to TFCC or LT injuries.

Other cases of extrinsic ligament injuries can be identified in distal radius fractures. For instance, in distal radius fracture there can be an associated injury not only of the SL ligament but also of the RSC, LRL, and SRL ligaments with ulnar translocation of the carpus, which means high-energy trauma and severe damage (▶ Fig. 7.41). However, in most of the cases there may be partial extrinsic ligament tears associated to distal radius fracture that can heal spontaneously without a specific treatment apart from the immobilization.

The DRC ligament damage is often found associated to LT injury and may need a proper repair.

Another wide extrinsic ligament injury that has been described is the PARC injury, i.e., proximal avulsion of radiocarpal capsule and capsuloligamentous structures. It is a cause of persisting wrist pain. This can develop on the radial side of the wrist, complicating SL and DCSS injuries, or on the ulnar side associated to TFCC injuries.

This can be frequently unnoticed as the lesion is covered by synovial or scar tissue.[33]

Another classification has been described to grade DCSS injuries.[33] According to some authors, DCSS injuries may have a role in predynamic instability especially when the dorsal portion of SL ligament is damaged (EWAS stage 3B SL ligament injuries), even if no proper biomechanical studies are available about its resistance strength.[33] This classification identifies four stages of dorsal capsule-scapholunate septum injuries (S).

S0: If the DCSS is intact, the fibers can be palpated with a probe and are correctly tensioned.

S1: DCSS is partially loosened when tested with a probe and > 50% of fibers are intact.

S2: DCSS is loosened and less than 50% of fibers are intact.

S3: DCSS is completely ruptured or disappeared.

7.6 Conclusions

The arthroscopic exploration of the wrist, both in the radiocarpal and midcarpal joints, is an essential tool to identify and classify all carpal ligament injuries and chondral lesions. The knowledge of different portals and exploration of all wrist ligaments and arthroscopic signs of carpal instabilities are extremely important for an accurate diagnosis and thus choosing the best treatment option in every stage of the disease.

References

[1] Grunz JP, Gietzen CH, Grunz K, Bley T, Schmitt R. Imaging of carpal instabilities. Röfo Fortschr Geb Röntgenstr Neuen Bildgeb Verfahr. 2021; 193(2):139–150

[2] Ramamurthy NK, Chojnowski AJ, Toms AP. Imaging in carpal instability. J Hand Surg Eur Vol. 2016; 41(1):22–34

[3] Van Overstraeten L, Camus E, Wahegaonkar A, et al. Anatomical description of the dorsal capsulo-scapholunate septum (DCSS)—arthroscopic staging of scapholunate instability after DCSS sectioning. J Wrist Surg. 2013; 2(3):284–284

[4] Corella F, Ocampos M, del Cerro M. Arthroscopic scaphoid 3D test for scapholunate instability. J Wrist Surg. 2018; 7(1):89–92

[5] Badia A, Khanchandani P. The floating lunate: arthroscopic treatment of simultaneous complete tears of the scapholunate and lunotriquetral ligaments. Hand (N Y). 2009; 4(3):250–255

[6] Herzberg G. Perilunate injuries, not dislocated (PLIND). J Wrist Surg. 2013; 2(4):337–345

[7] Corella F, Del Cerro M, Ocampos M, Larrainzar-Garijo R. The "rocking chair sign" for floating lunate. J Hand Surg Am. 2015; 40(11):2318–2319

[8] Watson HK, Ballet FL. The SLAC wrist: scapholunate advanced collapse pattern of degenerative arthritis. J Hand Surg Am. 1984; 9(3):358–365

[9] Terzis A, Klinger A, Seegmüller J, Sauerbier M. Inter-rater reliability of magnetic resonance imaging in comparison to computed tomography and wrist arthroscopy in SLAC and SNAC wrist. J Clin Med. 2021; 10(16):3592

[10] Asaad AM, Andronic A, Newby MP, Harrison JWK. Diagnostic accuracy of single-compartment magnetic resonance arthrography in detecting common causes of chronic wrist pain. J Hand Surg Eur Vol. 2017; 42(6):580–585

[11] Hjelle K, Solheim E, Strand T, Muri R, Brittberg M. Articular cartilage defects in 1000 knee arthroscopies. Arthroscopy. 2002;18(7):730–734

[12] Garcia-Elias M, Lluch AL, Stanley JK. Three-ligament tenodesis for the treatment of scapholunate dissociation: indications and surgical technique. J Hand Surg Am. 2006; 31(1):125–134

[13] Garcia-Elias M, Lluch AL. Wrist instabilities, misalignments, and dislocations. 2016

[14] Dautel G, Goudot B, Merle M. Arthroscopic diagnosis of scapholunate instability in the absence of X-ray abnormalities. J Hand Surg [Br]. 1993; 18(2):213–218

[15] Dreant N, Dautel G. Development of a arthroscopic severity score for scapholunate instability. Chir Main. 2003; 22(2):90–94

[16] Lindau T, Arner M, Hagberg L. Intraarticular lesions in distal fractures of the radius in young adults. A descriptive arthroscopic study in 50 patients. J Hand Surg [Br]. 1997; 22(5):638–643

[17] Geissler WB. Arthroscopically assisted reduction of intra-articular fractures of the distal radius. Hand Clin. 1995; 11(1):19–29

[18] Messina JC, Van Overstraeten L, Luchetti R, Fairplay T, Mathoulin CL. The EWAS classification of scapholunate tears: an anatomical arthroscopic study. J Wrist Surg. 2013; 2(2):105–109

[19] Viegas SF, Wagner K, Patterson R, Peterson P. Medial (hamate) facet of the lunate. J Hand Surg Am. 1990; 15(4):564–571

[20] Slutsky DJ. The use of a volar ulnar portal in wrist arthroscopy. Arthroscopy. 2004; 20(2):158–163

[21] Corella F, Ocampos M, Cerro MD, Larrainzar-Garijo R, Vázquez T. Volar central portal in wrist arthroscopy. J Wrist Surg. 2016; 5(1):80–90

[22] Reagan DS, Linscheid RL, Dobyns JH. Lunotriquetral sprains. J Hand Surg Am. 1984; 9(4):502–514

[23] Harley BJ, Werner FW, Boles SD, Palmer AK. Arthroscopic resection of arthrosis of the proximal hamate: a clinical and biomechanical study. J Hand Surg Am. 2004; 29(4):661–667

[24] Palmer AK. Triangular fibrocartilage complex lesions: a classification. J Hand Surg Am. 1989; 14(4):594–606

[25] Mayfield JK. Wrist ligamentous anatomy and pathogenesis of carpal instability. Orthop Clin North Am. 1984; 15(2):209–216

[26] Viegas SF. Ulnar-sided wrist pain and instability. Instr Course Lect. 1998; 47:215–218

[27] Shin AY, Battaglia MJ, Bishop AT. Lunotriquetral instability: diagnosis and treatment. J Am Acad Orthop Surg. 2000; 8(3):170–179

[28] Berger RA. The anatomy of the ligaments of the wrist and distal radioulnar joints. Clin Orthop Relat Res. 2001; 383(383):32–40

[29] Nagao S, Patterson RM, Buford WL, Jr, Andersen CR, Shah MA, Viegas SF. Three-dimensional description of ligamentous attachments around the lunate. J Hand Surg Am. 2005; 30(4):685–692

[30] Garcia-Elias M. Soft-tissue anatomy and relationships about the distal ulna. Hand Clin. 1998; 14(2):165–176

[31] Moritomo H. Anatomy and clinical relevance of the ulnocarpal ligament. J Wrist Surg. 2013; 2(2):186–189

[32] Bonte F, Mathoulin CL. The PARC lesion: a proximal avulsion of the radiocarpal capsule. J Wrist Surg. 2017; 6(1): 80–86

[33] Van Overstraeten L, Camus EJ. A systematic method of arthroscopic testing of extrinsic carpal ligaments: implication in carpal stability. Tech Hand Up Extrem Surg. 2013; 17(4):202–206

7

8 Imaging of the Wrist

Luis Cerezal and Diogo Roriz

Abstract

Standard imaging of the wrist consists of a posteroanterior and lateral radiographs. Three normal Gilula's lines should be smoothly identifiable on the posteroanterior radiograph. Additional views, such as the clenched fist or radial and ulnar deviation, might be valuable in patients suspected to have carpal instability with normal standard radiographs. Dynamic imaging, either with fluoroscopy or kinematic 4D computed tomography, should demonstrate a normal alignment and smooth movement of bones within a carpal row and between different rows, through the entire range of motion of the wrist. Asynchronous motion or "snapping" can be a sign of dynamic instability, before static abnormalities are established. Computed tomography and conventional magnetic resonance imaging, especially if done with arthrography, allow the diagnosis of partial or complete tears of the intrinsic and to some extent the extrinsic ligaments of the wrist.

Keywords: Radiography, dynamic imaging, MR arthrography, intrinsic ligaments, extrinsic ligaments, carpal instability

8.1 Imaging Techniques

8.1.1 Conventional Radiographs

Imaging of the wrist in patients suspected to have carpal instability should begin with conventional radiographs. Standard radiographic studies are the first line for assessing carpal alignment and signs of degenerative disease and should include a standardized posteroanterior (PA) and a lateral view of the wrist. The study should compare both wrists to assess anatomical variants or ligament laxity that should not be confused with pathology.[1]

In the evaluation of wrist pathology, especially in carpal instability, correct positioning of the radiographic projections is essential (▶ Fig. 8.1, ▶ Fig. 8.2). Evaluation of the carpal alignment and measurement of distances and angles of the carpal axes can be greatly altered by poor positioning of the patient.

The space between the carpal bones must be 2 mm or less. An increased distance of 3 mm or more, or asymmetry to the contralateral side could indicate static instability. In the case of the scapholunate space, it is not uncommon in patients with ligamentous laxity without frank instability to have an enlarged scapholunate interval. The bilateral comparative study and clinical history are key to avoid false diagnoses of scapholunate dissociation.

On the PA view, three smooth arcs must be normally identified—the Gilula's lines (▶ Fig. 8.1). The first arc is drawn along the proximal convex borders of the scaphoid, lunate, and triquetrum, whereas the second line is made by the distal concave surfaces of these bones. The third arc links the proximal convex borders of the capitate and hamate. A normal lunate exhibits a trapezoidal configuration. Any disruption of these arcs, bone overlap, or cortical asymmetry to the contralateral wrist might indicate instability.[2]

Nevertheless, two particular step-offs can be considered normal variants: a decreased height of the triquetrum relative to the lunate bone originating a step-off of the first arc, while preserving the second arc[3] and a step-off of the second arc when there is a medial lunate facet in type II lunate.[4]

On the lateral view of the wrist, the distal radius, lunate, capitate, and third metacarpal base should be colinear. The scapholunate angle is formed by the intersection of lines along the long axis of the scaphoid and the short axis of the lunate (▶ Fig. 8.3). It is normal between 30 and 60 degrees.[5] The capitolunate angle is drawn along the long axis of the capitate and the short axis of the lunate. The normal angle is between 0 and 30 degrees.[6]

If the initial radiographic studies are normal, but the clinical suspicion persists, additional views are recommended. PA views in ulnar and radial deviation allows an initial approach to the kinematics of the wrist (▶ Fig. 8.4). The distances between the carpal bones should be similar and unchanged at these studies.[5] Any disturbance in the normal alignment or displacement of the carpal bones may indicate underlying instability. The clenched fist is one of the most commonly used additional views. It forces the capitate proximally and the scapholunate space to widen in case of scapholunate instability.[7]

Multiple series of dynamic or selective stress radiographic views have been described. Currently they are used less frequently and in case of suspicion of instability, sectional imaging methods are usually required, especially magnetic resonance imaging (MRI).

8.1.2 Fluoroscopy

Fluoroscopy can be occasionally used in the diagnosis of dynamic instability if static studies are normal. Stability is then assessed in a PA study during active wrist motion, such as radial and ulnar deviation and with provocative testing. Lateral projections are preferable if midcarpal instability is suspected, with radial and ulnar deviation, flexion and extension, or dart-throwing movements. If the patient has a painful "clunk," it is important for it to be reproduced during the examination.

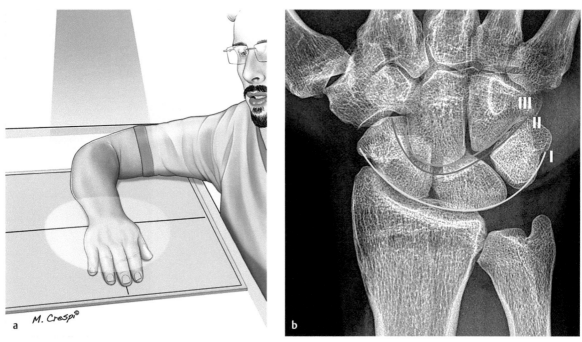

Fig. 8.1 **(a)** Standard posteroanterior (PA) projection of the wrist. The patient should be seated alongside the examination table with the shoulder abducted to 90 degrees, the elbow flexed to 90 degrees, and the forearm in pronation. The hand should be placed palm down on the image receiver with fingers extended. The shoulder, elbow, and wrist should all be in the transverse plane, perpendicular to the central beam. The long axes of the third metacarpal, capitate, and radius should fall in a straight line. **(b)** Image technical evaluation. On an adequately positioned PA view, the ulnar styloid process is visualized to its full extent on the medial aspect of the ulna, with the ulnar fovea visible and the extensor carpi ulnaris groove lying radial to the ulnar styloid process. The articular surfaces of the carpal bones should be parallel, and the joint spaces should be about 2 mm wide. Gilula's arcs should be parallel without discontinuity. Any change in joint spaces, the shape of a carpal bone, or disruption of Gilula's arcs on the PA view commonly indicates carpal subluxation or dislocation.

8

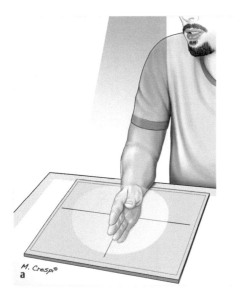

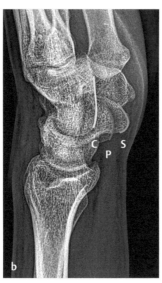

Fig. 8.2 **(a)** Standard lateral projection of the wrist. The arm should be adducted against the trunk and the elbow flexed to 90 degrees so that the ulnar edge of the forearm and hand rest on the image receptor. The forearm should be midprone, and the wrist should be in a neutral position. The shoulder, elbow, and wrist align perpendicular to the central beam in the same sagittal plane. **(b)** Image technical evaluation. The pisoscaphocapitate (PSC) relationship confirms the correct positioning of the lateral view of the wrist. The palmar cortex of the pisiform should lie centrally between the scaphoid's distal pole and the capitate's anterior surface, ideally in the central third of this interval.

Throughout the range of motion, matching smooth carpal movements should be seen, and the distance from the capitate to the radius should be preserved.[8] Asynchronous motion between the carpal bones, "snapping," and interval gapping are indicative of loss of stability. The possibility to evaluate bone movement through the entire range of motion shows advantage over stress views.[9]

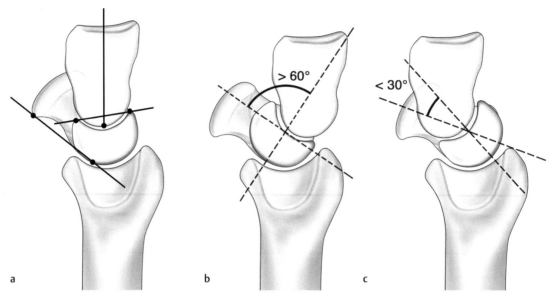

Fig. 8.3 **(a)** Measurement method of scapholunate (SL) and capitolunate (CL) angles. The SL and CL angles are critical measurements in evaluating carpal alignment and instability on a lateral radiograph of the wrist. The scaphoid line (S) is drawn tangential to the scaphoid along the palmar aspects of the proximal and distal poles of the bone, the lunate line (L) is perpendicular to a line drawn tangential to the palmar and dorsal distal margins of the lunate, and the capitate line (C) following the long axis of the capitate. The SL angle has an average value ranging from 30 to 60 degrees and the CL angle should be less than 30 degrees. **(b)** Dorsal-intercalated segment instability (DISI) pattern of carpal instability. Fixed carpal deformity after combined injury of SL ligament and secondary scaphoid stabilizers. On the lateral radiograph, DISI typically demonstrates dorsal tilt of the lunate with SL angle > 60 degrees and CL angle > 30 degrees. **(c)** Carpal misalignment after combined injury of lunotriquetral ligament and secondary lunotriquetral joint stabilizers. On the lateral radiograph, volar-intercalated segment instability (VISI) typically demonstrates volar tilt of the lunate with SL angle < 30 degrees and CL angle > 30 degrees.

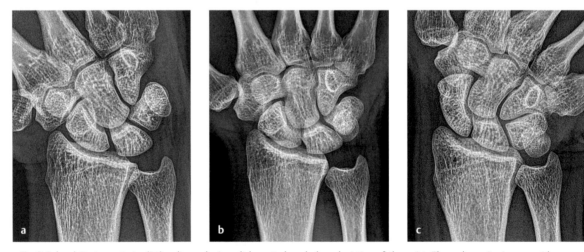

Fig. 8.4 **(a–c)** Posteroanterior (PA) radiographs in radial, neutral, and ulnar deviation of the wrist. These dynamic views provide information about carpal mobility and instability. The distances between the carpal bones are usually equal throughout and unchanged by radial or ulnar deviation.

8.1.3 Ultrasound

Ultrasound has a limited role in the assessment of wrist instability. High-frequency ultrasound probes (higher than 15 mHz) allows a good evaluation of the dorsal component of the scapholunate ligament (▶ Fig. 8.5). The examination of this ligament could be improved with dynamic or stress maneuvers such as radial and

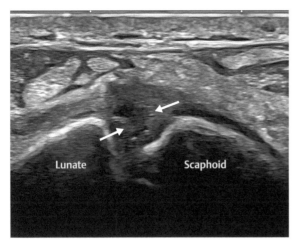

Fig. 8.5 Acute tear of the dorsal component of the scapholunate ligament. Ultrasound image of the dorsal wrist with a high-frequency transducer reveals a complete rupture of the dorsal component of the scapholunate ligament (*arrows*) and a slight widening of the interosseous space.

ulnar deviation or forceful grip. Ultrasound examination also makes it possible to detect small bone avulsions or hidden fractures. The assessment of the remaining intrinsic and extrinsic ligaments is very limited.

8.1.4 Computed Tomography

Computed tomography (CT) can have a diagnostic role in the later phases of instability, demonstrating static carpal subluxation and providing a high-resolution assessment of subchondral bone plate irregularities, cysts, and sclerosis as initial signs of osteoarthritis. Its role is also important in the evaluation of associated fractures, such as scaphoid fracture.

Kinematic 4D-CT allows the association of high-resolution three-dimensional bone assessment with the data given from a dynamic study,[10] but the use of a higher radiation dose should be taken into consideration.

CT arthrography allows the complementary evaluation of interosseous ligaments and, for this purpose, might be relevant in the early disease. It demonstrated an accuracy similar to MRI to evaluate scapholunate ligament (SLL) and lunotriquetral ligament (LTL) injuries.[11,12] It also appears to be superior to the MRI for the detection of articular cartilage defects.[13]

8.1.5 Magnetic Resonance Imaging

The role of MRI for evaluating carpal stability depends mostly on its ability to depict carpal ligaments. The use of multichannel phased–array coils and 3 Tesla (3T) scanners has dramatically improved, over the past few years, the diagnostic performance of MRI for ligament injuries. For optimal visualization of the intrinsic and extrinsic ligaments, a high–field-strength magnet, dedicated wrist coil, narrow field of view, and thin image slices are required.

The presence of joint effusion increases the sensitivity of the MRI to detect ligament injuries. Partial tears can be identified on MRI as incomplete discontinuity, elongated but intact ligament, focal thinning, irregularity, or high signal intensity within a portion of the ligament. Complete tears of a carpal ligament appear as a discontinuity within the ligament or complete absence of the ligament.

Both MRI and MR arthrography demonstrate high diagnostic accuracy for detecting SLL tears.[14] A meta-analysis for detecting SLL injury determined a sensitivity of 82% and specificity of 93% for MR arthrography compared to surgery or gross pathology as standard of reference.[15]

However, detection of LTL tears with conventional MRI only has 55 to 60% accuracy when compared to arthroscopy.[16] A 3 T MRI may increase the sensitivity in the detection of LTL tears. MR arthrography shows a much better performance with 80 to 95% accuracy for tears of LTL ligament.[16]

8.2 Imaging in Carpal Instability Dissociative

Carpal instability dissociative (CID) is the most common form of carpal instability. It is characterized by a dissociation of bones in the same carpal row. The proximal row is the most affected, with scapholunate dissociation (STD) and lunotriquetral dissociation (LTD) being the most frequent.

8.2.1 Scapholunate Dissociation

Intrinsic ligaments of the proximal carpal row, the SLL and LTL, are C-shaped structures with three components: dorsal, proximal, and volar. Dorsal and volar portions are true ligaments, whereas the proximal portions are thin fibrocartilaginous membranes with no stabilizing role. The dorsal component of SLL is the strongest part and the main stabilizer of the scapholunate joint. SLL tears are most often secondary to trauma, occurring mostly near the scaphoid insertion. However, they can also be caused by rheumatoid arthritis, calcium pyrophosphate dihydrate (CPPD) arthropathy, and Kienböck disease.[16,18] Its injury leads to independent moves of the scaphoid and lunate in opposing directions. The scaphoid follows its nature to flexion and migrates away from the lunate (▶ Fig. 8.6).

Axial and coronal MR images are better suited for the assessment of the SLL. Partial tears are demonstrated by irregularity, thinning, or focal discontinuity of the ligament. They are most often seen at the central or volar portions, which are also the weakest parts of the ligament. A full-thickness gap and lack of visualization of the ligament with the appropriate imaging are indicative of a

8

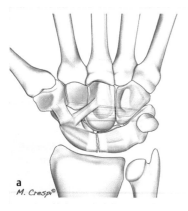 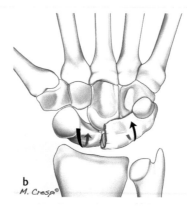

a
M. Cresp©

b
M. Cresp©

Fig. 8.6 (a) Diagram illustrating a static form of scapholunate dissociation. Scapholunate ligament tear and integrity of the main secondary stabilizers (dorsal intercarpal ligament, scaphotrapezial and scaphocapitate ligaments). (b) Diagram illustrating the static form of scapholunate dissociation or dorsal-intercalated segment instability (DISI) deformity. Scapholunate ligament tear and associated failure of the secondary scaphoid stabilizers. The scaphoid, devoid of proximal constraints, adopts a flexed posture, and the lunate follows its natural tendency toward extension with the triquetrum (arrows).

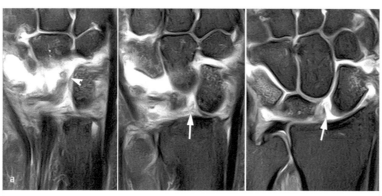

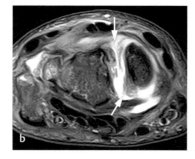 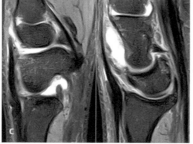

a

b

c

Fig. 8.7 Chronic scapholunate ligament tear (a static form of scapholunate dissociation). (a) Consecutive coronal proton density (PD) fat-suppressed magnetic resonance (MR) images show a detachment of the dorsal intercarpal ligament from the scaphoid (arrowhead), and a complete tear of the dorsal and volar components of the scapholunate ligament (arrows). (b) Axial PD fat-suppressed MR image shows a complete tear of the dorsal and volar components of the scapholunate ligament (arrows). (c) Sagittal PD fat-suppressed MR images demonstrate a dorsal-intercalated segment instability (DISI) pattern of wrist instability with an extension of the lunate and dorsal translation and flexion of the scaphoid.

complete tear (▶ Fig. 8.7). CT and MR arthrography are more accurate in detecting ligament injuries, allowing the contrast to outline the damaged structure in partial tears and free communication of contrast between the midcarpal and radiocarpal compartments in complete tears (▶ Fig. 8.8).

Four stages of progressive severity have been considered in scapholunate dissociation (SLD).[19] In Stage I (predynamic) a partial tear occurs at the SLL while the extrinsic carpal ligaments, which act as second stabilizers, remain intact, most importantly the volar scaphotrapezial, dorsal intercarpal, and scaphocapitate ligaments.

A complete tear for the SLL is the hallmark of Stage II (dynamic), showing increased distance between the two bones with dynamic or stress studies. The clenched pencil view is considered the most sensitive stress view.[20] From

flexion to extension of the wrist, the long axis of the lunate bone rotates from dorsal to palmar. Failure to do so is a sign of dynamic instability, which can be demonstrated on lateral view fluoroscopy.[9]

Combined intrinsic and extrinsic ligament tear leads to Stage III instability (static). Scaphoid rotatory subluxation develops, leading to flexion of the distal pole of the scaphoid, while the lunate initially preserves its neutral position. On PA radiograph, the distal pole of the scaphoid overlaps its waist, resembling a ring—"scaphoid cortical ring sign"[21]—and the distance between the "ring" and the proximal pole becomes inferior than 7 mm.[22] However, this can also be observed in normal wrists.[23] A scapholunate diastasis is established when this articular space becomes greater than 4 mm (Terry-Thomas sign) and interruption may be seen in Gilula's arcs I and II on the PA view.

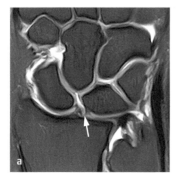 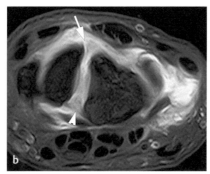

Fig. 8.8 Partial tear of the scapholunate ligament with involvement of the dorsal component (predynamic form of scapholunate dissociation). **(a,b)** Coronal and axial T1 fat-suppressed magnetic resonance (MR) arthrographic images show a tear of the dorsal component of the scapholunate ligament (*arrows*). Note the normal volar component in **b** (*arrowhead*).

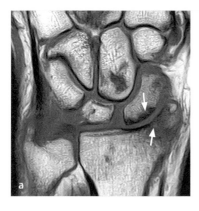 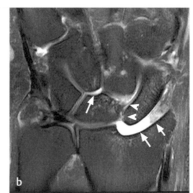

Fig. 8.9 Scapholunate advanced collapse (SLAC) wrist. **(a)** SLAC Stage II, osteoarthritis involving the whole radioscaphoid articulation (*arrows*). **(b)** SLAC Stage III, osteoarthritis of the radioscaphoid and midcarpal joints (*arrows*). Note a marked remodeling of the distal radius secondary to dynamic disturbances of the scaphoid and the rupture of the Gilula's arcs 1 and 2 (*arrowheads*).

A scapholunate angle greater than 60 degrees on the lateral view can also present on this stage. Later, the lunate extends (dorsal tilt) and dorsal-intercalated segment instability (DISI) is reached. At this moment, it assumes a triangular morphology on the PA radiographs. This fixed extension of the lunate may be maintained during wrist flexion.

Finally, in Stage IV disease, osteoarthritis develops and carpal height is lost, named scapholunate advanced collapse (SLAC) (▶ Fig. 8.9). It also develops in several stages described by Watson and colleagues,[19] from affecting only the radial styloid-scaphoid joint (SLAC I), then the entire radioscaphoid joint (SLAC II) and later the capitolunate joint (SLAC III). Chondromalacia at the radial styloid-scaphoid joint is the earliest sign of SLAC.[10] Importantly, the radiolunate joint is not affected until advanced disease is reached.[24] Later, a new stage was added to the initial classification (Stage IV SLAC), consisting of midcarpal osteoarthritis.[24]

MRI allows an accurate assessment of progressive joint damage in the SLAC wrist. It is of special relevance in the presurgical assessment of the status of the large lunate articular cartilage (SLAC Stage II vs III) in patients in whom proximal carpectomy or carpal arthrodesis are considered.

8.2.2 Lunotriquetral Dissociation

The volar band of the LTL is the most important for stability (▶ Fig. 8.10). On conventional MRI, ligament injury is typically best seen on fat-suppressed T2-weighted images obtained in the coronal plane and is manifested as either a complete disruption of the ligament or a focal linear defect (▶ Fig. 8.11). However, nonvisualization of the ligament is not a very reliable sign of ligament injury because this ligament is not as well seen on routine, in contrast to the SLL. The imaging modality of choice for visualizing the LTL is CT arthrography or MR arthrography. In complete tears, the contrast injected will freely provide communication between the radiocarpal and midcarpal joints (▶ Fig. 8.12).

Lunotriquetral dissociation (LTD) is less frequent than SLD and involves injuries of not only the LTL but also the extrinsic ligaments, particularly the dorsal radiolunotriquetral ligament (dRLTL).[25] With injuries of these structures, the lunate and, to a lesser extent, the scaphoid rotate in a palmar direction, while the triquetrum follows the opposite direction. The scapholunate angle decreases to less than 30 degrees[26] and a volar-intercalated segment instability (VISI) is established. The lunotriquetral angle is the angle between the axis of the lunate and triquetrum, evaluated in the lateral view radiograph. Normally it opens dorsally with a mean of 14 degrees. In LTD, the angle turns palmar with a mean of 16 degrees. Importantly, the lunotriquetral distance in the PA radiograph is not necessarily increased in STD. In addition, increased range of motion at this joint can be found in asymptomatic individuals with hyperlaxity.[27]

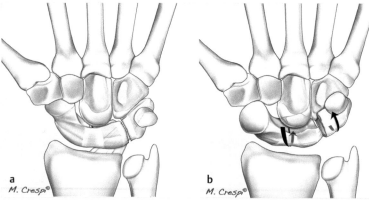

Fig. 8.10 (a) Diagram illustrating a static form of lunotriquetral dissociation. Lunotriquetral ligament tear and integrity of the main secondary stabilizer (dorsal radiocarpal ligament). **(b)** Diagram illustrating the static form of lunotriquetral dissociation or volar-intercalated segment instability (VISI) deformity. Lunotriquetral ligament and dorsal radiocarpal ligament disruption results in a VISI instability pattern. The triquetrum is translated proximally and adopts an extended posture. The lunate, by contrast, follows the scaphoid in flexion (*red arrows*).

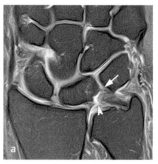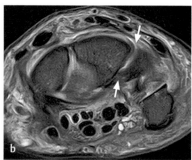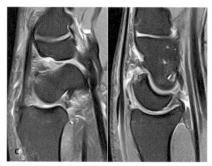

Fig. 8.11 Chronic ulnocarpal impaction with Palmer class 2D lesion, involvement of the lunotriquetral ligament, and volar-intercalated segment instability (VISI) pattern of instability. **(a,b)** Coronal and axial proton density (PD) fat-suppressed magnetic resonance (MR) images show an extensive central perforation of the triangular fibrocartilage (TFC) (*arrowhead* in **a**), and a complete tear of the lunotriquetral ligament (*arrows*). **(c)** Sagittal PD fat-suppressed MR images demonstrate a VISI pattern of wrist instability with flexion of the scaphoid and lunate.

8.3 Imaging in Carpal Instability Nondissociative

In carpal instability nondissociative (CIND) the proximal carpal row alignment is maintained, but there is a misalignment with the distal forearm or with the distal carpal row. Injury/insufficiency of the extrinsic ligaments is usually the cause.

8.3.1 Extrinsic Ligaments

CINDs are characterized by joint malalignment between the forearm and the proximal carpal row (radiocarpal CIND) or between the proximal and distal rows (midcarpal CIND) while the articular function is preserved within each row. Unfortunately, the specific extrinsic ligaments involved or the degree of injury in each form of instability remain controversial.

Radiocarpal CIND can be further divided in ulnar or radial translocation. The radioscaphocapitate ligament (RSCL), palmar radiolunotriquetral ligament (pRLTL), and dRLTL are obliquely oriented ligaments inserted proximally on the radius that antagonize the natural forces of the carpus for ulnar deviation, based on the

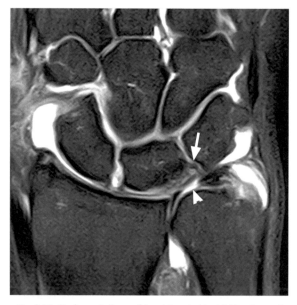

Fig. 8.12 Predynamic form of lunotriquetral instability. Coronal T1 fat-suppressed magnetic resonance (MR) arthrographic image demonstrates a central perforation of the triangular fibrocartilage (TFC) (*arrowhead*), and a complete tear of the lunotriquetral ligament (*arrow*).

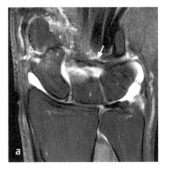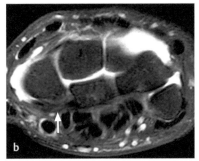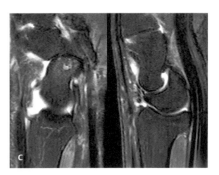

Fig. 8.13 Dorsal type of midcarpal instability. **(a–c)** Proton density (PD) fat-suppressed magnetic resonance (MR) images show a nondissociative pattern of wrist instability with dorsal subluxation of the capitate and dorsal tilting of the scaphoid and lunate. Note the thickening and increased signal in the triquetrohamatecapitate ligament (*arrow* in **a**), and radioscaphocapitate (*arrow* in **b**).

coronal inclination of the distal radius.[16] Trauma, rheumatoid arthritis, or CPPD arthropathy can lead to ligament injuries and ulnar translocation of the carpus. Depending on the status of the SLL, ulnar translocation can be seen in the entire proximal carpal row (intact ligament) or with the scaphoid remaining in place and the remaining proximal carpus moving to the ulnar side (torn ligament).[22] Radial translocation is usually secondary to loss of inclination of the radial articular surface, due to radial styloid fractures or loss of bone to friction, such as in SLAC or SNAC wrist.[19]

Midcarpal CIND is a dynamic disorder of the proximal carpal row and can be also divided in palmar, dorsal, combined, or adaptive forms. In the dart-throwing movement, the proximal carpus changes from a flexed position in radial deviation to extension in ulnar deviation of the wrist. The entire proximal carpal row moves as a functional unity, while the distal carpal row rotates in the opposite direction.[28] Insufficiency due to tears or attenuation of the extrinsic ligaments might affect this smooth and balanced movement, producing a painful snapping or "clunk" in extremes of movement.

In palmar CIND (or CIND-VISI), the most common form of midcarpal instability, the proximal carpal row remains flexed during the radial to ulnar wrist deviation until the triquetrohamate joint engages and a sudden, abrupt movement into proximal carpal extension is seen, producing a painful "clunk."[29] Arcuate ligament on the palmar side and the dRLTL on the dorsal side are believed to be involved. Fluoroscopy or kinematic 4D-CT will typically reveal these findings. Lateral view radiographs might reveal an increased capitate-lunate angle (>30 degrees), with a normal scapholunate angle (30–60 degrees) in static CIND-VISI.

In dorsal or CIND-DISI, the "clunk" occurs in ulnar deviation due to capitate dorsal subluxation (▶ Fig. 8.13). There is no consensus regarding the exact ligaments that are responsible for this instability. Dynamic imaging is usually recommended to establish the diagnosis.

In patients with combined CIND, signs of both palmar and dorsal CIND are identified, due to palmar and dorsal

extrinsic ligaments insufficiency. Features of radiocarpal instability might also be found.[30]

The usefulness of both conventional MRI and arthrographic techniques (CT arthrography and MR arthrography) in the evaluation of the extrinsic ligaments of the wrist is not well established. On the one hand, there are technical difficulties in dealing with small-sized ligaments, with an oblique pathway and common anatomical variants. On the other hand, the ligaments injured in the different forms of CIND are not clearly defined. In addition, injuries to these ligaments are associated with distension or dysfunction rather than rupture and discontinuity, as occurs in other ligaments (disturbance of ligament mechanoreceptors).

8.4 Conclusions

Posteroanterior and lateral wrist radiographs remain the primary imaging modality for routine imaging work-up in patients with suspected carpal instability.

Radiographic stress views and dynamic fluoroscopy of the wrist allow accurate diagnosis of dynamic carpal instability.

MRI is an accurate method in diagnosing SLL injuries but is limited in evaluating LTL tears.

CT and MR arthrography is the most accurate imaging methods for determining SLL and LTL injuries.

The usefulness of MRI, CT arthrography, and MR arthrography in assessing extrinsic ligaments injuries seems limited.

References

[1] Dietrich TJ, Toms AP, Cerezal L, et al. Interdisciplinary consensus statements on imaging of scapholunate joint instability. Eur Radiol. 2021; 31(12):9446–9458

[2] Garcia-Elias M. The treatment of wrist instability. J Bone Joint Surg Br. 1997; 79(4):684–690

[3] Gilula LA. Carpal injuries: analytic approach and case exercises. AJR Am J Roentgenol. 1979; 133(3):503–517

8

[4] Viegas SF, Wagner K, Patterson R, Peterson P. Medial (hamate) facet of the lunate. J Hand Surg Am. 1990; 15(4):564–571

[5] Loredo RA, Sorge DG, Garcia G. Radiographic evaluation of the wrist: a vanishing art. Semin Roentgenol. 2005; 40(3):248–289

[6] Sarrafian SK, Melamed JL, Goshgarian GM. Study of wrist motion in flexion and extension. Clin Orthop Relat Res. 1977(126):153–159

[7] Gilula LA, Yin Y, eds. Imaging of the wrist and hand. Philadelphia, PA: Saunders; 1996:373–384

[8] Kani KK, Mulcahy H, Chew FS. Understanding carpal instability: a radiographic perspective. Skeletal Radiol. 2016; 45(8):1031–1043

[9] Sulkers GSI, Strackee SD, Schep NWL, Maas M. Wrist cineradiography: a protocol for diagnosing carpal instability. J Hand Surg Eur Vol. 2018; 43 (2):174–178

[10] White J, Couzens G, Jeffery C. The use of 4D-CT in assessing wrist kinematics and pathology: a narrative view. Bone Joint J. 2019; 101-B (11):1325–1330

[11] Crema MD, Zentner J, Guermazi A, Jomaah N, Marra MD, Roemer FW. Scapholunate advanced collapse and scaphoid nonunion advanced collapse: MDCT arthrography features. AJR Am J Roentgenol. 2012; 199(2):W202–7

[12] Schmid MR, Schertler T, Pfirrmann CW, et al. Interosseous ligament tears of the wrist: comparison of multi-detector row CT arthrography and MR imaging. Radiology. 2005; 237(3):1008–1013

[13] Haims AH, Moore AE, Schweitzer ME, et al. MRI in the diagnosis of cartilage injury in the wrist. AJR Am J Roentgenol. 2004; 182(5): 1267–1270

[14] Lee RK, Ng AW, Tong CS, et al. Intrinsic ligament and triangular fibrocartilage complex tears of the wrist: comparison of MDCT arthrography, conventional 3-T MRI, and MR arthrography. Skeletal Radiol. 2013; 42(9):1277–1285

[15] Hafezi-Nejad N, Carrino JA, Eng J, et al. Scapholunate interosseous ligament tears: diagnostic performance of 1.5 T, 3 T MRI, and MR arthrography-a systematic review and meta-analysis. Acad Radiol. 2016; 23(9):1091–1103

[16] Grunz JP, Gietzen CH, Grunz K, Bley T, Schmitt R. Imaging of carpal instabilities. Röfo Fortschr Geb Röntgenstr Neuen Bildgeb Verfahr. 2021; 193(2):139–150

[17] Resnick D, Niwayama G. Carpal instability in rheumatoid arthritis and calcium pyrophosphate deposition disease. Pathogenesis and roentgen appearance. Ann Rheum Dis. 1977; 36(4):311–318

[18] Schmitt R, Heinze A, Fellner F, Obletter N, Strühn R, Bautz W. Imaging and staging of avascular osteonecroses at the wrist and hand. Eur J Radiol. 1997; 25(2):92–103

[19] Watson H, Ottoni L, Pitts EC, Handal AG. Rotary subluxation of the scaphoid: a spectrum of instability. J Hand Surg [Br]. 1993; 18(1): 62–64

[20] Lee SK, Desai H, Silver B, Dhaliwal G, Paksima N. Comparison of radiographic stress views for scapholunate dynamic instability in a cadaver model. J Hand Surg Am. 2011; 36(7):1149–1157

[21] Nathan R, Blatt G. Rotary subluxation of the scaphoid. Revisited. Hand Clin. 2000; 16(3):417–431

[22] Taleisnik J. Classification of carpal instability. Bull Hosp Jt Dis Orthop Inst. 1984; 44(2):511–531

[23] Abe Y, Doi K, Hattori Y. The clinical significance of the scaphoid cortical ring sign: a study of normal wrist X-rays. J Hand Surg Eur Vol. 2008; 33(2):126–129

[24] Peterson B, Szabo RM. Carpal osteoarthrosis. Hand Clin. 2006; 22(4): 517–528, abstract vii

[25] Theumann NH, Pfirrmann CWA, Antonio GE, et al. Extrinsic carpal ligaments: normal MR arthrographic appearance in cadavers. Radiology. 2003; 226(1):171–179

[26] Shin AY, Battaglia MJ, Bishop AT. Lunotriquetral instability: diagnosis and treatment. J Am Acad Orthop Surg. 2000; 8(3):170–179

[27] Garcia-Elias M, Ribe M, Rodriguez J, Cots M, Casas J. Influence of joint laxity on scaphoid kinematics. J Hand Surg [Br]. 1995; 20(3): 379–382

[28] Ramamurthy NK, Chojnowski AJ, Toms AP. Imaging in carpal instability. J Hand Surg Eur Vol. 2016; 41(1):22–34

[29] Lichtman DM, Wroten ES. Understanding midcarpal instability. J Hand Surg Am. 2006; 31(3):491–498

[30] Wolfe SW, Garcia-Elias M, Kitay A. Carpal instability nondissociative. J Am Acad Orthop Surg. 2012; 20(9):575–585

III

9 Scapholunate Ligament Injury Etiology and Classification

Alex Lluch, Ana Scott-Tennent, Mireia Esplugas, and Marc Garcia-Elias

Abstract

Traumatic damage to the carpus may cause different degrees of scapholunate ligament (SLL) injury that can produce wrist impairment. Nevertheless, not every SLL injury generates an unstable wrist. Some patients may have a partial lesion, others a complete but balanced lesion, while others may have a complete symptomatic lesion. Even more, some of them can evolve into a carpal collapse or an arthropathy. Because of this, the term *scapholunate dysfunction* has been proposed to define the whole spectrum of SLL pathology, since the term "instability" only applies to a narrow range of SLL afflictions.

The degree and severity of injury, the time from initial trauma, the individual configuration of the carpus, the presence of other associated injuries, and the status of the other SL joint (SLj) stabilizers are factors that will influence the evolution of a carpal dysfunction and its prognosis and treatment.

The aims of this chapter are: (1) to help the surgeon better understand the spectrum of SLL dysfunction, (2) review the mechanisms of injury and types of ligament lesion, and (3) recognize where to place each individual in the staging of SL disorder, which is the first step in management.

Keywords: carpal instability, scapholunate instability, scapholunate dysfunction, wrist ligament injury, scapholunate ligament injury, scapholunate ligament tear scapholunate injury classification, scapholunate injury staging

9.1 Introduction

"Carpal instability" has been broadly used to depict wrist pathologies that have been caused by any grade of ligament injury, with scapholunate ligament (SLL) being the most commonly affected. In the same way, the term "SL instability" has also been indistinctly and widely used to describe any degree of SLL injury, and many times wrongly applied to asymptomatic carpal malalignments.

A low-energy trauma may cause a partial ligament injury, which could be initially compensated by secondary stabilizers. On the contrary, a more severe trauma may provoke a complete ligament lesion, which can also be initially stable but is more likely to become unstable and evolve to a carpal collapse with time.

Therefore, the authors believe that the term *SL dysfunction* is more appropriate as it includes all these different scenarios, different from the term *SL instability* which defines just some of them.[1,2]

9.2 Natural History of Scapholunate Dysfunction

After a significant wrist trauma, a spectrum of SL ligament injuries can occur and secondary adaptations may develop. This depends on the severity and time from initial trauma, the individual configuration of the wrist, possible associated injuries, and the competence of secondary stabilizers of the SL joint (SLj) (▶ Fig. 9.1).

An in vitro study carried out by Werner and Short showed that carpal loading after sectioning the SLL induces a scaphoid internal rotation (intracarpal pronation) and a lunate external rotation (intracarpal supination). These opposed rotations increase the SLj gap. Authors also found that the severity of this SLj gap is related to the amount of SLL secondary stabilizing ligaments that were sectioned. Accordingly, this reinforces the concept that there are different functional types of SLL injuries

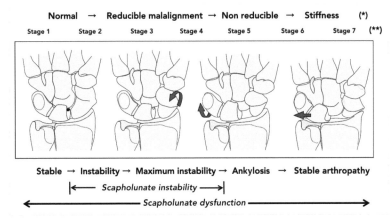

Fig. 9.1 The spectrum of scapholunate ligament (SLL) injuries. SL dysfunction includes significantly different situations, from partial and stable lesions (*left*) to arthropathy (*right*). SLL instability is only part of this spectrum. (*) Correct carpal alignment or easiness to achieve carpal reduction in cases of complete unrepairable lesions has an influence on treatment. (**) Considering six different variables, staging of SLL dysfunction is possible. (See ▶ Table 9.1.)

9

Table 9.1 Staging of SL dysfunction

	I	II	III	IV	V	VI	VII
Partial lesion	Yes	No	No	No	No	No	No
Reparable	Yes	Yes	No	No	No	No	No
Normal radiolunate angle	Yes	Yes	Yes	No	No	No	No
Stable lunate	Yes	Yes	Yes	Yes	No	No	No
Reducible	Yes	Yes	Yes	Yes	Yes	No	No
Normal cartilage	Yes	Yes	Yes	Yes	Yes	Yes	No

Based on Carreño et al.[1]

and that secondary stabilizers play an important role on these injuries.[3]

Secondary SLj stabilizers can be static (ligaments) or dynamic (muscles). The former is a complex of ligaments that work together to constrain carpal displacements, while the latter is a group of muscles crossing the wrist that are connected to proprioceptors located in carpal ligaments and tuned by a sensorimotor system (SMS) (as already stated in Chapter 3). Dynamic stabilizers can compensate for some SLL lesions and maintain normal SL alignment, preventing the appearance of symptoms.[4,7] However, and especially if static stabilizers remain untreated, dynamic stabilizers may give up at the end. If this happens, carpal biomechanics is significantly altered under loading (kinetics) or with motion (kinematics), becoming a dysfunctional wrist.

There are several different clinical scenarios depending on the degree of SLL lesion and the competence of secondary stabilizers. If dynamic stabilizers can't compensate for a complete SLL disruption or an incomplete lesion that progresses, secondary changes in the carpus are quite predictable. The scaphoid flexes, internally rotates (pronation), and becomes dorsally displaced, creating an abnormal contact of the proximal pole on the dorsal aspect of the radial scaphoid fossa. The disconnected lunate follows the triquetrum toward an excessive extension, external rotation (supination), and ulnar translation defining the so-called "dorsal-intercalated segment instability" (DISI) deformity (▶ Fig. 9.2). If left untreated, this malalignment can promote a subsequent carpal degeneration with the development of a scapholunate advanced collapse (SLAC) pattern.[2]

Hyperlax individuals need special consideration when talking about carpal instability and dysfunction, as their ligaments behave mechanically differently. Normally these individuals present with a hypermobile (and many times malaligned) but asymptomatic wrist. Different from ligament competent wrists, they may become symptomatic

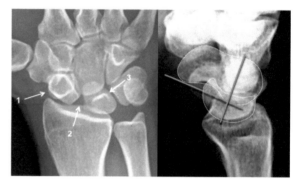

Fig. 9.2 X-ray showing evidence of dorsal-intercalated segment instability (DISI) and static radiological signs of an advanced scapholunate (SL) dysfunction (Stages IV and V). **(a)** In the posteroanterior (PA) view[1]: Shortened scaphoid with a "ring sign,"[2] widened SL interval or SL gap ("Terry Thomas sign")[3] and obliquely oriented ovoid or quadrangular configuration of the lunate, due to the distal placement of the wider volar area, suggesting bone extension. **(b)** In the lateral view: Dorsally tilted lunate (DISI) leading to an increased SL angle (*blue lines* showing an angle of more than 60 degrees).

after a relatively minor trauma that can disbalance the previous compensating effect of secondary SLj stabilizers. Their basis of treatment is specific hand therapy programs, and surgery is only indicated in selected cases.

9.3 Scapholunate Ligament Injury Pathomechanics

9.3.1 Injury Mechanisms

SLL injury usually occurs after a fall on an outstretched hand, forcing the wrist into extension, combined with some variable degrees of radioulnar inclination and/or intracarpal rotation. When ulnar inclination prevails, the scaphoid is pulled distally by the scaphocapitate and the

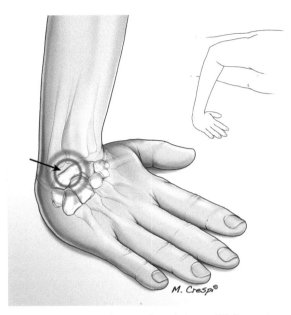

Fig. 9.3 Common mechanism of scapholunate (SL) ligament injury. SL ligament rupture after a fall on an outstretched hand, with hyperextension and ulnar deviation. Scaphotrapeziotrapezoidal ligaments pull the scaphoid distally, while palmar radiolunate ligaments maintain the lunate fixed to the radius.

scaphotrapeziotrapezoidal ligaments while the lunate remains solidly constrained against the radius by the two volar radiolunate ligaments. In this condition, the SLj is under tension and its ligaments start to disrupt (▶ Fig. 9.3). Normally, the volar scapholunate ligament is the first to rupture, followed then by the interosseous membrane and finally by the dorsal ligament if the trauma energy is severe enough. This could be described as an "SL dissociation" or as Stage I of the so-called "progressive perilunate instability," according to Mayfield et al.[8]

Nevertheless, this is not the only injury mechanism that has been described for SLL lesions. Hyperflexion with impact, traction, and intracarpal hyperpronation forces have also been reported by patients suffering from SL tears. The latter has been recognized in some patients with isolated dorsal SLL ligament injury, after an unexpected blockage of a drill, for example. This would induce an intracarpal pronation that may rupture the dorsal ligament keeping the volar region intact,[9] contrary to the pathophysiology that classically has been described.[2,8]

9.3.2 Associated Injuries to SLL Tears

Furthermore, some other injuries may be associated with SLL tears: (A) fractures (scaphoid and distal radius

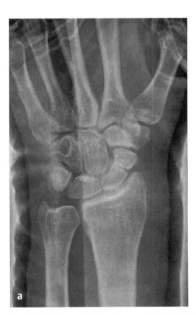
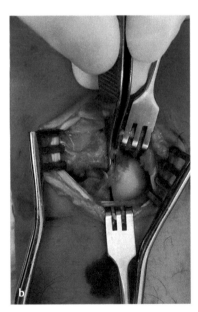
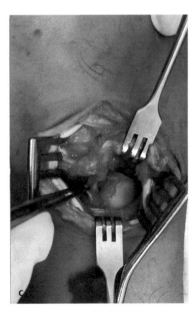

Fig. 9.4 Example of acute scapholunate (SL) injury with associated scaphoid fracture: **(a)** X-ray (posteroanterior [PA] view) showing a reduced transscaphoid perilunate injury in the left wrist. **(b,c)** Intraoperative clinical image showing evidence of SL ligament avulsion from scaphoid—Type 1A Andersson–Garcia-Elias classification (Adson forceps)—with an associated scaphoid fracture in a left wrist. (Courtesy of Pau Forcada, MD.)

9

fractures being the most common) and (B) other ligament injuries (lunotriquetral ligament, perilunate dislocations, etc.). They all need to be taken into account when facing the treatment of SLL dysfunction (▶ Fig. 9.4).[1,2]

9.4 Scapholunate Ligament Injury Classifications

There is a wide spectrum of SLL lesions, and there are many factors influencing SL dysfunction, such as the severity and time from the initial trauma, the individual configuration of the wrist, possible associated injuries, and secondary stabilizer competence. Because of this, several SL injury classifications have been described. Geissler and European Wrist Arthroscopy Society (EWAS) classifications[10,11] are focused on the degree to which the components of the SLL complex are injured, whereas the Andersson–Garcia-Elias classification[12] is focused on how the ligament complex is broken. Apart from that, SLL injury is a dynamic condition that may evolve with time. Accordingly, and based on six prognostic factors, seven stages (I–VII) can be defined in the spectrum of SL dysfunction.

9.4.1 Scapholunate Ligament Injury Classifications

Aside from the already mentioned factors influencing SLj pathology, the localization of the injury and the amount

of damage to the SL ligament have also critical influence on SLj dysfunction. In relation to that and as noted before, there are three classifications with relevant clinical implications.

Geissler and EWAS Classifications

Depending on the amount of ligament damage, SLL injury can be classified as partial or total. The degree of injury has been classically classified by arthroscopic evaluation according to Geissler.[10] However, more recently, a modified classification including the site of the attenuation or tear has been proposed by the European Wrist Arthroscopy Society (EWAS).[11] This classification was done by sectioning the different portions of the SLL, followed by the volar and dorsal extrinsic ligaments in 13 different cadavers, and then describing the subsequent arthroscopic and anatomopathological findings. It includes seven possible types of SL injury (I–V), in which type III is unfolded in IIIA-B-C depending on the localization of the damage within the SLL. The EWAS classification shares some similarities with SLL staging (▶ Table 9.2). In this regard, arthroscopy is an essential tool in SLL dysfunction diagnosis nowadays.

Andersson–García-Elias Classification

Dorsal SLL does not always rupture in the same way. Andersson and Garcia-Elias retrospectively reviewed 45 patients with dorsal SLL ruptures and were able to identify

Table 9.2 Arthroscopic EWAS (European Wrist Arthroscopy Society) classification and correlation with SL dysfunction stages

Arthroscopic stage (EWAS)	Arthroscopic testing SLL from standard midcarpal portals	Correlation with SL dysfunction stage (▶ Table 9.1, ▶ Fig. 9.1)
I	No passage of the probe	Stage I
II: lesion of membranous SLL	Passage of the tip of the probe in SL space with no widening (stable)	Stage I
IIIA: partial lesion volar SLL	Volar widening on dynamic testing from midcarpal joint (anterior laxity)	Stage II
IIIB: partial lesion dorsal SLL	Dorsal widening on dynamic testing from midcarpal joint (dorsal laxity) or evidence of rupture after dorsal SLL probe hook testing	Stage III
IIIC: complete SLL tear	Complete widening of SL space on dynamic testing	Stage IV
IV: complete SLL tear with SL gap	SL gap with passage of arthroscope from midcarpal to radiocarpal joint. No radiographic abnormalities	Stage IV-V
V	SL gap with passage of arthroscope from midcarpal to radiocarpal joint. Radiographic abnormalities (SL gap, DISI)	Stage VI

DISI, dorsal-intercalated segment instability; SL, scapholunate; SLL, scapholunate ligament.
Based on Messina et al.[11]
Note: EWAS classification appears in the first and second columns and the relation with SL staging in the third column (see ▶ Table 9.1 and ▶ Fig. 9.1).

four different types of injury. This finding allowed them to classify complete dorsal SLL lesions[12]: *Type 1* (42%) are complete avulsions from the scaphoid. *Type 2* (16%) are complete avulsions from the lunate, with the scaphoid portion of the ligament intact. Both type 1 and 2 can be subclassified into (*a*) for pure ligament avulsions or (*b*) for bony avulsions, and require reattachment of the avulsed ligament with anchors or transosseous sutures. *Type 3* (20%) are midsubstance ruptures that may allow an end-to-end repair of the two ligament stumps. *Type 4* (22%) are elongations of partially ruptured SL ligaments that can be treated by shortening and augmentation of the repair. This classification can be done by open or arthroscopic manners and allows the surgeon to decide the most appropriate repairing technique, if repairable (▶ Fig. 9.5).

9.4.2 Stages of Scapholunate Joint Dysfunction

Apart from that, and based on six prognostic factors, seven stages (I–VII) can be defined in the spectrum of SL dysfunction. Although this is not a classification by itself, treatment and prognosis may vary from one stage to another. Staging helps where to place a particular injury within the spectrum, and which treatment may be suitable for each individual. The six factors are (1) extent of ligament rupture, (2) repairability of the ligament tear, (3) defined presence of static radiological changes, (4) ulnar translocation of the lunate, (5) reducibility of carpal malalignment, and (6) status of the cartilage (▶ Table 9.1). From the seven stages, only stages from II to IV describe true unstable conditions (▶ Fig. 9.1). Failure of treatment of SLL injuries, such as ligament repairing or reconstruction surgical techniques, is likely to happen if one is unable to correctly recognize which type of SLL lesion a patient has within this spectrum (▶ Fig. 9.6). Therefore, being able to define its stage is decisive in SL dysfunction management.[1,13]

9.5 Conclusion

Because of the wide variety of lesions and the inherent complexity of this disorder, treatment of SL injuries is still a challenge. Knowing its natural history, being able to understand the mechanism of injury, and identifying the type of lesion and its stage are essential in SL dysfunction management.

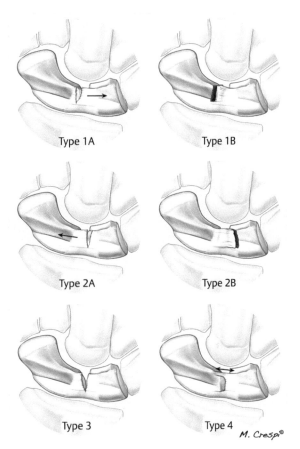

Fig. 9.5 Classification of dorsal scapholunate (SL) injury according to Andersson–Garcia-Elias.[12] Type 1A ligament avulsion from scaphoid. Type 1B bony avulsion from scaphoid. Type 2A ligament avulsion from lunate. Type 2B bony avulsion from lunate. Type 3 are midsubstance ruptures. Type 4 are elongation of a partially ruptured SL ligament. (Adapted with permission from Andersson JK, Garcia-Elias M. Dorsal scapholunate ligament injury: a classification of clinical forms. J Hand Surg Eur Vol. 2013;38(2):165–169.[12])

9

III

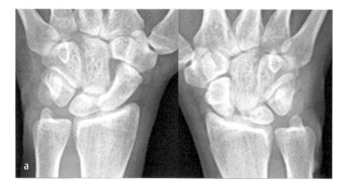
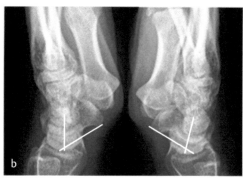

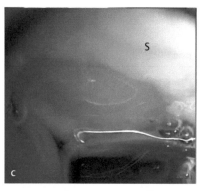
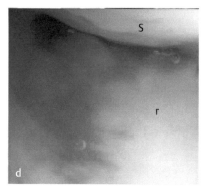
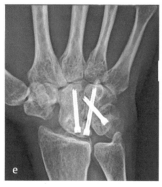

Fig. 9.6 Example of a clinical practice of treatment based on staging in scapholunate joint (SLj) dysfunction. *Clinical case showing treatment decision based on staging system. The authors of this chapter decided to scope the wrist before making treatment decisions in order to better identify SLj dysfunction of the patient. Both X-ray findings and the evidence of cartilage damage confirmed by the arthroscopic findings suggest this is Stage VII of SLj dysfunction (▶ Table 9.1). In the face of such findings, the authors decided to use salvage treatment, as SLL reconstruction techniques are more prone to fail in the face of advanced SLj dysfunction.* **(a)** X-ray (bilateral posteroanterior [PA] view) showing increased SL gap in right wrist suggesting SLj dysfunction. **(b)** X-ray (bilateral lateral view) showing increased SL angle in right wrist compared to its contralateral. **(c)** Evidence of cartilage damage in proximal pole of the scaphoid **(s)** while scoping the wrist before making treatment decision (from 3–4 radiocarpal arthroscopy portal). **(d)** Evidence of cartilage damage in dorsal rim of distal radius **(r)** (from 3–4 radiocarpal arthroscopy portal). **(e)** Postoperative X-ray (PA view) showing four-corner fusion.

References

[1] Carreño A, Lluch A, Esplugas M, García-Elías M. Disfunciones sintomáticas del Carpo. In: Traumatología y ortopedia. Miembro superior. 1.ª ed. Barcelona: Elsevier; 2021:259–270

[2] Garcia-Elias M, Lluch AL. Wrist instabilities, misalignments and dislocations. In: Wolfe SW, Hotchkiss RN, Pederson WC, et al. Green's operative hand surgery. 7th ed. Vol. 1. Philadelphia, PA: Elsevier; 2017:418–478

[3] Werner FW, Short WH. Carpal pronation and supination changes in the unstable wrist. J Wrist Surg. 2018; 7(4):298–302

[4] Hagert E, Lluch A, Rein S. The role of proprioception and neuromuscular stability in carpal instabilities. J Hand Surg Eur Vol. 2016; 41(1):94–101

[5] Salva-Coll G, Garcia-Elias M, Hagert E. Scapholunate instability: proprioception and neuromuscular control. J Wrist Surg. 2013; 2(2): 136–140

[6] Salva-Coll G, Garcia-Elias M, Leon-Lopez MT, Llusa-Perez M, Rodríguez-Baeza A. Effects of forearm muscles on carpal stability. J Hand Surg Eur Vol. 2011; 36(7):553–559

[7] Esplugas M, Garcia-Elias M, Lluch A, Llusá Pérez M. Role of muscles in the stabilization of ligament-deficient wrists. J Hand Ther. 2016; 29 (2):166–174

[8] Mayfield JK, Johnson RP, Kilcoyne RK. Carpal dislocations: pathomechanics and progressive perilunar instability. J Hand Surg Am. 1980; 5(3):226–241

[9] Cromheecke M, Lluch A, Verstreken F. Isolated injury of the dorsal scapholunate ligament caused by intracarpal pronation. J Hand Surg Eur Vol. 2021; 46(8):891–892

[10] Geissler WB, Freeland AE, Savoie FH, McIntyre LW, Whipple TL. Intracarpal soft-tissue lesions associated with an intra-articular fracture of the distal end of the radius. J Bone Joint Surg Am. 1996; 78(3):357–365

[11] Messina JC, Van Overstraeten L, Luchetti R, Fairplay T, Mathoulin CL. The EWAS classification of scapholunate tears: an anatomical arthroscopic study. J Wrist Surg. 2013; 2(2):105–109

[12] Andersson JK, Garcia-Elias M. Dorsal scapholunate ligament injury: a classification of clinical forms. J Hand Surg Eur Vol. 2013; 38(2): 165–169

[13] Garcia-Elias M, Lluch AL, Stanley JK. Three-ligament tenodesis for the treatment of scapholunate dissociation: indications and surgical technique. J Hand Surg Am. 2006; 31(1):125–134

10 The "4R" Algorithm of Treatment

Riccardo Luchetti and Fernando Corella

Abstract

Scapholunate dysfunction is not a unique injury but a spectrum of them, which includes acute and chronic injuries, partial and complete tears, reducible and nonreducible instabilities, etc. This spectrum of injuries can be treated with a myriad of techniques both openly and arthroscopically.

The election of a specific technique depends on the preference and experience of the surgeon, but there are general rules for a correct indication.

The aim of this chapter is to group all the techniques in four major groups called the "4R." They are Repair, Reinforcement, Reconstruction, and Resection and define how and when to choose between this major groups.

Keywords: scapholunate, carpal instability

10.1 Introduction

The first important topic to discuss, as explained in the previous chapter, is that "SL dysfunction" is not synonymous with "SL instability." For example, there are pathologies that should not be considered as an unstable carpus but a collapsed one, when there are degenerative changes. Furthermore, a wrist without degenerative changes but with a nonreducible scaphoid and lunate should not be understood as an unstable wrist either, but rather fixed and prearthritic.

Also, it is important to take into consideration that a carpal instability is not synonymous with "malalignment," because some wrists may not have normal carpal kinematics, but may function painlessly. In conclusion, carpal instability should be only used synonymously with symptomatic carpal dysfunction and as just one portion of the SL pathology.[1]

As mentioned earlier, the authors propose to organize the different SL treatments for all ranges of SL dysfunction in the four major groups called the "4R." The meaning of each "R" is as follows:

First "R": Repair. This group includes all techniques used to repair a fresh and acute injury of the ligament or to repair a ligament with a subacute injury but with healing capacity.

Second "R": Reinforcement. This group includes all techniques used to reinforce an SL ligament and the soft tissue around it. These techniques are indicated when there is a partial or a complete tear, with a ligament remnant damaged but in continuity.

Third "R": Reconstruction. This group includes all techniques that replace an injured ligament with a new tissue (usually a tendon graft) that resemble its function. In these techniques the SL ligament is completely torn and there is no remnant of the ligament.

Fourth "R": Resection. This group includes all techniques used when the SL injury evolves into a fixed and collapsed carpus with or without arthritic changes.

The specific advantages, disadvantages, and technical details of every possible technique will be discussed in the upcoming chapters of this book.

10.2 Defining the Type and Stage of Injury Through the Arthroscopic Exploration

In order to choose the best possible treatment, several aspects should be taken into consideration in every specific patient, such as age, medical history, dominance, level of pain, work, and leisure activities. Preoperatively, both the clinical and radiological explorations are essential for the decision. All these essential topics have been discussed in previous chapters.

Hereafter, the focus will be on how to classify the different stages of SL pathology.

One of the best ways to define the injury is by asking six questions (which are explained in the previous chapter), as proposed by Garcia-Elias[1]:

1. Is the dorsal scapholunate interosseous ligament (dSLIL) intact and functional?
2. If the ligament has ruptured, does it have good integrity for repair?
3. Is the scaphoid alignment normal?
4. Is radiolunate (RL) alignment still retained?
5. Are abnormal carpal alignments easily reducible?
6. Is the articular cartilage normal?

By answering them, each case could be subdivided into one of the seven different stages, with each stage having a different kind of treatment.

But the answers to these questions are not always easy during the preoperative clinical and radiological evaluations. None of the radiological tools such as X-rays, ultrasound, magnetic resonance imaging (MRI), computed tomography (CT) can definitely provide the exact type, portion, grade, and healing potential of the SL ligament or the reducibility of the instability, the grade and location of the cartilage loss, etc. The evaluation of all these facts would completely change the stage of injury and the group of treatment to choose. Thus, the only way for obtaining an accurate answer is to check them intraoperatively.

The development of wrist arthroscopy and the simplicity of a diagnostic arthroscopy should preclude the performance of an open approach to answer these questions. An open approach causes a great amount of scar tissue and could injure secondary stabilizers as well as the proprioception.[2] That is why, the authors encourage all surgeons to arthroscopically explore the wrist for defining the stage of the SL dysfunction and then pick the applicable specific technique from the 4R groups. These techniques can be done openly or arthroscopically, depending on the preference and experience of the surgeon.

As explained, wrist arthroscopy gives all the information, but several explorations should be performed. These explorations are grouped in the 7-items arthroscopic exploration which is explained in detail in Chapter 7.

10.2.1 Gap Between the Bones

This is the most common exploration, as most of the classifications use a probe that is inserted in the SL joint and is twisted to define the stage of instability. The classification that the authors recommend to use is the EWAS classification.[3]

However, it is important to remark that in the midcarpal joint, there is no ligament in the SL joint (different from the radiocarpal [RC] joint, where the membranous portion covers the joint). So, the SL ligament is not directly tested but the state of the ligament is interpreted with the laxity of the joint. That is why it is essential to have a direct visualization and testing as will be explained later.

10.2.2 Acute vs Chronic

Most of the times the suspicion of an acute or chronic injury is easy, considering when the trauma occurred. However, there can be doubts when evaluating injuries associated to distal radius fractures or carpal bone fractures. In these cases, old and chronic injuries can be found, and no specific treatment is needed.

It is important to look for signs of acute injury, which are a hemorrhagic ligament along with fresh torn stumps.

10.2.3 Quality of the Ligament

The evaluation of the quality of the ligament should be done by direct visualization and testing of the three different portions, having in mind that the injury usually occurs and progresses from volar to dorsal.

In the RC joint the membranous portion of the SL ligament could be checked and visualized if it is detached from the scaphoid or lunate. Remaining in the RC joint the dorsal portion of the SL ligament could be also checked as well as the dorsal capsuloscapholunate septum (DCSS).[4] The volar portion of the SL ligament could also be checked from the RC joint using the 1/2 portal passing the scope between the palmar RC ligaments and the scaphoid.

In the midcarpal joint the volar portion of the ligament can be visualized and tested if the synovial tissue over this portion is removed.

However, the most important portion to evaluate is the dorsal one, as a complete injury with no remnant or a bad quality ligament will lead to a reconstruction, while lesions in continuity could be treated with a reinforcement.

To evaluate the dorsal portion of the SL ligament, a "hook test" can be performed. The probe is introduced in the SL joint, and a dorsal traction is performed, capturing the dorsal portion of the ligament. If there is a competent ligament, the probe is caught in the dorsal SL ligament (positive hook test), if not there will be no capture (negative hook test) (▶ Fig. 10.1).

10.2.4 Dorsal Displacement of the Scaphoid

Patients with SL dysfunction complain of pain in the dorsal side of the wrist. This may occur due to the dorsal displacement and impingement between the proximal pole of the scaphoid and the dorsal edge of the radius. When exploring, this pain appears when the scaphoid is displaced over the dorsal edge of the radius (Watson's test, ballottement test, or in hyperextension of the wrist).

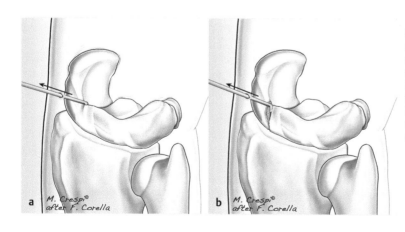

a M. Crespi® after F. Corella b M. Crespi® after F. Corella

Fig. 10.1 Hook test. The probe is introduced in the scapholunate (SL) joint, and a dorsal traction is performed, capturing the dorsal portion of the ligament. **(a)** Positive hook test. There is a ligament in continuity; the probe is caught in the dorsal SL ligament. **(b)** Negative hook test. There is no ligament in continuity, as there is no capture of the ligament.

This dorsal displacement can be explored with the "arthroscopic scaphoid 3D (dorsal, dynamic, displacement) test."[5] This test can be useful if there are doubts about the mechanical repercussions of an SL tear (partial, complete, volar, dorsal, etc.) and it will help in the decision making of the kind of treatment to be used (▸ Fig. 10.2).

10.2.5 Reducibility

This is one of the key points when deciding the treatment in SL pathologies. If the scaphoid cannot be easily reduced to its normal position, salvage surgeries (resection group) are recommended. If it is reducible, reconstructions techniques can be performed.

Arthroscopically this reducibility can be checked easily. The scaphoid should be easily reduced and positioned to the height of the lunate only by pushing with the arthroscopic probe (▸ Fig. 10.3).

If it is not reduced, the authors clearly recommend not to perform ligamentoplasties or other reconstruction techniques. However, an alternative is to remove scar tissue around the scaphoid with the help of a dissector, and after this removal, it could be checked again if the scaphoid can be reduced.

10.2.6 Combined Injuries

The concurrence of tears of the SL and lunotriquetral (LT) ligaments is not unusual and can also occur without an apparent perilunate dislocation. Badia and Khanchandani called this combined lesion a "floating lunate."[6] More recently Herzberg has described this pathology as perilunate dislocations in which there was no dislocation of the capitate from the lunate on the initial radiographs and called them "perilunate injuries, not dislocated (PLIND)."[7]

As the image studies can underestimate this combined injury (specially the LT instability), it is important to always check, before deciding the kind of treatment, the presence of a floating lunate. This can be done with the "rocking chair sign"[8] (▸ Fig. 10.4). An oscillating movement of the probe is performed, from the posterior to the anterior horn of the lunate and back again. If there is a combined injury the lunate would make a movement similar to a "rocking chair," whereas the scaphoid and lunate would remain static.

10.2.7 Degenerative Changes

As a nonreducible instability precludes the performance of a reconstruction technique, the presence of cartilage damage can also modify the type of treatment.

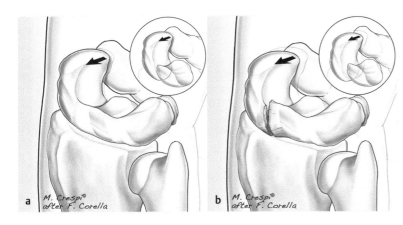

Fig. 10.2 Arthroscopic scaphoid 3D test. The scaphoid is pushed dorsally from the scaphoid tubercle. **(a)** Negative test. There is no scapholunate (SL) dysfunction; the proximal row moves dorsally together. **(b)** Positive test. There is an SL dysfunction; the scaphoid moves dorsally while the lunate remains in the same position.

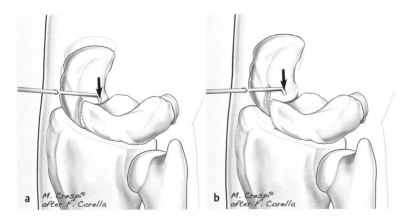

Fig. 10.3 Scaphoid reducibility. The probe is introduced through the radial midcarpal portal (RMC) and push the scaphoid. **(a)** Easily reducible instability: the scaphoid should be reduced and positioned to the height of the lunate. **(b)** Not easily reducible instability: the scaphoid cannot be positioned to its normal height in the midcarpal joint.

10

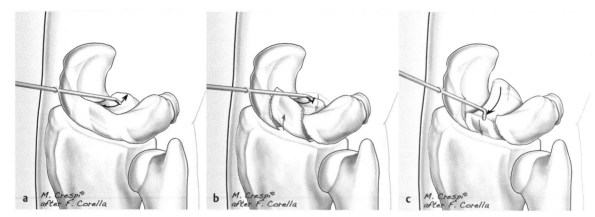

Fig. 10.4 Rocking chair sign. An oscillating movement of the probe is performed, from the posterior to the anterior horn of the lunate and back again. **(a)** Negative test. The lunate bone remains static when this oscillating movement is performed. **(b)** Positive test. The lunate makes a movement that resembles a rocking chair, whereas the scaphoid and lunate would remain static.

Watson and Ballet have described that degenerative processes of an SL ligament injury can be developed, which has been called a scaphoid lunate advanced collapse (SLAC) of the wrist.[9]

The three stages of SLAC can be distinguished on radiographs. In Stage I, there is damage only to the most radial aspect of the radioscaphoid joint. In Stage II, narrowing of the whole radioscaphoid joint occurs, and in Stage III, there is in addition narrowing of the midcarpal joint.

During the decision-making process, defining the exact stage of osteoarthritis plays a central role. The gold standard for assessing the status of the cartilage is wrist arthroscopy. The correlation between cartilage lesions, classified by arthroscopy and MRI, is low and the level of cartilage lesion may be more severely classified in an MRI than during arthroscopy.[10] Furthermore, MRI in detecting wrist chondral loss, despite a high specificity of 97%, has a low sensitivity of 65%.[11]

Different locations should be explored arthroscopically for the cartilage loss in order to define correctly the stage of the collapse: the radius scaphoid fossa (specially its dorsal aspect), the midcarpal joint, and the radiolunate joint.

10.3 Organizing the Treatments: The 4R

To initially summarize and simplify the treatments, the algorithm in ▶ Fig. 10.5 is proposed.

However, not everything is so definitive, and it is important to understand that sometimes the treatments can be overlapped and a similar technique can be used for two groups specially the repair and reinforcement of the ligament.

10.3.1 Repair

As explained at the beginning of the chapter, repair means to treat an acute and freshly torn ligament. This

can be done in the first 3 to 6 weeks of the traumatic event. As most of the times the initial X-rays are normal and there is a delay in the MRI it is not common to find an acute injury in such a short period of time. However, these fresh injuries are commonly seen associated to a distal radius fractures and carpal bone fractures or perilunate injuries.

Many techniques can be used for the treatment of an acute injury; most of these techniques are performed along with the stabilization of the joint with K-wires. In fact, one way of treatment is only to pin the joint after an anatomical reduction has been achieved under arthroscopic control and maintain the immobilization until the ligaments has healed. Furthermore, a suture of the dorsal or volar portion of the ligament can be also performed under arthroscopic control. In these techniques the dorsal capsule can be included in the repair.

The pinning and suturing of the ligament can be also performed by open surgery. In these cases, many surgeons include a capsulodesis to increase the resistance of the ligament.

So, some arthroscopic and open techniques, along with the repair of the ligament, perform a reinforcement by including the dorsal capsule in the repair.

All these techniques will be explained in detail in further specific chapters.

10.3.2 Reinforcement

The reinforcement of the ligament consists of a suture of the torn ligament along with the capsule and soft tissues around it. The ligament remnant should be in continuity and with enough quality.

One of the most challenging decisions in the algorithm is to decide where a reconstruction or a reinforcement should be done. In order to decide, two arthroscopic explorations should be considered: the quality of the ligament and the dorsal displacement of the scaphoid.

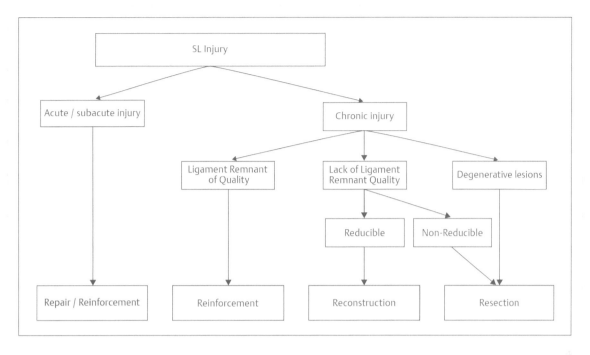

Fig. 10.5 The 4R algorithm.

When there is a ligament in continuity with a positive hook test and the dorsal displacement is limited or at least with an end-point resistance, the ligament has enough quality. In this case, a reinforcement technique could be done.

On the other hand, when the hook test is negative, there is no remnant of the ligament with retracted edges and an important dorsal displacement; with lack of end-point resistance, the ligament doesn't have enough quality. In this case, a reconstruction technique should be considered.

The different open and arthroscopic techniques used to perform a reinforcement of the ligament will be explained in detail in the next chapters.

10.3.3 Reconstruction

The reconstruction of the ligament consists in the substitution of a completely torn ligament without a healing capacity. This substitution is usually performed with a tendon graft, but also with a bone-ligament-bone graft and other techniques.

It is also a challenge to decide between a reconstruction or a palliative technique. For helping in this decision making two arthroscopic explorations can be used: the reducibility and the presence of cartilage loss and its extension.

If the instability is easily reducible with the probe as explained before and there is no cartilage loss, or it is limited to a small portion of the dorsal rim of the radius, a reconstruction technique can be performed.

However, if the instability is not easily reducible or the cartilage loss include more than the dorsal rim, a salvage procedure is indicated. The first scenario usually corresponds with Grade IV of the EWAS classification or Grade V, but with a slight radiological misalignment. The second scenario corresponds with Grade V (especially if the gap is too open) with an important misalignment. Nevertheless, despite the initial radiological study, the last decision should be taken after the arthroscopic exploration.

All the different reconstruction techniques will be explained in further chapters.

10.3.4 Resection

This last group of techniques will be performed when the possibility of reconstruction has been discarded. So, the group of resection consists in removal of bone, partial fusions or even total fusions, or arthroplasties.

The type of surgery depends on the joint affected. So once more, the arthroscopic visualization of all the locations where cartilage loss occur is essential.

If only the dorsal portion of the radius is affected (SLAC I) a partial resection of the radial styloid and the dorsal border of the distal radius can be performed.

If most of the radial fossa presents degenerative lesions (SLAC II) a partial fusion such as a four-corner arthrodesis

10

or scaphoidectomy and midcarpal tenodesis[12] should be considered along with a proximal row carpectomy.

If the midcarpal joint is affected (SLAC III) a partial four-corner arthrodesis is the most extended treatment.

All the techniques that could be done considering the location of the cartilage loss will be explained in a further chapter.

10.4 Conclusion

The spectrum of SL injuries can be treated with a myriad of techniques both openly and arthroscopically. The authors have grouped all of them in four major groups called the "4R," which are Repair, Reinforcement, Reconstruction, and Resection.

The best selection of a specific technique depends both on the preference and experience of the surgeon and on the answer to several questions to accurately define the grade of the injury. The arthroscopic exploration is one of the best tool to define how and when to choose between these major groups.

References

[1] Garcia-Elias M, Lluch AL. Wrist instabilities, misalignments and dislocations. In: Wolfe SW, Hotchkiss RN, Pederson WC et al. Green's Operative Hand Surgery, 7th ed. Vol. 1, Philadelphia: Elsevier, 2017; 418-478

[2] Hagert E, Lluch A, Rein S. The role of proprioception and neuromuscular stability in carpal instabilities. J Hand Surg Eur Vol. 2016; 41(1):94–101

[3] Messina JC, Van Overstraeten L, Luchetti R, Fairplay T, Mathoulin CL. The EWAS classification of scapholunate tears: an anatomical arthroscopic study. J Wrist Surg. 2013; 2(2):105–109

[4] Overstraeten LV, Camus EJ, Wahegaonkar A, et al. Anatomical description of the dorsal capsulo-scapholunate septum (DCSS): arthroscopic staging of scapholunate instability after DCSS sectioning. J Wrist Surg. 2013; 2(2):149–154

[5] Corella F, Ocampos M, Cerro M. Arthroscopic scaphoid 3D test for scapholunate instability. J Wrist Surg. 2018; 7(1):89–92

[6] Badia A, Khanchandani P. The floating lunate: arthroscopic treatment of simultaneous complete tears of the scapholunate and lunotriquetral ligaments. Hand (N Y). 2009; 4(3):250–255

[7] Herzberg G. Perilunate injuries, not dislocated (PLIND). J Wrist Surg. 2013; 2(4):337–345

[8] Corella F, Del Cerro M, Ocampos M, Larrainzar-Garijo R. The "Rocking Chair Sign" for floating lunate. J Hand Surg Am. 2015; 40(11):2318–2319

[9] Watson HK, Ballet FL. The SLAC wrist: scapholunate advanced collapse pattern of degenerative arthritis. J Hand Surg Am. 1984; 9 (3):358–365

[10] Terzis A, Klinger A, Seegmüller J, Sauerbier M. Inter-rater reliability of magnetic resonance imaging in comparison to computed tomography and wrist arthroscopy in SLAC and SNAC wrist. J Clin Med. 2021; 10(16):3592

[11] Asaad AM, Andronic A, Newby MP, Harrison JWK. Diagnostic accuracy of single-compartment magnetic resonance arthrography in detecting common causes of chronic wrist pain. J Hand Surg Eur Vol. 2017; 42(6):580–585

[12] Luchetti R. Proximal row carpectomy, scaphoidectomy with midcarpal arthrodesis or midcarpal tenodesis: when and how to use. J Hand Surg Eur Vol. 2018; 43(6):579–588

11 Acute "R"epair: Open Treatment

Riccardo Luchetti, Sara Montanari, Andrea Atzei, and Frank Nienstedt

Abstract

Two types of open surgical approaches and treatment for scapholunate (SL) ligament injuries are described. In SL ligament injuries with detachment, direct repair is indicated, while in intraligament injuries, repair associated with reinforcement is the best indication of treatment. The traditional approach with wide exposure is described and criticized. Through this approach it is possible to repair and reinforce the ligament, but the complete detachment of the dorsal capsule from the scaphoid, lunate, and triquetrum might destabilize the carpal complex. In order to spare the connection of the dorsal interosseous ligament from the scaphoid, lunate, and triquetrum, the double "window technique" is described. The SL ligament with lunate or scaphoid detachment can be repaired with an anchor screw using the proximal window. If the lesion is intraligamentous, it is necessary to associate the repair with a dorsal reinforcement by a dorsal capsulodesis technique using the second distal window approach. The capsule-ligamentous flap is harvested from the dorsal intercarpal ligament and is turned proximally and sutures to the lunate are passed through a tunnel under the spared dorsal capsule.

Keywords: scapholunate lesion, scapholunate instability, wrist, surgical approach wrist, ligament repair wrist

11.1 Introduction

Acute scapholunate interosseous ligament (SLIL) injuries occur frequently and are linked to sprained wrist trauma,[1,2] distal radius fractures,[3,4] carpal fracture-dislocations,[5] and less frequently associated with scaphoid fractures.[6,8,9,10]

Acute injuries are defined as those presented within 4 weeks after the initial trauma, subacute injuries from 4 weeks to 6 months, and chronic injuries at 6 months after the initial trauma.[11,12] Acute SL ligament injuries can be divided into complete or partial, associated or isolated. Acute complete SL ligament injuries need to be treated within few weeks after trauma with suture repair or reinsertion and/or pinning[12] and/or dorsal capsulodesis. If a complete SL ligament injury is confirmed, the location of the ligament injury must be identified to better define the treatment and the quality of the possible outcome. The term "partial" includes several conditions in which the SL ligament is involved in the injury: the ligament can be damaged in only one part of its components (volar, proximal, or dorsal) (▶ Fig. 11.1a–c) or in more than one of its components (volar, dorsal, and proximal) at the same time. It may be only elongated and/or not detached from its skeletal insertion, but damaged in its context like partial intraligamentous lacerations (▶ Fig. 11.2a–f).

The volar component of the SLIL may show the same patterns of ligament lesion. Detachment from the scaphoid (▶ Fig. 11.3a), from the lunate (▶ Fig. 11.3b), or intraligamentous lesion (▶ Fig. 11.3c).

It is important to consider the reparability of the SLIL lesion before starting the treatment. This depends on the site of the SLIL injury and on the quality of the tissue in terms of healing potential. This means that not all the types of SLIL injuries have the same healing potential or need the same type of surgical treatment.

Complete SLIL injuries where the ligament is detached from the scaphoid or lunate border have a higher potential of healing when sutured without delay. On the contrary, the intraligamentous lesion has a poor healing potential and needs different treatment and prognostic consideration. These data (site of injury, partial or complete, healing potential) are part of the algorithm parameters proposed by Garcia-Elias et al.[13] Other parameters that must be considered are the abnormality of the radioscaphoid and the radiolunate angle, the amount of the SL gap, the ease or difficulty to correct these pathologic parameters, and finally the evaluation of the state of the cartilage.

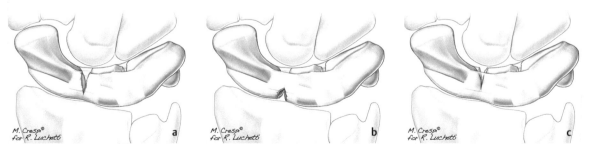

Fig. 11.1 (a) Tear of the dorsal component of the scapholunate ligament; **(b)** tear of the proximal (membranous) component of the scapholunate ligament; **(c)** tear of the anterior component of the scapholunate ligament.

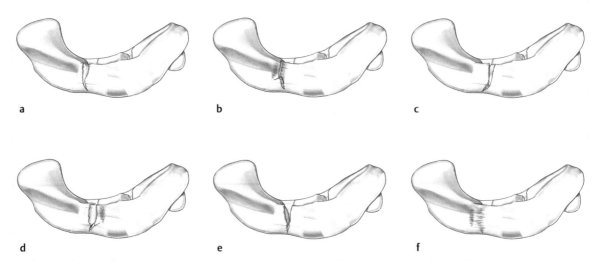

Fig. 11.2 Different types of scapholunate ligament dorsal component tears. **(a)** Lateral tear (close to the scaphoid); **(b)** ligament detached from the scaphoid; **(c)** medial tear (close to the lunate); **(d)** ligament detached from the lunate; **(e)** central intraligamentous tear; **(f)** ligament stretching.

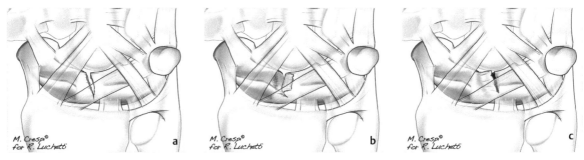

Fig. 11.3 Different types of scapholunate ligament volar component tears. **(a)** Intraligamentous tear; **(b)** detachment from the scaphoid; **(c)** detachment from the lunate.

Arthroscopy is the best method to obtain these information and guide the surgeons toward the correct method of treatment. Arthroscopic staging of the SLIL injury should follow the EWAS classification according to Messina et al.[14] Arthroscopy might also show the presence of chondral and osteochondral damage of the carpal bones that may preclude surgical ligament repair.

11.2 Clinical Signs

Clinical symptoms are pain at the radial site of the wrist mainly dorsally, but also volarly, depending on the most affected component. Pain can be of variable intensity, sometimes it appears only under stress. The clinical signs are the sensation of snapping, instability in flexion-extension movements and radioulnar deviation of the wrist, especially under load, and swelling which is not always present. In severe cases, functional impairment of the wrist with loss of strength with

pain and the need for protection with a wrist splint is evident.

The typical clinical test is the shift test (or Watson's test), which evokes snap and pain. In cases of partial injury during this maneuver the pain is present but the click is not appreciated and there is a sort of positive "apprehension test" as for shoulder instabilities: the patient protects the wrist from the test maneuver by contracting the muscles or evading the maneuver itself. It is therefore necessary to distract him during the test to better appreciate any snap or the onset of pain.

11.3 Instrumental Diagnostics

Diagnostic investigations start with radiology. Standard wrist radiographs may be positive if they document SL diastasis more than 3 mm. If radiographs do not highlight signs of malalignment, you may perform comparative or dynamic X-rays: comparative clenched pencil view, ulnar and radial deviation of both wrists (see Chapter 8).[11] If these radiographic investigations show an opening of the SL joint space, the presence of a dynamic SL lesion is confirmed; if they are negative, but positive symptoms are present you may proceed toward a second level of investigation. For some authors[15] ultrasound can be useful to identify a lesion of the SL ligament. However, with this technique only the dorsal component of the SL ligament can be evaluated.[15,16] Therefore, if the lesion involves the volar component of the SL ligament, it is not possible to identify it.

Complete lesions of the SL ligament can be identified by magnetic resonance imaging (MRI).[17,18] The quality of the MRI is important: in fact, a 1.5 T MRI is required at least. MRI examinations of less than 1.5 T quality lose reliability. However, there are cases in which the MRI 1.5 T fails to identify the lesion. Our experience reports that MRI fails to identify 15% of complete lesions.[19] It is unlikely that MRI may detect partial SLL injuries. Our experience reports a failure rate of 70%.[19] Some authors report exceptional results using MRA (magnetic resonance arthrography) (100% positive responses in comparison with wrist arthroscopy).[20] However, in our experience this is not always the case. Both partial and complete lesions may give a negative response on MRA.

11.4 Arthroscopy

Arthroscopic staging of the SL ligament injury is of utmost importance for correct surgical treatment.[4,14,21] Arthroscopy also provides important data on the quality of the damaged ligament, the extent of the lesion (involvement of the various components), the presence of associated ligament injuries (intrinsic and extrinsic ligaments), and chondral or osteochondral lesions.

Once the type of lesion of the SL ligament has been established by instrumental examination and especially by arthroscopy, its treatment should be carried out. Open repair is the traditional method to treat such a lesion and

the dorsal approach is traditionally used to repair the dorsal component of the SLIL.[22] Only recently, the volar component of it has been considered amenable to be repaired,[23,24] but the literature reports aa few publications of open[25,26,27] and arthroscopic methods.[28] The open surgical repair of the volar component of the SLIL has been published by Marcuzzi et al.[26,27] They did not find a widespread use, maybe because it is not necessary for the reduced biomechanical importance of the volar component. Therefore, all the surgical efforts have been focused on the dorsal component of the SLIL.

The problem here is how to treat a complete or a partial SLIL injury and especially how to repair the SLIL injuries classified as type 2-a-c-e-f (that include the Andersson 3 and 4 type lesions) with the worst healing potential.[12]

We present the traditional standard technique with an extensive approach to the dorsum of the wrist and propose a less invasive technique with maximum respect for all structures both retinacular and ligamentous that are not involved in the SL injury. In particular conditions, such as in fracture dislocations of the carpus, the surgical approach will depend on the present damage (Video 11.1).

11.5 Traditional Surgical Technique

A longitudinal dorsal skin incision centered over the SL interval and the Lister's tubercle is used. The dorsal retinaculum of the third and fourth compartment, divided along the Lister's tubercle, is reflected ulnarly. The extensor pollicis longus (EPL) tendon is retracted radially, the extensor digiti communis tendons (EDC) ulnarly, and the posterior interosseous nerve (PIN) is resected. The wrist joint is exposed through a "ligament-sparing technique" according to Berger and Bishop[29] (▸ Fig. 11.4a–c).

The dorsal and proximal membranous portions of the SLIL are evaluated.

Surgical procedures like simple SL bone reinsertion with bone anchor (▸ Fig. 11.4a–c, ▸ Fig. 11.5a–d) or SL

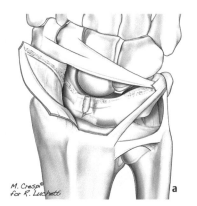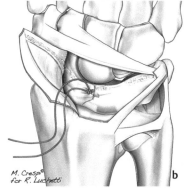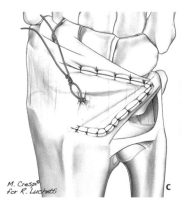

Fig. 11.4 Drawings showing the dorsal capsulodesis according to the Berger technique. **(a)** Dorsal radiocarpal approach according to the Berger-Bishop technique with exposition of the carpal bones in which the scapholunate ligament is detached from the lunate; **(b)** the ligament is repaired using an anchor screw; **(c)** the dorsal capsule if sutured to the incision margins and to the scapholunate ligament using the same suture passed through the capsule itself.

repair with dorsal capsulodesis (▶ Fig. 11.6a–c) depend on the type of SL injury.[30,31,32,33,34,35] Once the SL dissociation is reduced anatomically, percutaneous pin fixation from the scaphoid into the lunate and from the scaphoid into the capitate is performed[13,35] (▶ Fig. 11.7a, b). If the SL reduction is not needed no pin fixation by K-wires are required

(▶ Fig. 11.7c). The ligament is then repaired using bone anchor sutures if it is detached from the lunate or the scaphoid (▶ Fig. 11.4b, c) or an intraligamentous suture is used.

At the end the capsule is sutured, the extensor tendons are repositioned and the retinaculum is repaired. A volar splint is applied to maintain the wrist at 20 to 25 degrees

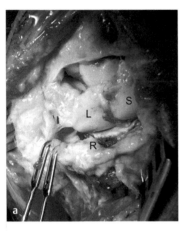
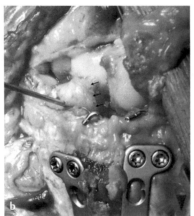
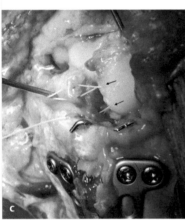
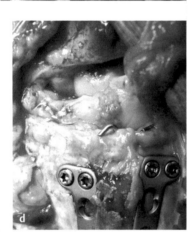

Fig. 11.5 **(a)** Dorsal approach: Intra-articular distal radius fracture with complete rupture of the scapholunate ligament. **(b)** Open reduction and internal fixation of the distal radius fracture with plates and pins. *Dark arrows* indicate the scapholunate ligament detached from the scaphoid. **(c)** *Dark arrows* indicate the entry points of two bone anchors in the proximal pole of the scaphoid with their suture threads passing through the detached scapholunate ligament. **(d)** The scapholunate ligament after reinsertion and pinning of the scapholunate and scaphocapitate joint. L, lunate; S, scaphoid; R, radius.

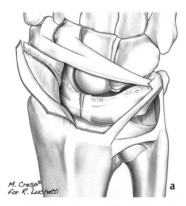
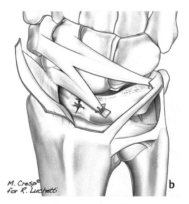
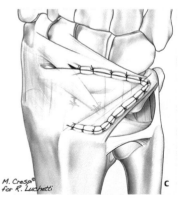

Fig. 11.6 Dorsal capsulodesis for intraligamentous scapholunate ligament injury. **(a)** Dorsal radiocarpal approach according to the Berger-Bishop technique with exposition of the intraligamentous injury of the scapholunate ligament; **(b)** a radially based flap is detached from the dorsal intercarpal ligament and is attached to the lunate using an anchor screw; **(c)** at the end the dorsal capsule is sutured to the margins.

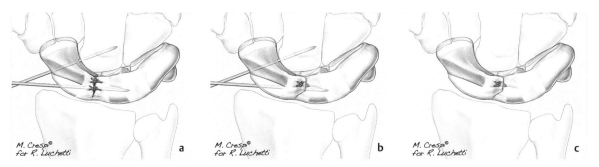

Fig. 11.7 **(a)** Drawings showing the correct position of the K-wires in the scapholunate (SL) ligament repair for an intraligament injury; **(b)** the same procedure of bones temporary fixation with two K-wires is used in SL ligament repair; **(c)** the same lesion can be treated without stabilization of the SL bones after SL ligament is repaired without involvement of the secondary ligaments' stabilizers.

of extension. The wrist is immobilized for 6 weeks. Digits are free to move actively. Daily medication permits to check the wrist condition and prevent infection. A hand therapist will help the patient constantly.

Pertinent protocol of wrist rehabilitation will start after K-wires removal at 6 to 8 weeks and continues for 2 months.

11.5.1 Advantages and Limits of the Traditional Technique

This technique has the advantage to expose the wrist completely from the dorsal side, to make a correct assessment of the damage and to allow an appropriate repair.

However, such an extensive surgical access exposes to various risks. (1) The opening of the retinaculum and its suture at the end of the surgery precludes any movement of the wrist for 4 weeks causing stiffness in the flexion-extension of the wrist and occasionally of the fingers due to adhesions of the extensor tendons. If immediate wrist mobilization is allowed, loss of restraint of the extensor tendons (bowstring) may occur. (2) The Berger-Bishop flap for the exposure of the carpus is conceptually great, but it might determine destabilization of the carpal bones due to the partial detachment of the secondary stabilizers, like the radiotriquetral (RT) and the dorsal intercarpal (DIC) ligaments. The proximal part of the DIC ligament that runs and is attached to the dorsal profile of the scaphoid and on the distal margin of the lunate is an important reinforcement of the SL ligament (▶ Fig. 11.8) and the dorsal capsule scapholunate septum (DCSS)[36] is part of this complex.[37,38] In this traditional technique a radially based ligament-capsular flap is detached from the dorsal crest of the scaphoid, and the dorsal margin of the lunate and the triquetrum. When repositioning the Berger-Bishop flap,[29] only the peripheral part is sutured and one may forget to reinsert the aforementioned part on the back of the scaphoid and lunate. This can be a possible factor of secondary SL instabilities.

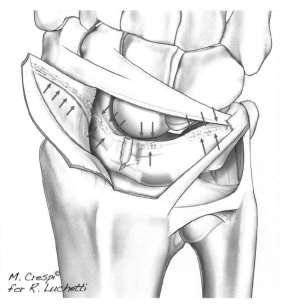

Fig. 11.8 The dorsal carpal bones are exposed through the Berger-Bishop flap. Note the insertion of the proximal part of the dorsal intercarpal (DIC) ligament from the dorsal border of the scaphoid, and the distal margin of the lunate and the triquetrum (*red arrows*). In this traditional technique, in which the DIC ligament is detached from the dorsal crest of the scaphoid, and the dorsal margin of the lunate and the triquetrum, a secondary carpal instability might occur.

For this reason, a more conservative surgical approach to the carpal bones was proposed that we are going to describe.

11.6 Preferred Method[39,40]

A dorsal approach with transverse or short longitudinal skin incision ("window approach") is used sparing the extensor retinaculum (▶ Fig. 11.9a, b).

If necessary, a small incision is made along the distal edge of the retinaculum on the course of the EPL tendon without reaching Lister's tubercle. The septum separating the third from the fourth extensors compartment is incised and the dorsal radial carpal capsule is exposed by retracting the extensor tendons: the EDC to the ulnar side and the EPL and wrist extensors to the radial side. A PIN neurectomy is performed and the dorsal capsule is incised from the edge of the distal radius and continued ulnarly between the fibers of the RT ligament for 2 cm (▶ Fig. 11.9a, b).

The capsule is turned over distally, and the carpal bones are accessed (▶ Fig. 11.10a–c): the SL ligament with the lunate and the proximal part of the scaphoid are then visualized (▶ Fig. 11.11a–c). SLIL injuries can have various patterns involving also the dorsal capsule attaching on the edge of the scaphoid and lunate (DCSS) and/or the scapholunotriquetral (SLT) ligament component of the DIC. If these components are intact, it is sufficient to repair the SL ligament according to the location of the rupture (▶ Fig. 11.10c). It is usually detached from the proximal pole of the scaphoid. A suture anchor is inserted here after having roughened the insertional edge and then the ligament is sutured. The proximal part of the damaged SLIL is usually debrided. If the lesion is on the lunate side, the same procedure is performed, but the suture anchor is applied to the lunate (▶ Fig. 11.10c).

If the lesion is intraligamentous a dorsal capsulodesis may be useful to reinforce the SL complex (▶ Fig. 11.12a–c) and can be performed in this way: the DIC ligament is identified and engraved at full thickness along the course of its fibers over the neck of the capitate, from the scaphoid margin to the hamate. This creates a complex of two ligaments: one distal and one proximal. The proximal portion is detached from the triquetrum creating a

radial-based ligamentous flap. This ligamentous flap is passed under the capsule by carving a small tunnel between the bone edge and the structure of the dorsal SLL distally and it is inserted on the dorsum of the lunate with a suture anchor (▶ Fig. 11.12a–c). In this way, the DCSS is only partially detached allowing the passage of the ligamentous flap, which is used as reinforcement of the SL ligament.

Finally, the dorsal radiocarpal (RC) capsule is resutured to the edge of the radius and to the RT ligament. The retinaculum, even if distally open, is not sutured and the skin incision is closed with nylon stitches. A drainage is always applied for hematoma prevention and removed on the first day. A volar wrist splint protects the wrist postoperatively and it is removed after 20 days.

11.7 Discussion

It is really difficult to diagnose acute SLIL lesions and the decision regarding the best surgical treatment is even more difficult.[1,2,11,32] Acute injuries of the SLIL are often missed because clinical diagnosis is difficult and only plain radiographs are usually performed in the acute setting. Bergh et al[1] demonstrated that MRI performed in acute lesion in patients with negative radiographs was positive for SLIL lesion in 4% of the cases. Moreover, in cases where an acute injury is diagnosed and treated, it is possible to find the ligament avulsed from the bone and retracted or you may find an intraligamentous lesion. In both cases it is difficult to reinsert or to suture the ligament.

Under load the SLIL complex must resist against considerable forces of tension and torsion, and a failure of

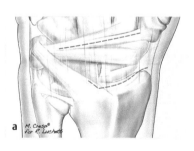
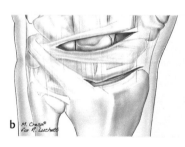

Fig. 11.9 The double window approach at the carpal joints. **(a)** Proximal and distal position of the capsular incision (*dotted red lines*); **(b)** the two approaches with exposition of the radiocarpal and midcarpal joint.

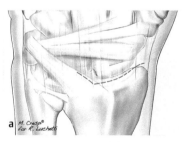
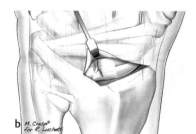
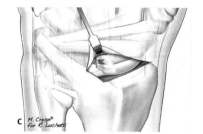

Fig. 11.10 (a) Design of the proximal skin incision (*dotted red line*); **(b)** exposition of the scapholunate (SL) ligament detached from the lunate; **(c)** the SL ligament is repaired using an anchor screw.

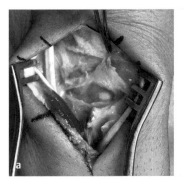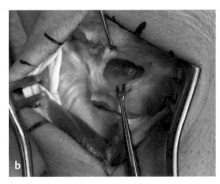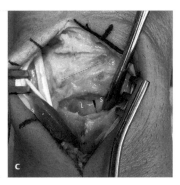

Fig. 11.11 Anatomical demonstrations of the windows approaches. **(a)** Proximal capsular window approach exposing the radiocarpal joint and scapholunate (SL) ligament; **(b)** distal capsular window approach exposing the midcarpal joint; **(c)** intraligamentous SL ligament shown through the proximal window approach.

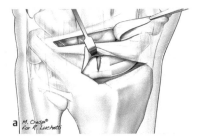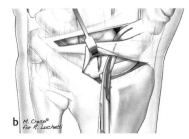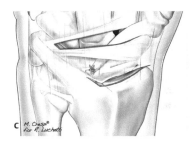

Fig. 11.12 Technique of dorsal Berger capsulodesis using the double window approach. **(a)** Exposition of the scapholunate (SL) ligament injury through the proximal window approach and a distal dissection of a capsule-ligamentous radially based flap. **(b)** The flap is turned proximally passing under the capsular bridge; **(c)** the capsule-ligamentous flap is sutured to the lunate with an anchor screw.

the repaired ligament can occur over time, causing secondary SL dissociation. Consecutive radiographic degenerative changes in the long-term outcome occur in one-third of patients.[12]

Nevertheless, the most promising treatment for SLIL injury is surgical repair as soon as possible, and there is no better moment to regain anatomic conditions. Otherwise, the SLIL structure will deteriorate within a few weeks. This implies that in subacute and chronic injuries the direct repair may become impossible or inadequate.[41]

In acute injuries, the first step is to assess and to classify the lesions. The type of SLIL injury (complete or partial, dorsal and/or volar) and the quality of the tissue of the ruptured ligament and associated ligaments and/or chondral lesions need to be known before starting open surgery. Arthroscopy is the gold standard in the diagnostic path of all carpal ligament lesions, and it is of utmost importance for the diagnosis of partial lesions of the SLIL, which would otherwise be very difficult to obtain. Open surgical approach is guided by the arthroscopic findings. The dorsal approach is the traditional way to manage the lesion of the SLIL ligament injury repairing the dorsal part of it according to the type of lesion found in arthroscopy. Traditional or short incisions are adopted due to the experience of the surgeon. However, we strongly suggest to

use the window approach[39,40] to the SLIL preserving the attachment of all the extrinsic ligaments and capsule to the dorsal part of the scaphoid, lunate, and triquetrum.[39,40] If the extrinsic ligaments are damaged, they have to be repaired, too.

The procedures used for the treatment of acute lesions of SLIL are direct ligament sutures or reinsertion with bone anchors and/or pin fixation.[12,41] All these procedures are based on the repair of the strong dorsal part of the SLIL, which is the most important portion from the biomechanical point of view. Fixation by bone anchors is the most frequent method to repair the SLIL, when it is detached from the lunate or scaphoid bone. Transosseous sutures have been almost abandoned and even if used they should be reinforced by a dorsal capsulodesis.[11,41,42] Pin fixation is used to reduce and maintain the correction of SLIL reduction and to protect the suture especially when the SL gap is wide, the scaphoid is flexed, and a dorsal intercalated segment instability (DISI) deformity is present.

In this situation one should consider associated ligament lesions. They need to be found and repaired. In partial or complete SLIL injuries without SL gap, a simple repair without pin fixation should be enough. The operated wrist is always splinted for 4 weeks in 25 degrees of extension.

11

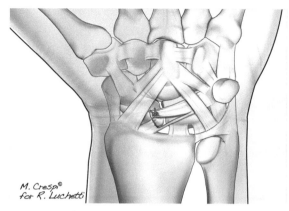

M. Crespi©
for R. Luchetti

Fig. 11.13 Volar capsulodesis of a volar scapholunate (SL) ligament injury according to van Kampen et al[44] using a ulnarly based flap harvested from the long radiolunate (LRL) ligament.

The most important dorsal component of the SLIL can most often be repaired directly. Its importance, however, should not be overemphasized. In low-demand patients, good status of the secondary stabilizers with compensatory effects from the adjacent capsule-ligamentous structures and the dynamic strength of "SL friendly" muscles[43] may sometimes effectively ensure good carpal stability, at least for some years.[43] However, in subjects with high functional demand, such as in athletes or hard workers, even a partial injury may have important consequences; therefore, a reparative procedure must be considered.

Mid-term follow-up showed good functional result after open SLIL repair: more than 70% of the patients had a significant improvement of pain and grip strength.[12]

Contemporary dorsal augmentation with capsulodesis after direct repair in a SLIL lesion also appears to be favorable in the short term in some patients.[30,31] However, the results appear to deteriorate both clinically and radiographically with time in patients who have high demands on their wrist.

The volar component of the SLL might be damaged only or associated with the dorsal part. Instrumental examinations like radiographs or MRI fail to demonstrate the lesion of the volar part of the ligament. Arthroscopy allows to recognize this lesion and to treat it correctly.[28] No open surgical procedures have been described and published for the management of an isolated volar SL lesion but only when associated with the dorsal SLIL component.[25,26,27] Marcuzzi et al[26,27] described 12 consecutive acute repairs of the palmar SLIL detached from the scaphoid (in association with the dorsal one) using bone anchors. An open volar approach, however, would require the access through important radiocarpal ligaments (radioscaphocapitate [RSC] and long radiolunate [LRL]). Thus, an arthroscopic or hybrid technique (arthroscopic assisted) should be suggested as a better and more anatomic solution[28] to treat this lesion. The volar capsulodesis proposed by van

Kampen et al[44] might be an optimal solution of reinforcement or augmentation in partial or complete SLIL injury with bad healing potential (▶ Fig. 11.13).

References

[1] Bergh TH, Lindau T, Bernardshaw SV, et al. A new definition of wrist sprain necessary after findings in a prospective MRI study. Injury. 2012; 43(10):1732–1742

[2] Jones WA. Beware the sprained wrist. The incidence and diagnosis of scapholunate instability. J Bone Joint Surg Br. 1988; 70(2):293–297

[3] Mudgal C, Hastings H. Scapho-lunate diastasis in fractures of the distal radius. Pathomechanics and treatment options. J Hand Surg [Br]. 1993; 18(6):725–729

[4] Geissler WB, Freeland AE, Savoie FH, McIntyre LW, Whipple TL. Intracarpal soft-tissue lesions associated with an intra-articular fracture of the distal end of the radius. J Bone Joint Surg Am. 1996; 78(3):357–365

[5] Herzberg G. Perilunate injuries, not dislocated (PLIND). J Wrist Surg. 2013; 2(4):337–345

[6] Schädel-Höpfner M, Junge A, Böhringer G. Scapholunate ligament injury occurring with scaphoid fracture: a rare coincidence? J Hand Surg [Br]. 2005; 30(2):137–142

[7] Caloia MF, Gallino RN, Caloia H, Rivarola H. Incidence of ligamentous and other injuries associated with scaphoid fractures during arthroscopically assisted reduction and percutaneous fixation. Arthroscopy. 2008; 24(7):754–759

[8] Ho PC, Hung LK, Lung TK. Acute ligament injury in scaphoid fracture. J Bone Joint Surg. 2000; 82B Suppl 1

[9] Jørgsholm P, Thomsen NOB, Björkman A, Besjakov J, Abrahamsson SO. The incidence of intrinsic and extrinsic ligament injuries in scaphoid waist fractures. J Hand Surg Am. 2010; 35(3):368–374

[10] Messina JC, Luchetti R. Combined scaphoid fractures and scapholunate ligament lesion. In: Herzberg G, ed. Scaphoide carpien 2010. Fractures and pseudoarthroses. Lyon: Sauramps Medical; 2010:135–139

[11] Linscheid RL, Dobyns JH. Treatment of scapholunate dissociation. Rotatory subluxation of the scaphoid. Hand Clin. 1992; 8(4):645–652

[12] Andersson JK. Treatment of scapholunate ligament injury: current concepts. EFORT Open Rev. 2017; 2(9):382–393

[13] Garcia-Elias M. Classification of SL instability. In: Shin & Day, eds. Advances in scapholunate ligament treatment. Chicago, IL: American Society for Surgery of the Hand; 2014

[14] Messina JC, Van Overstraeten L, Luchetti R, Fairplay T, Mathoulin CL. The EWAS Classification of scapholunate tears: an anatomical arthroscopic study. J Wrist Surg. 2013; 2(2):105–109

[15] Dao KD, Solomon DJ, Shin AY, Puckett ML. The efficacy of ultrasound in the evaluation of dynamic scapholunate ligamentous instability. J Bone Joint Surg Am. 2004; 86(7):1473–1478

[16] Ramamurthy NK, Chojnowski AJ, Toms AP. Imaging in carpal instability. J Hand Surg Eur Vol. 2016; 41(1):22–34

[17] Andersson JK, Andernord D, Karlsson J, Friden J. Efficacy of MRI and clinical test in diagnostics of wrist ligament injuries: a systematic review. Arthroscopy. 2015; 31:2014–2020

[18] Hafezi-Nejad N, Carrino JA, Eng J, et al. Scapholunate interosseous ligament tears: diagnostic performance of 1.5 T, 3 T MRI and MR arthrography—a systematic review and meta-analysis. Acad Radiol. 2016; 23(9):1091–1103

[19] De Santis S, Cozzolino R, Luchetti R, Cazzoletti L. Comparison between MRI and arthroscopy of the wrist for the assessment of posttraumatic lesions of intrinsic ligaments and the triangular fibrocartilage complex. J Wrist Surg. 2021; 11(1):28–34

[20] Cherian BS, Bhat AK, Rajagopal KV, Maddukuri SB, Paul D, Mathai NJ. Comparison of MRI & direct MR arthrography with arthroscopy in diagnosing ligament injuries of wrist. J Orthop. 2019; 19:203–207

[21] Geissler WB, Haley T. Arthroscopic management of scapholunate instability. Atlas Hand Clin. 2001; 6:253–274

III

[22] Swanstrom MM, Lee SK. Open treatment of acute scapholunate instability. Hand Clin. 2015; 31(3):425–436

[23] Short WH, Werner FW, Sutton LG. Dynamic biomechanical evaluation of the dorsal intercarpal ligament repair for scapholunate instability. J Hand Surg Am. 2009; 34(4):652–659

[24] Nikolopoulos FV, Apergis EP, Poulilios AD, Papagelopoulos PJ, Zoubos AV, Kefalas VA. Biomechanical properties of the scapholunate ligament and the importance of its portions in the capitate intrusion injury. Clin Biomech (Bristol, Avon). 2011; 26(8):819–823

[25] Dunn MJ, Johnson C. Static scapholunate dissociation: a new reconstruction technique using a volar and dorsal approach in a cadaver model. J Hand Surg Am. 2001; 26(4):749–754

[26] Marcuzzi A, Leti Acciaro A, Caserta G, Landi A. Ligamentous reconstruction of scapholunate dislocation through a double dorsal and palmar approach. J Hand Surg [Br]. 2006; 31(4):445–449

[27] Marcuzzi A, Ozben H, Russomando A. Experience chirurgicale de 12ans sur la reparation des ligaments scapholunaire dorsal et palmaire dans traitment chirurgical de la dissociation scapholunaire. Chir Main. 2013; 32:430–440

[28] Del Piñal F. Arthroscopic volar capsuloligamentous repair. J Wrist Surg. 2013; 2(2):126–128

[29] Berger RA, Bishop AT. A fiber-splitting capsulotomy technique for dorsal exposure of the wrist. Tech Hand Up Extrem Surg. 1997; 1(1): 2–10

[30] Cohen MS, Taleisnik J. Direct ligamentous repair of scapholunate dissociation with capsulodesis augmentation. Tech Hand Up Extrem Surg. 1998; 2(1):18–24

[31] Lavernia CJ, Cohen MS, Taleisnik J. Treatment of scapholunate dissociation by ligamentous repair and capsulodesis. J Hand Surg Am. 1992; 17(2):354–359

[32] Moran SL, Garcia-Elias M. Acute scapholunate injuries. In: Cooney WP III, ed. The wrist: diagnosis and operative treatment. 2nd ed. Philadelphia, PA: Wolters Kluwer, Lippincott, Williams & Wilkins; 2010:617–641

[33] Luchetti R, Pegoli I, Papini Zorli I, Garcia-Elias M. Le instabilità del carpo. In: Landi A, Catalano F, Luchetti R, eds. Trattato di Chirurgia della Mano. Roma. Verduci Editore, 2007:117–158

[34] Rosati M, Parchi P, Cacianti M, Poggetti A, Lisanti M. Treatment of acute scapholunate ligament injuries with bone anchor. Musculoskelet Surg. 2010; 94(1):25–32

[35] Haerle M, Wahegaonkar A, Garcia-Elias M, Bain G, Luchetti R. Part 2: Management of scapholunate dissociation. IFSSH Scientific Committee on Carpal Instability. 2016 https://docplayer.net/52308182-Ifssh-scientific-committee-on-carpal-instability.html

[36] Overstraeten LV, Camus EJ, Wahegaonkar A, et al. Anatomical description of the dorsal capsulo-scapholunate septum (DCSS)-arthroscopic staging of scapholunate instability after DCSS sectioning. J Wrist Surg. 2013; 2(2):149–154

[37] Elsaidi GA, Ruch DS, Kuzma GR, Smith BP. Dorsal wrist ligament insertions stabilize the scapholunate interval: cadaver study. Clin Orthop Relat Res. 2004(425):152–157

[38] Viegas SF, Yamaguchi S, Boyd NL, Patterson RM. The dorsal ligaments of the wrist: anatomy, mechanical properties, and function. J Hand Surg Am. 1999; 24(3):456–468

[39] Luchetti R, Atzei A, Cozzolino R, Fairplay T. Current role of open reconstruction of the scapholunate ligament. J Wrist Surg. 2013; 2 (2):116–125

[40] Loisel F, Wessel LE, Morse KW, Victoria C, Meyers KN, Wolfe SW. Is the dorsal fiber-splitting approach to the wrist safe? A kinematic analysis and introduction of the "window" approach. J Hand Surg Am. 2021; 46(12):1079–1087

[41] Garcia-Elias M. Carpal instability. In: Wolfe SW, Hotchkiss RN, Pederson WC, Kozin SH, eds. Green's operative hand surgery. Vol. 1. 6th ed. New York: Elsevier Churchill Livingstone; 2011:465–522

[42] Wolfe SW, Kakar P. Carpal instability. In: Wolfe SW, Pederson WC, Kozin SH, Cohen MS, eds. Green's operative hand surgery. 8th ed. New York: Elsevier; 2021:488–562

[43] Esplugas M, Garcia-Elias M, Lluch A, Llusá Pérez M. Role of muscles in the stabilization of ligament-deficient wrists. J Hand Ther. 2016; 29 (2):166–174

[44] van Kampen RJ, Bayne CO, Moran SL. A new technique for volar capsulodesis for isolated palmar scapholunate interosseous ligament injuries: a cadaveric study and case report. J Wrist Surg. 2015; 4(4): 239–245

11

12 Acute "R"epair: Arthroscopic Treatment

Vicente Carratalá Baixauli, Fernando Corella, Francisco J. Lucas García, Eva Guisasola Lerma, and Cristóbal Martínez Andrade

Abstract

Scapholunate ligament (SLL) injury is the most frequent injury of the intrinsic carpal ligaments. The dorsal part of the SLL is the most important part for the stability of the scapholunate joint. The reattachment of the SLL is indicated in acute injuries. Arthroscopy is the gold standard for diagnosing scapholunate injuries and allows to perform a repair/reattachment of the SLL with dorsal and volar capsular reinforcement, reproducing the treatment conducted by open surgery, but avoiding injury to the soft tissue caused by damage to the secondary dorsal stabilizers; the dorsal blood supply; and in many cases, the proprioceptive innervation of the posterior interosseous nerve. The techniques described in this chapter can be performed to repair the dorsal and volar parts of the SLL on acute isolated injuries and those associated with distal radius fractures, carpal fractures, or perilunate injuries.

Keywords: arthroscopy, scapholunate ligament, acute injury, reinsertion, dorsal scapholunate septum

12.1 Introduction

Scapholunate ligament (SLL) injury is the lesion that most commonly occurs in the intrinsic ligaments of the carpus.[1]

The dorsal aspect of the SLL is the thickest and most resistant and plays the most important role in scapholunate stability, mainly due to its attachment to the dorsal capsule.[2] The dorsal capsuloligamentous scapholunate septum (DCSS) is also part of the scapholunate complex, joining the ligament to the dorsal capsule and the dorsal intercarpal ligament, and it has been demonstrated that it plays an important role in scapholunate stability.[3]

However, the injury of the scapholunate goes from volar to dorsal, so in several cases an isolated rupture of the volar side can be found (a Grade IIIA of the EWAS classification[2]) or combined with a dorsal injury (a Grade IIIC, IV, and V of the EWAS classification[2]).

The reattachment of the SLL is indicated in acute injuries. Unfortunately, an early diagnosis of SLL injury is uncommon because this injury is diagnosed as wrist pain in most of the patients, which delays the use of a magnetic resonance imaging (MRI) and/or arthroscopy by 6 to 8 weeks. However, this condition can be found frequently associated to other lesions such as bone fractures (scaphoid, distal radius, etc.) and perilunate injuries.

SLL injuries are reportedly common with distal radius fractures (16–40%)[4] and are also associated to scaphoid fractures.[5] The use of arthroscopy in the treatment of the distal radius fractures and carpal fractures allows us to make this diagnosis, among other advantages. The healing potential of scapholunate injuries is limited, and treatment must be done during the acute phase of the injury to achieve better results.[6]

- The arthroscopy is the gold standard for diagnosing scapholunate injuries and allows to perform a repair/reattachment of the SLL with dorsal and volar capsular reinforcement reproducing the treatment conducted by open surgery but avoiding the damage of the soft tissues and blood supply that is inherent to the open approach.[7,8]

Several arthroscopic or arthroscopy-assisted treatments have been described for SLL injuries, but only a few are aimed at primary repair of the ligament, especially its dorsal and volar aspect.

Arthroscopy-assisted reduction and temporary fixation with Kirschner wires (K-wire) is indicated for acute, Geissler II-III injuries. Fixation should be maintained for a minimum of 6 to 8 weeks.[9,10]

This technique has given varying results. The best results were observed in a series of patients with Geissler Grade II-III acute or subacute injuries and incomplete scapholunate tears.[11] The results of complete SLL injuries and those of patients who were not treated during the acute phase were considerably worse.[12]

In cases of an acute complete rupture of the SLL (Geissler Grade IV) with a repairable dorsal ligament, the recommended conventional treatment is direct repair using an open dorsal approach, with direct suture, transosseous suture, or reinsertion with bone anchors, sometimes in combination with capsular reinforcement or dorsal capsulodesis.[7,13] This repair can be performed in combination with temporary fixation with K-wire or with fixation by placing a screw between the scaphoid and semilunar bones, thereby allowing for earlier recovery of movement.[6] Satisfactory results have been published with open SLL repair techniques[7,13,14] but they are associated with significant wrist stiffness.

In addition to damaging soft tissues and increasing fibrosis and joint rigidity, the dorsal wrist approach used for treating scapholunate injuries almost always injures the posterior interosseous nerve (PIN), which is involved in the proprioception of the SLL[15] and can be fundamental for dynamic stability and functional recovery. Moreover, during the approach and the dorsal and volar capsulotomy, there is also a significant aggression on the vascular supply to the SLL, which impairs its healing capacity. Finally, the secondary stabilizers are also affected by this surgical approach.[16]

There are reports of dorsal and palmar arthroscopic capsuloligamentous suturing techniques.[3,17] After publication of their studies, Mathoulin et al[3] demonstrated that arthroscopy-guided dorsal capsuloplasty gave promising results in the short term with regard to improving pain, mobility of the wrist, strength, and reduction in the scapholunate angle. There is only one arthroscopic technique to perform a volar reinforcement, which has been published by del Piñal.[17] In this technique, an all-inside arthroscopic suture of the volar SLL and capsule is performed without suture anchors, that is, by means of a needle inserted just ulnar to flexor carpi radialis.

With the development of arthroscopy techniques, it is now possible to perform a treatment similar to that described for open surgery, with reinsertion of the dorsal portion of the SLL, and to add a dorsal capsular reinforcement over the repair performed,[8] thereby reproducing the dorsal capsuloligamentous union (DCSS) which has been described as an important element in scapholunate stability.[18]

12.2 Indications

- The ideal candidates are patients with a partial or complete injury, whether acute or subacute, with competent secondary stabilizers and without chondral involvement. In such cases the SLL still preserves some potential for healing and the state of the tissue permits direct repair or reinforcement.
- This technique can be performed on acute isolated injuries of the SLL and those associated with distal radius fractures,[7] carpal fractures, or perilunate injuries.

12.3 Technique

As the reattachment is performed to the bone, small anchors are needed. No specific implant is required and it can be performed with any type of small anchor with 2/0 threads. Along with the anchor, a lasso to recover the threads is needed (it can be a lasso from a commercial company or a16-G Abbocath loaded with a thread loop). Finally, a small knot pusher is needed to retrieve the threads from volar to dorsal.

12.4 Scapholunate Dorsal Capsuloligament Reattachment

The arthroscopic portals used for this technique are: 3–4, 6 R, midcarpal ulnar (MCU), and midcarpal radial (MCR).

12.4.1 Step 1: Insertion of the Anchor and Ligamentous Suture

With the scope in the 6 R portal, 3–4 portal is used as a working portal to introduce a bone anchor into the dorsal and proximal edge of the scaphoid or lunate bone, depending on where the SLL has been detached (▶ Fig. 12.1).

A TFCC SutureLasso 70° (Arthrex, Naples, FL) is used from the 3–4 portal, to pass through the dorsal part of the SLL, recovering the Nitinol loop through the same portal (▶ Fig. 12.1, ▶ Fig. 12.2). Using the loop, one of the sutures' ends of the implant is passed through the detached edge of the ligament and is pulled out again through the 3–4 portal (▶ Fig. 12.3).

Sometimes more than one anchor is needed to repair the dorsal part of the SLL. The position of the implants in the scaphoid, the lunate, or both will depend on the location and characteristics of the injury.

Using a knot pusher, we tie both sutures in a sliding knot over the implant, leaving a simple stitch through the SLL with the sutures tied and uncut because these sutures will be used for the following dorsal plication (▶ Fig. 12.4).

Sometimes there is not enough ligament tissue to complete the reinsertion, in that situation the anchor can be placed in the midcarpal space, performing a Mathoulin-like capsuloligamentous plication but using a bone anchor to strengthen the reconstruction.

12.4.2 Step 2: Dorsal Capsulodesis (Dorsal Capsular Reinforcement)

With the scope in the 6 R portal, a 18G needle is introduced with one of the implant's sutures inside through

12

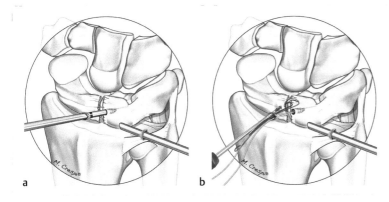

a b

Fig. 12.1 (a) Introduction of the anchor through the 3–4 portal. **(b)** Recovering one of the implant's suture through the 3–4 portal using the nitinol loop of the SutureLasso 70° (Arthrex, Naples, FL).

III

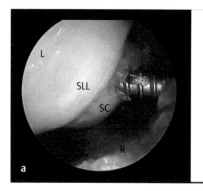 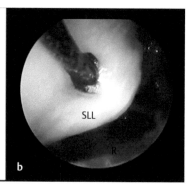

Fig. 12.2 View from the 6 R portal. **(a)** A 2.2 mm Micro Corkscrew suture anchor (Arthrex, Naples, FL) is introduced in the dorsal and proximal margins of the scaphoid or lunate bone, depending on where the SLL has detached. **(b)** A TFCC Sutur-eLasso of 70° (Arthrex, Naples, FL) from 3–4 is used to cross the remains of the SLL from dorsal to proximal, recovering the Nitinol loop through the same portal. L, lunate); R, radius); SC, scaphoid; SLL, scapholunate ligament.

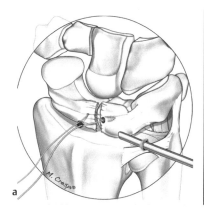 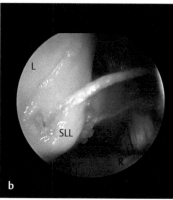

Fig. 12.3 (a) One of the sutures' ends of the implant is passed through the detached edge of the ligament and is pulled out through the 3–4 portal. **(b)** View from the 6 R portal. Passing one of the sutures through the detached ligament. L, lunate; R, radius; SLL, scapholunate ligament.

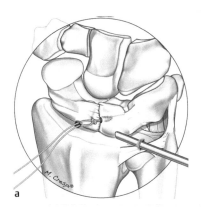 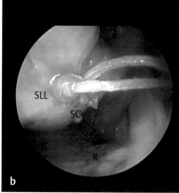

Fig. 12.4 (a) The two ends of the suture are tied with a sliding knot over the implant, leaving a simple stitch through the SLL with the suture end uncut. L, lunate; R, radius); SC, scaphoid; SLL, scapholunate ligament. **(b)** View from the 6 R portal. The sliding knot is performed through the 3–4 portal using a knot pusher.

the 3–4 portal, passing through the ligament's tissue toward the midcarpal joint (▶ Fig. 12.5).

Changing the arthroscope to the MCU portal, the suture introduced through the needle is recovered, using a grasper, through the MCR portal.

As a result, one of the implant's suture will enter the 3–4 portal, crossing the SLL from the radiocarpal space through to the midcarpal joint and exiting through the MCR portal.

The MCR suture is recovered from the 3–4 portal incision through the space in between the dorsal capsule and

the extensor tendons. The risk of trapping the EDC tendons in the suture is very low because these portals are created in the radial edge of the extensor digitorum communis (EDC) and the suture is recovered parallel to the tendons.

With the scope in the 6 R portal, the implant sutures are tied again, withdrawing traction. The closure of the dorsal interval of the scapholunate with the capsular plication performed by reconstructing the dorsal capsuloligamentous union of the SLL complex can be seen.

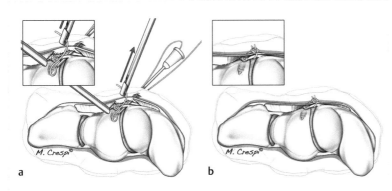

Fig. 12.5 **(a)** A 18G needle is used to pass one of the implant's sutures through the 3–4 portal, passing through the ligament's tissue toward the midcarpal joint. The suture is recovered through the midcarpal radial (MCR) portal. The MCR suture is recovered from the 3–4 portal incision through the space in between the dorsal capsule and the extensor tendons. **(b)** The implant sutures are tied again. The closure of the dorsal interval of the scapholunate with the capsular plication reconstructs the dorsal capsuloligamentous union of the scapholunate ligament complex.

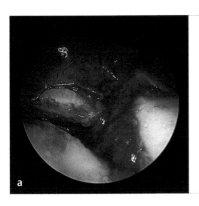
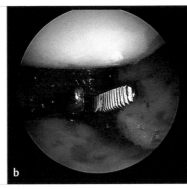

Fig. 12.6 **(a)** View from the ulnar midcarpal (UMC) portal. There is an acute injury of the volar portion of the scapholunate ligament, with a small fragment of the volar ulnar corner of the lunate bone. **(b)** The capsular portal is made just over the scapholunate joint, through the tear of the injury.

12.5 Scapholunate Volar Capsuloligament Reattachment (Video 12.1)

Apart from the four common dorsal wrist portals, 3–4, 6 R, ulnar midcarpal (UMC), and radial midcarpal (RMC), to perform volar repair, the volar radial (VR) portal popularized by Slutsky[19] is required. This portal may be used to perform the volar reattachment or reinforcement of the volar portion of the SLL and the reattachment of the radioscaphocapitate ligament.

12.5.1 Step 1: Volar Portal Establishment

After the performance of the dorsal portals and with the scope located in the dorsal side, the volar radial portal is performed.

Once the capsular plane has been reached through the approach of the portals, the "capsular portal" should be performed. It is useful to locate the light of the arthroscope just over the position where the portal is to be performed. With transillumination, it is easier to achieve an exact position for the portal.

In some acute cases, the detachment of the volar ligaments can be used as the capsular portal (▶ Fig. 12.6).

12.5.2 Step 2: Anchor Placement

In acute cases the anchor is positioned in the bone area, where the ligament has been detached. Normally the introduction of the K-wire (if necessary) and anchor is performed under direct visualization, looking with the scope through the MCR portal (▶ Fig. 12.7).

Sometimes, if there is a midsubstance injury, or the avulsion is not easily identified, the anchor can be placed in either the lunate or the scaphoid bones.

12.5.3 Step 3: Capsuloligamentous Suture and Knotting

The arthroscope is placed in the ulnar midcarpal portal. A knot pusher is introduced inside the joint from the dorsal portal located in front of the portion to repair and then advanced through the volar capsule portal. This way the knot pusher can be advanced inside the volar approach (VR) where the threads of the anchor are also located.

The knot pusher is loaded with the two threads and retrieved to the dorsal portal (▶ Fig. 12.8).

A 16G Abbocath loaded with a loop is used to pierce the volar ligament that needs to be reattached. The loop is captured from the dorsal portal, where the threads are located, and then loaded with the first thread. Now the

12

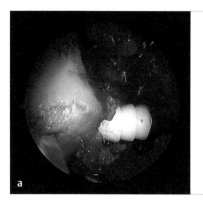
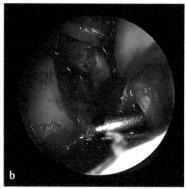

Fig. 12.7 (a,b) View from the radial mid-carpal (RMC) portal. The anchor is introduced through the volar radial (VR) portal, in the detached area of the ligament in the lunate. The threads remain inside the volar portal.

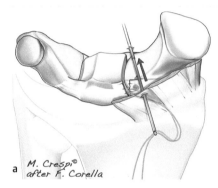
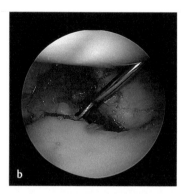
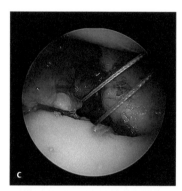

M. Crespi®
after F. Corella

Fig. 12.8 (a) Drawing for explaining how the threads of the anchor are captured from the RMC portal with the knot pusher. **(b)** The arthroscope is in the ulnar midcarpal (UMC) portal. The knot pusher is introduced from the radial midcarpal (RMC) portal, advanced inside the volar radial (VR) portal and loaded with the threads of the anchor. **(c)** The threads are retrieved to the RMC portal.

loaded loop is taken to the volar portal. This way the first limb of the "U" capsuloligamentous suture is performed (▶ Fig. 12.9).

The same procedure is performed again for the second limb of the "U" capsuloligamentous suture (▶ Fig. 12.10).

Finally, both threads are knotted; this way the volar capsuloligamentous tissue is reattached or reinforced to the bone, maintaining the knot out of the wrist (▶ Fig. 12.11).

If K-wires are needed for the pathology (for example in perilunate injuries), they should be positioned before the anchor, while maintaining the traction of the wrist. But if there is no need of K-wires, traction should be removed before the knot is performed.

12.6 Postoperative Period

After surgery, a forearm splint is placed that allows the patient to move fingers and elbow. After 2 weeks, the stitches are removed, maintaining the forearm splint up to 4 weeks, when the secondary K-wireis removed and a removable wrist brace is placed. Four weeks postoperatively, after removing the forearm splint, the patient starts specific rehabilitation treatment.[20]

12.7 Discussion

Scapholunate dissociation is the most common cause of acquired carpal instability. The natural course of scapholunate dissociation without treatment is still unclear.

Restoration with preservation of the anatomy and function of the SLL after traumatic dissociation is a formidable challenge for hand surgeons. The literature contains innumerable references in this respect, relating to a great variety of surgical procedures that aim to restore the interrupted carpal architecture.

What has been demonstrated by several studies is that the treatment of acute SLL injuries generally yields better results than treatment of chronic lesions.[9] The ideal time for performing a repair in the acute phase is not well defined: the intercarpal ligaments degenerate rapidly in the first 2 to 6 weeks, after which primary repair or reinsertion may be difficult, and with an often poor result due to poor tissue quality and poor healing capacity.[6] Although isolated acute SLL injures are diagnosed late, this condition is usually associated to other lesions like distal radius fractures or scaphoid fractures. In these cases, an arthroscopic repair can be performed.

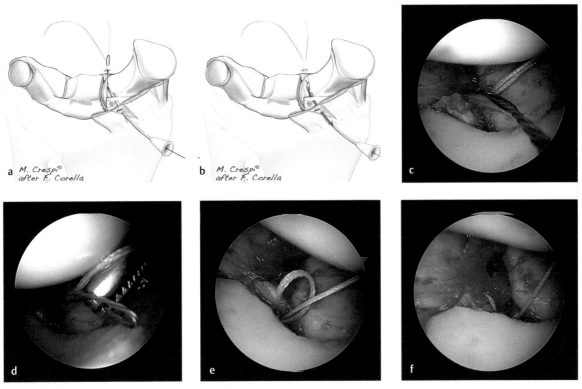

Fig. 12.9 **(a,b)** Drawing for explaining how the first limb of the "U" suture is performed. **(c)** The Abbocath loaded with a loop is introduced just over the avulsed fragment. **(d)** The loop is captured and taken to the radial midcarpal (RMC) portal, where it is loaded with the first thread. **(e,f)** The loop is recovered to the volar portal along with the first thread, capturing the ulnar portion of the detached ligaments. The first limb of the "U" suture is completed.

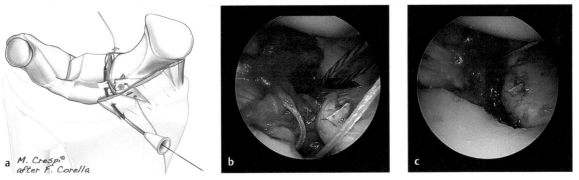

Fig. 12.10 **(a)** Drawing for explaining how the second limb of the "U" suture is performed. **(b)** The Abbocath pierces the volar ligaments from a more radial position. The loop is taken to the radial midcarpal (RMC) portal and loaded with the second thread. **(c)** The loop and thread are retrieved to the volar portal, so the second limb of the "U" suture is completed.

The dorsal portion of the SLL is the thickest and the strongest one.[21,22] For this reason, most surgical treatments to repair acute injuries are focused on this portion. Several arthroscopic techniques have been described for the treatment of acute SLL injuries such as thermal shrinkage, debridement and reduction, and K-wire fixation.[23]

The authors described an arthroscopic repair of the dorsal portion of the SLL using bone anchors associated to a dorsal arthroscopic capsulodesis.[8]

The volar scapholunate reattachment allows a direct repair to bone of an acute torn volar ligament. It is usually performed along with a dorsal repair and K-wires for sta-

12

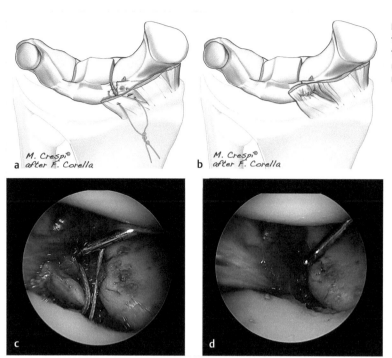

a M. Crespi® after F. Corella

b M. Crespi® after F. Corella

c

d

Fig. 12.11 (a,b) Drawing for explaining the final position of the threads. **(c,d)** The two threads are knotted outside of the joint, reattaching the avulsed capsule and ligament to the detached area of the lunate.

bilizing the scapholunate joint if an acute and complete lesion is found.

The preferred open surgery method for treating acute injuries is direct repair of the ligament using bone anchors or transosseous tunnels, sometimes in combination with dorsal capsulodesis and fixation with K-wire.[24] In the survey by Zarkadas et al[25] more than two-thirds of the interviewees preferred direct repair with (44%) or without (33%) associated dorsal capsulodesis. However, the arthroscopic techniques described to date for acute injuries did not reproduce the open surgery treatment and in many cases were limited to arthroscopic reduction and fixation with K-wire.[1] The results of this technique in complete SLL injuries and those of patients who were not treated during the acute phase were poor with satisfactory results being achieved only in 55% of cases.[12]

With the development of arthroscopy techniques, it is now possible to perform a treatment similar to that described for open surgery, with reinsertion of the dorsal portion of the scapholunate ligament, and to add dorsal capsular reinforcement over the repair performed,[8,26] thereby reproducing the dorsal capsuloligamentous union (DCSS) described as an important element in scapholunate stability.

The results published on scapholunate reinsertion using open surgery have been satisfactory regarding scapholunate stability when the treatment was performed in the acute phase of the lesion.[27,30] However, the treatment has been linked to greater joint stiffness and restricted motion due to the surgical approach, scarring, and association of dorsal capsulodesis.[28,29]

The authors studied 19 patients with acute SLL injury treated with this technique.[26] Prospective follow-up of the patients was performed with systematic collection of data preoperatively and at 6 and 12 months.

At 12 months, 79% of patients presented with good or excellent results according to the Mayo Wrist Score, with significant improvement in grip strength and QuickDASH score.

The reduction in range of motion was markedly lower than that published after open surgery, with a mean loss of only 10 degrees (0–20 degrees) compared with the contralateral wrist, probably due to the lower degree of soft tissue aggression, less scar tissue, and the fact that the dorsal reinforcement performed is much more selective and limited in space than that performed using open capsulodesis techniques.

Only two patients had a poor outcome and needed a second operation. In both cases, an arthroscopy-assisted scapholunate ligamentoplasty was performed. These cases that required a second surgery due to a poor outcome with the initial suture corresponded to patients who were treated at a later stage, probably related to loss of healing capacity after the first weeks.

12.8 Conclusions

The arthroscopic technique for repair/reattachment of the SLL with dorsal/volar capsular reinforcement allows a reliable and stable primary repair of the dorsal aspect of the ligament in acute or subacute scapholunate injuries where there is tissue that can potentially be repaired, thus achieving an anatomical repair similar to that obtained with open surgery, but without the complications and stiffness secondary to the injury of the soft tissues that is inherent to the open dorsal and volar approach.

References

[1] Manuel J, Moran SL. The diagnosis and treatment of scapholunate instability. Hand Clin. 2010; 26(1):129–144

[2] Bednar JM. Acute scapholunate ligament injuries: arthroscopic treatment. Hand Clin. 2015; 31(3):417–423

[3] Mathoulin CL, Dauphin N, Wahegaonkar AL. Arthroscopic dorsal capsuloligamentous repair in chronic scapholunate ligament tears. Hand Clin. 2011; 27(4):563–572, xi

[4] Desai MJ, Kamal RN, Richard MJ. Management of intercarpal ligament injuries associated with distal radius fractures. Hand Clin. 2015; 31 (3):409–416

[5] Jørgsholm P, Thomsen NO, Björkman A, Besjakov J, Abrahamsson SO. The incidence of intrinsic and extrinsic ligament injuries in scaphoid waist fractures. J Hand Surg Am. 2010; 35(3):368–374

[6] Garcia-Elias M. Carpal instability. In: Wolfe SW, Hotchkiss RN, Pederson WC, Kozin SH, eds. Green's operative hand surgery. Vol. 1. 6th ed. New York: Elsevier Churchill Livingstone; 2011:465–522

[7] Luchetti R, Atzei A, Cozzolino R, Fairplay T. Current role of open reconstruction of the scapholunate ligament. J Wrist Surg. 2013; 2(2): 116–125

[8] Carratalá V, Lucas FJ, Miranda I, Sánchez Alepuz E, González Jofré C. Arthroscopic scapholunate capsuloligamentous repair: suture with dorsal capsular reinforcement for scapholunate ligament lesion. Arthrosc Tech. 2017; 6(1):e113–e120

[9] Geissler WB. Arthroscopic management of scapholunate instability. J Wrist Surg. 2013; 2(2):129–135

[10] Whipple TL. The role of arthroscopy in the treatment of scapholunate instability. Hand Clin. 1995; 11(1):37–40

[11] White NJ, Rollick NC. Injuries of the scapholunate interosseous ligament: an update. J Am Acad Orthop Surg. 2015; 23(11):691–703

[12] Darlis NA, Kaufmann RA, Giannoulis F, Sotereanos DG. Arthroscopic debridement and closed pinning for chronic dynamic scapholunate instability. J Hand Surg Am. 2006; 31(3):418–424

[13] Szabo RM. Scapholunate ligament repair with capsulodesis reinforcement. J Hand Surg Am. 2008; 33(9):1645–1654

[14] Kalainov DM, Cohen MS. Treatment of traumatic scapholunate dissociation. J Hand Surg Am. 2009; 34(7):1317–1319

[15] Hagert E, Persson JK. Desensitizing the posterior interosseous nerve alters wrist proprioceptive reflexes. J Hand Surg Am. 2010; 35(7): 1059–1066

[16] Elsaidi GA, Ruch DS, Kuzma GR, Smith BP. Dorsal wrist ligament insertions stabilize the scapholunate interval: cadaver study. Clin Orthop Relat Res. 2004(425):152–157

[17] Del Piñal F. Arthroscopic volar capsuloligamentous repair. J Wrist Surg. 2013; 2(2):126–128

[18] Tommasini Carrara de Sambuy M, Burgess TM, Cambon-Binder A, Mathoulin CL. The anatomy of the dorsal capsulo-scapholunate septum: a cadaveric study. J Wrist Surg. 2017; 6(3):244–247

[19] Slutsky DJ. Wrist arthroscopy through a volar radial portal. Arthroscopy. 2002; 18(6):624–630

[20] Lerma EG, Baixauli VC, Selma FC, Garcia FL. The role of rehabilitation after repair of wrist injuries. Revista Iberoamericana de Cirugía de la Mano. 2016; 44:131–142

[21] Berger RA. The gross and histologic anatomy of the scapholunate interosseous ligament. J Hand Surg Am. 1996; 21(2):170–178

[22] Sokolow C, Saffar P. Anatomy and histology of the scapholunate ligament. Hand Clin. 2001; 17(1):77–81

[23] Rohman EM, Agel J, Putnam MD, Adams JE. Scapholunate interosseous ligament injuries: a retrospective review of treatment and outcomes in 82 wrists. J Hand Surg Am. 2014; 39(10):2020–2026

[24] Swanstrom MM, Lee SK. Open treatment of acute scapholunate instability. Hand Clin. 2015; 31(3):425–436

[25] Zarkadas PC, Gropper PT, White NJ, Perey BH. A survey of the surgical management of acute and chronic scapholunate instability. J Hand Surg Am. 2004; 29(5):848–857

[26] Carratalá V, Lucas FJ, Miranda I, Prada A, Guisasola E, Miranda FJ. Arthroscopic reinsertion of acute injuries of the scapholunate ligament: technique and results. J Wrist Surg. 2020; 9(4):328–337

[27] Pomerance J. Outcome after repair of the scapholunate interosseous ligament and dorsal capsulodesis for dynamic scapholunate instability due to trauma. J Hand Surg Am. 2006; 31(8):1380–1386

[28] Bickert B, Sauerbier M, Germann G. Scapholunate ligament repair using the Mitek bone anchor. J Hand Surg [Br]. 2000; 25(2):188–192

[29] Rosati M, Parchi P, Cacianti M, Poggetti A, Lisanti M. Treatment of acute scapholunate ligament injuries with bone anchor. Musculoskelet Surg. 2010; 94(1):25–32

[30] Minami A, Kato H, Iwasaki N. Treatment of scapholunate dissociation: ligamentous repair associated with modified dorsal capsulodesis. Hand Surg. 2003; 8(1):1–6

12

13 Chronic "R"einforcement (Capsulodesis): Open Treatment of Chronic SL Injury

Weston Ryan and Robert M. Szabo

Abstract

Capsulodesis for the treatment of chronic scapholunate (SL) injury can be a valuable method for restoring carpal stability. The goal of capsulodesis involves reduction of the SL interval by adding a restraint to scaphoid flexion and reinforcement using local capsuloligamentous tissue to counter the pathomechanics of carpal instability. There have been mixed reported outcomes in the literature over time, though technical modifications have yielded results as good as any other current option and confirmed capsulodesis as a viable surgical option for patients with chronic SL injury. The authors describe their preferred surgical technique of the dorsal intercarpal capsulodesis.

Keywords: capsulodesis, carpal instability, dorsal intercarpal ligament, scapholunate, SLAC, DISI

13.1 Introduction and Historical Perspective

13.1.1 Scapholunate Injury Overview

Wrist injuries are common, can be caused by a variety of mechanisms, and represent a significant number of patients evaluated in the clinical and acute care setting. Ligamentous wrist injury can be seen in 20 to 30% or more[1,3] of patients with traumatic wrist injuries and frequently can be missed initially when a more obvious fracture is present.[4] Importantly, carpal ligament injury can manifest as carpal instability, which if not treated in a timely manner, can trigger the progression of early arthritis. Several types of carpal instability have been described and classified, characterized by carpal kinematics, alignment, and predictable patterns of joint arthrosis. Scapholunate interosseous ligament (SLIL) injury is the most common cause of carpal instability.[5,6]

It is important to note that instability does not imply misalignment on radiograph, or vice versa. Many iterations and classification systems have been proposed over the past 50 years to encompass the complex nature of carpal instability.[7,11] Instability is present when there is aberrant kinematics through the carpus' arc of motion, inability to bear load in a stable position, or malalignment associated with symptoms.[11] A widely accepted classification of scapholunate (SL) instability originally described by Watson et al further outlines the behavior of the carpus with SL injury; the detailed mechanics of which are discussed elsewhere.[12] In brief, if malalignment is apparent on standard radiographs, then the instability is

termed "static." If instability is only present with stress examination or stress imaging studies, then it is termed "dynamic." Additionally, differentiating if the static SL dissociation is reducible will guide decision making further. It is essential to recognize the nature of the instability being referenced both when treating patients and when reviewing literature, as often it can be unclear or unreported by grouping dynamic and static patients together which clouds the interpretation of reported outcomes.

Overall, the SL ligament represents an important centerpiece for carpal stability, and when injured and left untreated, it can lead to scapholunate advance collapse (SLAC) with chronic pain and progressive loss of function. A stereotypical pattern of joint arthrosis develops that is well described. The goals of treating SLIL injury is to: (1) alleviate pain; (2) restore the anatomic intercarpal relationships, and thus articular kinematics (3) be durable; (4) maintain motion; (5) have low morbidity; (6) prevent premature arthritic changes that may become painful and necessitate wrist salvage procedures. This review will focus on chronic SL instability and its surgical management with open capsulodesis which satisfies the first five criteria above. No procedure described so far to the authors' knowledge satisfies the above fifth criteria over the long term.

13.1.2 Overview of Open Surgical Techniques and Indications

Direct SLIL repair alone and reconstruction with autograft, local tissue, and allograft has been well described, and predominately advocated for patients with intact repairable tissue, reducible articulations, and good healing potential.[13,18] Outside of the acute phase of injury, attempts at late ligamentous repair, soft tissue reconstruction, and augmentation have failed to maintain carpal alignment consistently and predictably over time.[18,21] This likely can be attributed to attenuation of the proximal row secondary stabilizing ligaments (scaphotrapezial [ST], scaphocapitate [SC], and radioscaphocapitate [RSC]) with chronic static SL dissociation, as well as the axial load from the capitate, slow healing, and prolonged postoperative immobilization.[22] Additionally, the scaphoid can assume a relatively fixed flexed and pronated position, further resisting direct SL reduction and creating a persistent dorsal intercalated segment instability (DISI) pattern. Therefore, proper patient selection and appropriate diagnosis (i.e., identifying subacute injury and static vs dynamic instability) is critical when considering the reported results of surgical intervention for symptomatic chronic SLIL injuries.

Many surgical options exist to address chronic SL dissociation, with continued modifications and technique adjustments described over time. However, there is a paucity of literature on surgical intervention producing reliable and favorable outcomes in long-term follow-up, indicating the difficult nature of treating this injury. Dynamic versus static instability is not the only factor in deciding surgical management as many procedures for chronic SL injury have reported good results in both populations. Procedures involve either arthrodesis or soft tissue reconstruction to counter the pathologic carpal motion believed to be associated with carpal arthrosis. Limited arthrodesis procedures sacrifice a lot of motion, and carpal contact pressures are altered and have been shown to precipitate arthrosis. Because of these limitations with arthrodesis, soft tissue reconstruction or reinforcement procedures have become the preferred option to restore SL kinematics in cases of flexible carpal instability. Soft tissue procedures can be in the form of ligament reconstruction, such as dorsal SLIL autograft, tendon ligamentoplasty such as the Brunelli procedure and its multiple variants, bone-ligament-bone grafts, and dorsal capsulodesis. Capsulodesis will be the focus of this section as other procedures are discussed in depth elsewhere in this book. In general, contraindications to capsulodesis or other "reinforcement"-type procedures are irreducible static SL dissociation and significant carpal arthrosis. This population is better served by arthrodesis or some other form of salvage procedure.

13.2 Capsulodesis: Literature Review and Surgical Considerations

The goal of dorsal wrist capsulodesis is to utilize local ligamentous tissues to restore carpal alignment and kinematics. To directly approach the problem of scaphoid flexion seen in chronic SL instability, Blatt described in 1987 a soft tissue tether using a flap of the dorsal radiocarpal wrist capsule (not ligamentous tissue) inserted onto the distal scaphoid pole.[23] Results using this capsulodesis as originally described were somewhat favorable,[19,23] though repeat studies and long-term follow-up showed progressive carpal collapse and SL widening.[24,26] The technique as originally described has fallen out of favor; however, the concept of capsulodesis has endured. Multiple modifications have been subsequently described, including utilizing the dorsal intercarpal ligament (DIL) across the radiocarpal joint,[27] and other different attachment points.

Capsulodesis should ideally address the pathomechanics of the SL injury, with the vector of resisted force aiding in SL interval reduction as well as the DISI deformity from scaphoid flexion. Attention must be paid to the origin, insertion, anchoring, and tension of any capsulodesis construct to ensure a durable carpal reduction while not substantially limiting motion. Berger described a technique utilizing a slip of the DIL originating from the triquetrum to the dorsal-proximal lunate in an attempt to maintain scaphoid reduction.[28] SL compression by the capsular flap after SL reduction is the primary mode of resistance of scaphoid flexion in this type of capsulodesis. The inherent pitfall with capsulodesis crossing the radiocarpal joint is restriction in range of motion (ROM). In Blatt's series, there was a 20-degree loss in wrist flexion. This was similarly seen in later studies, both with techniques similar to Blatt's and Berger's.[19,25,26,29,30] Moran et al reported on 14 patients who underwent Berger-type dorsal capsulodesis and found a significant decrease in wrist flexion-extension by about 30%, as well as no significant change in SL gap and scaphoid flexion at final follow-up compared to preoperative measures.[30] In the final analysis and long-term follow-up, dorsal capsulodesis for chronic SL instability by nearly all techniques had inconsistent results in preventing radiocarpal arthrosis. Pain, however, was typically improved postoperatively, though not fully relieved in all patients.

The dorsal intercarpal ligament capsulodesis (DILC) was proposed to adapt the capsulodesis concept to address scaphoid flexion more directly while avoid hindering radiocarpal motion.[31] As originally described by Slater and Szabo, the major portion of the DIL is taken from its trapezium insertion and attached to the distal and radial aspect of the scaphoid under tension, providing a dorsal and ulnar directed force to the scaphoid. Thus, scaphoid flexion and SL diastasis are addressed, respectively (► Fig. 13.1). Initial cadaveric biomechanical studies showed reduced SL gap, and improved scaphoid flexion with DILC when directly compared to a traditional Blatt capsulodesis.[32] In 2 years' follow-up of static SL instability patients, the DILC reconstruction maintained the SL reduction and had overall good clinical outcomes, making it a promising technique.[33] Since the introduction of this technique, the role of the DIL in SL stability has been robustly explored. Cadaveric dissections, along with further histologic and magnetic resonance imaging, have characterized the DIL attachments with the lunate and scaphoid, as well as areas of adherence to the dorsal SLIL.[34,36] Biomechanical study of cadavers with progressive ligamentous sectioning further maintained the structural role the DIL can play on both SL diastasis and lunate and scaphoid angulation. Mitsuyasu et al showed that radiolunate angle was unchanged with dorsal SLIL transection, though significantly increased with isolated release of the DIC from its lunate attachment (► Fig. 13.2).[37] Similarly, with better understanding of the key role the dorsal SLIL and DIL play in carpal stability, Viegas et al had described a transverse capsulodesis using the DIL for SLIL reconstruction which retains the anatomic origin and insertions, and directly attaches the DIL to both the scaphoid and the lunate.[38,39] Early 2 years' follow-up results were promising, with clinical results showing maintained

13

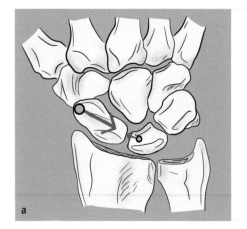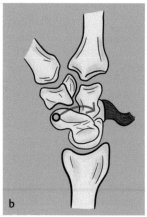

Fig. 13.1 Coronal **(a)** and sagittal **(b)** plane force vectors (*red arrows*) that can be applied by potential ligamentous attachment points (*green dots*) in capsulodesis. There are multiple possibilities for attachment depending on the technique; however, scapholunate compression and scaphoid extension forces are the most important to consider.

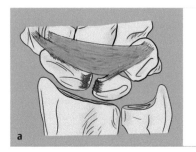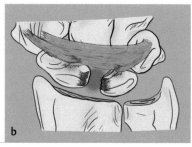

Fig. 13.2 (a) Even with scapholunate interosseous ligament (SLIL, *dark purple*) disruption, there can be a maintained scapholunate (SL) interval, supported in part by attachments of the dorsal interosseous ligament (DIL). **(b)** With disruption of the DIL's scaphoid and lunate attachments, static SL dissociation can readily occur.

preoperative ROM and SL reduction.[40] Long-term follow-up is yet to be published that establishes the durability and improved outcome of this operation,[41] though the use of these adaptations of the DIC for capsulodesis has favorable support from an anatomic and biomechanical perspective. Together, these studies have led the authors to incorporate both scaphoid and lunate fixation as a modification of their originally described method of the DILC.

Long-term follow-up is limited for many capsulodesis techniques. From the authors' original series, results at 5 to 15 years showed a similar trend to previous techniques over time: the SL interval widened, and a proportion of patients developed radiographic radiocarpal and intercarpal arthrosis. Importantly, there appeared to be a lack of correlation between radiographic arthrosis and clinical outcome measures, raising the question of how these factors were related, if at all.[34] There has been a trend in the literature showing the tendency of capsulodesis procedures to either lose fixation or stretch out, with slow diastasis of the SL interval and a relatively typical progression of arthrosis in some patients.[19,21,25,26,29,30] Pomerance evaluated 17 patients at an average of 66-month follow-up after undergoing dorsal radioscaphoid capsulodesis, again showing that initial postoperative reduction of the SL gap and scaphoid flexion was difficult to maintain, especially in higher demand patients.[14] If and how capsulodesis prolongs the natural progression of carpal arthrosis is not well understood. Nonetheless, there

appears to be a patient population that has good long-term outcomes after dorsal capsulodesis. A recent review of long-term results at minimum 5 years for DILC in chronic SL instability showed maintained SL gap reduction and promising clinical function scores.[42] In these patients, the authors attributed their success to technique modifications such as using two anchors for SLIL repair after careful reductions, as well as their technique in DILC reinforcement. The impact on surgical technique clearly plays a significant role in the outcome of patients undergoing capsulodesis. There is ample opportunity for developing and testing further modifications to consistently provide efficacious long-term clinical benefit.[43]

Another technique to address scaphoid flexion instability was proposed by Brunelli et al involving utilizing a slip of the flexor carpi radialis. A more thorough review of ligamentoplasty is described elsewhere, though a comparative discussion to capsulodesis is warranted. Originally described to pass through the scaphoid tuberosity and anchor to the dorsal-ulnar corner of the distal radius, it has been largely modified to anchor to the dorsal lunate and dorsal radiotriquetral ligament to avoid inhibiting motion implied with radial tethering as discussed earlier. This affords some level of SLIL reconstruction as well.[44,45] Certainly, many variations have been subsequently described and are included in this book. One concern of ours in favor of capsulodesis is that tendon weave ligamentoplasty inherently utilizes a biologically different tissue for soft tissue reconstruction that may be prone to attenuation and stretch over time.[27,45,46] Although ligament properties are stronger than tendon, ligamentoplasty may be prone to a similar mode of failure as capsulodesis. More recently, techniques using local tendon graft to reconstruct both dorsal and volar SLIL components have been introduced.[47] Early biomechanical comparison has shown minimal difference, and long-term outcomes of these modifications are yet to be reported.[48,49] Daly et al compared tenodesis-type procedures with capsulodesis and found improved SL gap and SL angle in the tenodesis group. Imada et al performed a meta-analysis focusing on longer-term outcomes of different reconstructive options including capsulodesis, tenodesis, and arthrodesis, and found no superiority between the procedures.[50,51] Again, inconsistent literature has yet to definitively show a clear benefit of one procedure. At this point in time, almost every procedure proposed for reconstruction of SL instability can claim "good results" at the 2-year mark and if followed longer has the similar fate of radiographic arthrosis in many cases but reduced clinical symptoms in most. Likely, as long as the described principles of fixation are obeyed, multiple construct types will be successful by these criteria if performed in a technically sound manner. So, the decision of what to choose depends on what potential complications the surgeon is willing to accept, what tissues are sacrificed in the process, and the technical difficulties encountered during the procedure. The authors still prefer capsulodesis for these reasons.

13.3 Author's Preferred Technique; The Dorsal Intercarpal Ligament Capsulodesis (Video 13.1)

13.3.1 Approach

The patient is positioned supine on the operating table with a hand table extension. A tourniquet is placed on the upper arm. General anesthesia or regional block with monitored anesthesia care is considered by patient and anesthesiologist choice. A dorsal approach to the carpus is performed. First, a dorsal longitudinal incision is made through skin, originating at Lister's tubercle, and extending 5 to 6 cm in length toward the third metacarpal. If additional exposure is needed, the incision can be extended proximally or distally. Full-thickness skin flaps are developed to allow sufficient retraction and exposure of the underlying retinacula and capsule. The radial sensory nerve is visualized and protected in the radial flap of skin. The interval between the third and fourth dorsal compartments is identified. The extensor retinaculum is divided and septum between the compartments is sharply split to free the tendons. The common extensor tendons are retracted ulnarly, while the extensor pollicis longus (EPL) is kept radial, exposing the dorsal wrist capsule and ligaments. A surgical sponge can be used to firmly wipe

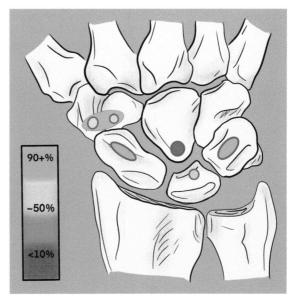

Fig. 13.3 The dorsal intercarpal ligament can have various bony attachments, with a universal origin at the dorsal triquetrum, and insertions at the trapezium, trapezoid, and dorsal scaphoid ridge. The dorsal lunate attachment has been more recently accepted.[34]

the field to better visualize the fiber orientation for correct structure identification. The DIL can be recognized by more transverse fibers originating from the triquetrum and inserting most radially in part onto the trapezium and trapezoid. Insertions are variable as described by many authors (▸ Fig. 13.3, DIL locations).[31,34,36] The dorsal radiocarpal ligament courses ulnarly and obliquely from the lip of the distal radius, and should be maintained intact. The midsubstance of the DIL is dissected and held with a vessel loop or umbilical tape. The ligament is then divided off its insertion on the trapezium and trapezoid. An approximately 5-mm strip of the ligament is isolated from the radial insertion and reflected ulnarly. The DIL has attachments along the dorsal scaphoid ridge, and care must be taken to avoid overaggressive resection at this area to not damage the vascular pedicle entering the scaphoid (▸ Fig. 13.4).

13.3.2 Scapholunate Reduction

Next, exposure and reduction of the SL interval is done. After reflection of the DIL, the scaphocapitate and scaphotrapezio-trapezoidal joints can be appreciated. This can help guide the surgeon to the SL interval. The dorsal wrist capsule is longitudinally incised in line with the SL joint. The second and fourth dorsal compartments are elevated subperiosteally as proximal as necessary. The SL interval is now fully exposed, and the remnant torn dorsal SLIL can be identified. This can be repaired if there is sufficient tissue stock, after the relationship of the

13

scaphoid and lunate has been provisionally reduced as follows. If primarily avulsed off the scaphoid, the authors' preferred method of dorsal SL ligament is to repair with a

mini-suture anchor in the scaphoid. A second suture anchor is placed in the lunate close to the SL interval. The suture from each of these anchors is later used to attach the DIL to the scaphoid and to the lunate to reinforce the SLIL repair. This is done by passing suture with a free needle while holding the DIL under tension radially.

Reduction of the scaphoid and lunate is done by joystick method, where 1.6 mm (0.062 in) K-wires are placed into the proximal scaphoid pole and lunate. Take care to place the wires to not interfere with later fixation pathways. The scaphoid is manipulated to reduce its flexed position and the lunate reduced out of extension and compressed together in a radial-ulnar direction to close the SL interval. In addition to inspecting the SL gap clinically and on PA fluoroscopy, scrutinizing the SL angle, scaphoid flexion, and scaphoid relation to the trapezium on lateral radiographs with comparison to the contralateral can help determine appropriate position. An additional one or two 1.2-mm (0.045-in) K-wires are driven across the SL joint percutaneously while the reduction is held. Bear in mind the dorsal radial sensory branches and extensor tendons when choosing a percutaneous path. Another K-wire is placed from the waist of the scaphoid into the capitate (▶ Fig. 13.5).

13.3.3 Dorsal Intercarpal Ligament Fixation

The DIL is then anchored to the distal pole of the reduced scaphoid. A decorticated trough is made on the dorsal distal scaphoid pole in line with the vector of pull from the ligament. A key aspect of the DIL capsulodesis lies in the attachment of the ligament distal to the scaphoid's axis of rotation, in order to provide an extension moment. A mini-suture anchor is placed at the base of the trough, and the tails used to secure the end of the DIL under tension. Additional nonabsorbable suture is used to reinforce the repair as well as secure the midsubstance

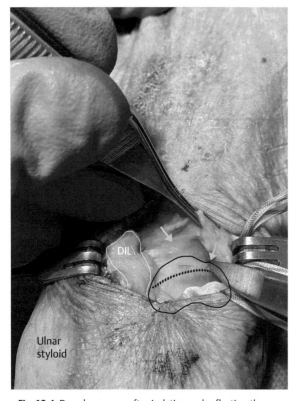

Fig. 13.4 Dorsal exposure after isolating and reflecting the dorsal intercarpal ligament (DIL, *white outline*) with extensor tendons retracted. The scaphoid (*outlined in black*), dorsal scaphoid ridge with some retained soft tissue (*dashed line*), site of DIL anchoring/insertion (*blue arrow*/scissor tips), and residual distal DIL with capsular tissue (*yellow arrow*) can be readily seen through this approach.

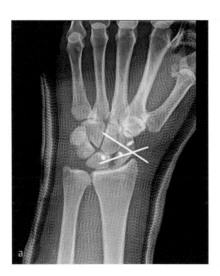
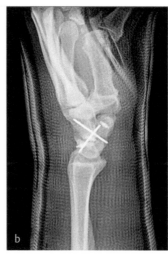

Fig. 13.5 PA **(a)** and lateral **(b)** radiographs of a postoperative dorsal intercarpal ligament capsulodesis (DILC), showing the distal scaphoid anchor and two anchors surrounding the scapholunate interval. Approximate K-wire positions are seen securing the scapholunate (SL) reduction and scaphoid position.

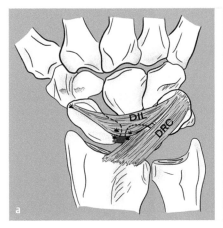

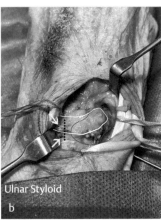

Fig. 13.6 (a) Representative depiction of final dorsal intercarpal ligament capsulodesis (DILC) construct by the authors' described technique. The DIL anchored attachments to scaphoid and lunate (*black star marks* represent anchors) can be seen, overlying and reinforcing scapholunate (SL) repair (*dark purple*). DRC, dorsal radiocarpal ligament. (b) Final cadaveric example of the DILC. DIL: *white*; scaphoid: *blue*; lunate anchors: *yellow*; scaphoid anchor: *green*; approximate location of SL interval: *dashed black line*.

of the ligament to the lunate for further augmentation. As discussed earlier, the lunate attachment plays an important role in carpal stabilization, as well as reinforcing the SLIL. When applicable and well approximated, the authors like to use the remaining tail suture from the SL repair anchors in the lunate and scaphoid to secure the proximal DIL (▶ Fig. 13.6). The capsular flaps can be closed over the SL repair, and the EPL is placed into its compartment. The extensor retinaculum is repaired over the extensor tendons, and skin is closed as usual. K-wires are cut beneath the skin, or left protruding with the patient instructed on pin care.

13.4 Essential Rehabilitation Points

The extremity is immobilized with a thumb spica plaster splint and dressing extending above the elbow. This is transitioned to an above-elbow thumb spica cast after suture removal for an additional 3 weeks. A below-elbow thumb spica cast is placed for 4 weeks more. At 8 weeks post-op, the authors remove the K-wires, continue casting for another 2 weeks, and then initiate gentle supervised range-of-motion exercises, with a removable wrist splint. Immobilization is terminated 3 months postoperatively, with restricted heavy lifting activities, particularly in wrist extension, until 6 months post-op.

13.5 Conclusion

There are many procedures to consider when dealing with SL instability. There continue to be modifications and new proposals as no one procedure has proven long-term superiority over another. Any procedure should be tested in the laboratory, designed with minimal potential complications, and be technically feasible for surgeons of all levels of talent. The DICL capsulodesis has these characteristics and a long track record of good clinical results.

References

[1] Richards RS, Bennett JD, Roth JH, Milne K, Jr. Arthroscopic diagnosis of intra-articular soft tissue injuries associated with distal radial fractures. J Hand Surg Am. 1997; 22(5):772–776

[2] Lindau T, Arner M, Hagberg L. Intraarticular lesions in distal fractures of the radius in young adults. A descriptive arthroscopic study in 50 patients. J Hand Surg [Br]. 1997; 22(5):638–643

[3] Stanley JK, Trail IA. Carpal instability. J Bone Joint Surg Br. 1994; 76 (5):691–700

[4] Pliefke J, Stengel D, Rademacher G, Mutze S, Ekkernkamp A, Eisenschenk A. Diagnostic accuracy of plain radiographs and cineradiography in diagnosing traumatic scapholunate dissociation. Skeletal Radiol. 2008; 37(2):139–145

[5] Kuo CE, Wolfe SW. Scapholunate instability: current concepts in diagnosis and management. J Hand Surg Am. 2008; 33(6):998–1013

[6] Rohman EM, Agel J, Putnam MD, Adams JE. Scapholunate interosseous ligament injuries: a retrospective review of treatment and outcomes in 82 wrists. J Hand Surg Am. 2014; 39(10):2020–2026

[7] Fisk GR. Carpal instability and the fractured scaphoid. Ann R Coll Surg Engl. 1970; 46(2):63–76

[8] Linscheid RL, Dobyns JH, Beabout JW, Bryan RS. Traumatic instability of the wrist. Diagnosis, classification, and pathomechanics. J Bone Joint Surg Am. 1972; 54(8):1612–1632

[9] Larsen CF, Amadio PC, Gilula LA, Hodge JC. Analysis of carpal instability: I. Description of the scheme. J Hand Surg Am. 1995; 20 (5):757–764

[10] Wolfe SW, Garcia-Elias M, Kitay A. Carpal instability nondissociative. J Am Acad Orthop Surg. 2012; 20(9):575–585

[11] Garcia-Elias M. Definition of carpal instability. The Anatomy and Biomechanics Committee of the International Federation of Societies for Surgery of the Hand. J Hand Surg Am. 1999; 24(866):7

[12] Watson HK, Weinzweig J, Zeppieri J. The natural progression of scaphoid instability. Hand Clin. 1997; 13(1):39–49

[13] Cohen MS. Scapholunate acute repair techniques. In: Shin AY, Day CS, eds. Epub-Advances in scapholunate ligament treatment. American Society for Surgery of the Hand; 2014:75–83

[14] Pomerance J. Outcome after repair of the scapholunate interosseous ligament and dorsal capsulodesis for dynamic scapholunate instability due to trauma. J Hand Surg Am. 2006; 31(8):1380–1386

[15] Beredjiklian PK, Dugas J, Gerwin M. Primary repair of the scapholunate ligament. Tech Hand Up Extrem Surg. 1998; 2(4):269–273

[16] Minami A, Kaneda K. Repair and/or reconstruction of scapholunate interosseous ligament in lunate and perilunate dislocations. J Hand Surg Am. 1993; 18(6):1099–1106

[17] Bickert B, Sauerbier M, Germann G. Scapholunate ligament repair using the Mitektmbone anchor: technique and preliminary results. J Hand Surg British & European. 2000; 25(2):188–192

13

[18] Kitay A, Wolfe SW. Scapholunate instability: current concepts in diagnosis and management. J Hand Surg Am. 2012; 37(10):2175–2196

[19] Lavernia CJ, Cohen MS, Taleisnik J. Treatment of scapholunate dissociation by ligamentous repair and capsulodesis. J Hand Surg Am. 1992; 17(2):354–359

[20] Glickel SZ, Millender LH. Ligamentous reconstruction for chronic intercarpal instability. J Hand Surg Am. 1984; 9(4):514–527

[21] Wyrick JD, Youse BD, Kiefhaber TR. Scapholunate ligament repair and capsulodesis for the treatment of static scapholunate dissociation. J Hand Surg [Br]. 1998; 23(6):776–780

[22] Wolfe SW, Neu C, Crisco JJ. In vivo scaphoid, lunate, and capitate kinematics in flexion and in extension. J Hand Surg Am. 2000; 25(5):860–869

[23] Blatt G. Capsulodesis in reconstructive hand surgery. Dorsal capsulodesis for the unstable scaphoid and volar capsulodesis following excision of the distal ulna. Hand Clin. 1987; 3(1):81–102

[24] Deshmukh SC, Givissis P, Belloso D, Stanley JK, Trail IA. Blatt's capsulodesis for chronic scapholunate dissociation. J Hand Surg [Br]. 1999; 24(2):215–220

[25] Moran SL, Cooney WP, Berger RA, Strickland J. Capsulodesis for the treatment of chronic scapholunate instability. J Hand Surg Am. 2005; 30(1):16–23

[26] Megerle K, Bertel D, Germann G, Lehnhardt M, Hellmich S. Long-term results of dorsal intercarpal ligament capsulodesis for the treatment of chronic scapholunate instability. J Bone Joint Surg Br. 2012; 94(12):1660–1665

[27] Linscheid RL, Dobyns JH. Treatment of scapholunate dissociation. Rotatory subluxation of the scaphoid. Hand Clin. 1992; 8(4):645–652

[28] Berger RA. A method of defining palpable landmarks for the ligament-splitting dorsal wrist capsulotomy. J Hand Surg Am. 2007; 32(8):1291–1295

[29] Wintman BI, Gelberman RH, Katz JN. Dynamic scapholunate instability: results of operative treatment with dorsal capsulodesis. J Hand Surg Am. 1995; 20(6):971–979

[30] Moran SL, Ford KS, Wulf CA, Cooney WP. Outcomes of dorsal capsulodesis and tenodesis for treatment of scapholunate instability. J Hand Surg Am. 2006; 31(9):1438–1446

[31] Slater RR, Jr, Szabo RM. Scapholunate dissociation: treatment with the dorsal intercarpal ligament capsulodesis. Tech Hand Up Extrem Surg. 1999; 3(4):222–228

[32] Slater RR, Jr, Szabo RM, Bay BK, Laubach J. Dorsal intercarpal ligament capsulodesis for scapholunate dissociation: biomechanical analysis in a cadaver model. J Hand Surg Am. 1999; 24(2):232–239

[33] Szabo RM, Slater RR, Jr, Palumbo CF, Gerlach T. Dorsal intercarpal ligament capsulodesis for chronic, static scapholunate dissociation: clinical results. J Hand Surg Am. 2002; 27(6):978–984

[34] Viegas SF, Yamaguchi S, Boyd NL, Patterson RM. The dorsal ligaments of the wrist: anatomy, mechanical properties, and function. J Hand Surg Am. 1999; 24(3):456–468

[35] Buijze GA, Dvinskikh NA, Strackee SD, Streekstra GJ, Blankevoort L. Osseous and ligamentous scaphoid anatomy: Part II. Evaluation of ligament morphology using three-dimensional anatomical imaging. J Hand Surg Am. 2011; 36(12):1936–1943

[36] Wessel LE, Kim J, Morse KW, et al. The Dorsal Ligament Complex: A Cadaveric, Histology, and Imaging Study. J Hand Surg Am. 2022; 47(5):480.e1–480.e9

[37] Mitsuyasu H, Patterson RM, Shah MA, Buford WL, Iwamoto Y, Viegas SF. The role of the dorsal intercarpal ligament in dynamic and static scapholunate instability. J Hand Surg Am. 2004; 29(2):279–288

[38] Viegas SF, Dasilva MF. Surgical repair for scapholunate dissociation. Tech Hand Up Extrem Surg. 2000; 4(3):148–153

[39] Camus E. Dorsal scapholunate capsulodesis: Viegas' technique. In: Carpal ligament surgery. Paris: Springer; 2013:235–241

[40] Camus EJ, Van Overstraeten L. Dorsal scapholunate stabilization using Viegas' capsulodesis: 25 cases with 26 months-follow-up. Chir Main. 2013; 32(6):393–402

[41] Gajendran VK, Peterson B, Slater RR, Jr, Szabo RM. Long-term outcomes of dorsal intercarpal ligament capsulodesis for chronic scapholunate dissociation. J Hand Surg Am. 2007; 32(9):1323–1333

[42] Shibayama H, Matsui Y, Kawamura D, Momma D, Endo T, Iwasaki N. Minimum 5-Year Outcomes of Dorsal Intercarpal Ligament Capsulodesis With Scapholunate Interosseous Ligament Repair for Subacute and Chronic Static Scapholunate Instability: A Clinical Series of 5 Patients. Journal of Hand Surgery Global Online. 2022; 4:162–165

[43] da Silva Gusmão Filho N, de Oliveira RK, Rios GT, de Sousa GGQ. Double dorsal capsulodesis in the treatment of chronic scapholunate instability: description of a new surgical technique and case report. Cirugía de Mano y Microcirugía. 2022; 2(1)

[44] Brunelli GA, Brunelli GR. A new technique to correct carpal instability with scaphoid rotary subluxation: a preliminary report. J Hand Surg Am. 1995; 20(3 Pt 2):S82–S85

[45] Talwalkar SC, Edwards ATJ, Hayton MJ, Stilwell JH, Trail IA, Stanley JK. Results of tri-ligament tenodesis: a modified Brunelli procedure in the management of scapholunate instability. J Hand Surg [Br]. 2006; 31(1):110–117

[46] Berger RA. The gross and histologic anatomy of the scapholunate interosseous ligament. J Hand Surg Am. 1996; 21(2):170–178

[47] Chae S, Nam J, Park IJ, Shin SS, McGarry MH, Lee TQ. Kinematic analysis of two scapholunate ligament reconstruction techniques. J Orthop Surg (Hong Kong). 2021; 29(2):23094990211025830

[48] Van Den Abbeele KL, Loh YC, Stanley JK, Trail IA. Early results of a modified Brunelli procedure for scapholunate instability. J Hand Surg [Br]. 1998; 23(2):258–261

[49] Chee KG, Chin AY, Chew EM, Garcia-Elias M. Antipronation spiral tenodesis: a surgical technique for the treatment of perilunate instability. J Hand Surg Am. 2012; 37(12):2611–2618

[50] Daly LT, Daly MC, Mohamadi A, Chen N. Chronic scapholunate interosseous ligament disruption: a systematic review and meta-analysis of surgical treatments. Hand (N Y). 2020; 15(1):27–34

[51] Imada AO, Eldredge J, Wells L, Moneim MS. Review of surgical treatment for chronic scapholunate ligament reconstruction: a long-term study. Eur J Orthop Surg Traumatol. 2022:1–7

14 Chronic "R"einforcement (Capsulodesis): Arthroscopic Scapholunate Repair

Max Haerle, Jean-Baptiste de Villeneuve Bargemon, Florian Lampert, and Lorenzo Merlini

Abstract

Scapholunate (SL) instability represents a wide range of possible lesions that can evolve over time. At first, the instability will be reducible during the predynamic or even dynamic stages to end up in a static lesion, where direct repair of the SL capsuloligamentous complex seems outdated, leaving room for ligamentoplasties or more palliative methods. The arrival of arthroscopy has allowed a better understanding of these lesions but also to propose mini-invasive solutions. Traditionally, the indications for arthroscopic repair are predynamic and dynamic instabilities with little visible radiological deformity. The authors report not only on their experience with these arthroscopic direct repairs, but also on their experience with modifications of this technique, expanding the indications for direct arthroscopic repairs.

Keywords: wrist, ligament, scapholunate, arthroscopy, carpus

14.1 Introduction

The scapholunate (SL) couple is a complex anatomical and biomechanical zone. Between these two bones there are two shearing forces, with a wrist flexion line crossing the wrist extension line.[1] A complex and subtle "dance" takes place accompanied by constant axial loads by the capitate that push the scaphoid and lunate apart. Many other capsuloligamentary entities are also essential to the proper functioning of the SL couple. This anatomical ensemble represents the scapholunate complex (SLC).

The dorsal portion of the scapholunate interosseous ligament (SLIOL) is the biomechanically most powerful part[2,3] and this portion is reinforced at its attachment to the dorsal capsuloscapholunate septum (DCSS) and dorsal intercarpal ligament (DIC). This dorsal assembly of a set of ligaments is very strong and thick, resisting rotation of the scaphoid. Instability and deformity typically attributed to an isolated SLIOL lesion range from SL gap and rotational subluxation of the scaphoid to instability of the dorsal intercalary segment (DISI). However, numerous cadaveric studies have used sequential transection of the carpal ligaments and cyclic loading to demonstrate that complete division of the SLIOL alone does not result in a significant change in static carpal posture and does not cause DISI-like deformity.[4,9]

In general, both the intrinsic and extrinsic systems must be damaged for complete SL diastasis to be visible on radiographs. In most cases, radiographic abnormalities are not visible immediately after an SLIOL injury but appear over time due to the progressive destruction of the ligament system. Biomechanical works suggest that detachment of the DCSS and DIC aggravates the dissociation.[10,11] In addition, Elsaidi et al conducted a cadaveric study by sequentially severing the different stabilizers of the SLC and subsequently applying an axial load on the wrists. They found that severe cases of SL instability (horizontalization of the scaphoid and dorsal tilt of the lunate) occur only when the dorsal attachments of the SLIOL are disrupted.[12] These assertions may have found some truth in the description of cases of SL instability without any SLIOL lesion.[13] These findings have significantly changed the treatment of SL dissociation and are the basis for the current approach to its arthroscopic repair. Similarly, in surgical practice, repair or reconstruction of the SLIOL following a traumatic injury achieves at best only 80 to 85% functional results, and radiological recurrence of the space between the scaphoid and lunate is frequently observed, sometimes worse than the original deformity.[14,15]

A nautical representation was described by Wolfe et al initially to describe the biomechanics of nondissociative injuries but is perfectly applicable to the description of dissociative injuries (such as SL instability) to allow understanding of the importance of extrinsic ligaments.[16,17] The various manifestations of dissociative instability of the carpus appear to result from a combination of injury to the SLIOL and acute injury to one or more critical stabilizers such as the DIC (on its semilunar insertion) and the scaphotrapeziotrapezoidal palmar ligament complex, or from progressive relaxation of the long radiolunate ligament for instability with significant flexion of the lunate (▶ Fig. 14.1).[18,19]

It is now accepted that repair of the SLIOL alone is not sufficient to maintain satisfactory biomechanics. Surgical treatment must also include reattachment of the SLIOL to the dorsal capsule that supports the dorsal carpal ligaments. Wrist arthroscopy therefore appears to be the treatment of choice in the management of SL instability.

14.2 Indications

In 2013, Messina and the European Wrist Arthroscopy Society group described an arthroscopic classification with a detailed description of the lesion[20] especially regarding stage 3 (3A, B, or C depending on the area affected). However, this classification only defines the lesion observed by the surgeon and does not take into account the SL instability as a whole. In the most common cases, dorsal capsuloligamentous arthroscopic repair (DCAR) described by Mathoulin et al[21] is suitable for instabilities in stage 1, 2, or even 3. Note that for stage

14

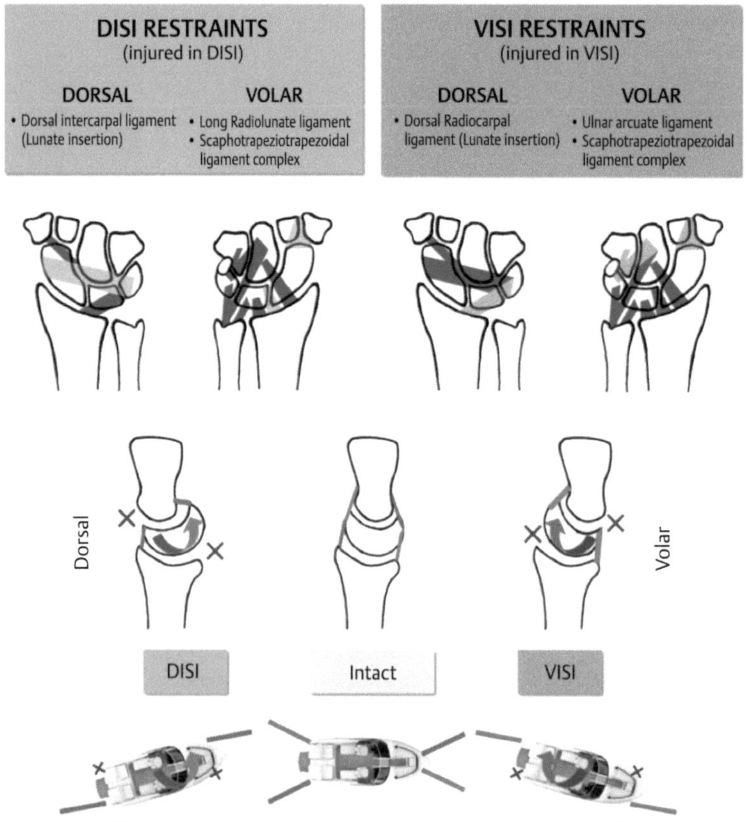

III

Fig. 14.1 The "mooring line" concept. (Reproduced with permission from Loisel F, Orr S, Ross M, et al. Traumatic Nondissociative Carpal Instability: A Case Series. J Hand Surg Am. 2022;47(3):285.e1-285.e11.)

3A, del Piñal described the possibility of a palmar reconstruction.[22] For stages starting from stage 3C, 4, to 5, reconstruction or ligamentoplasty is currently indicated. Ligamentoplasties can be performed under arthroscopy[23,24] but are surgically demanding, with potential complications that are not negligible. However, the authors propose a modification of the original technique by reporting their experience in the most advanced cases of SL instability.

14.3 Surgical Technique

14.3.1 Classic Arthroscopic Repair

A diagnostic arthroscopy is of best value in SL lesions. The scope is inserted through the 3–4 radiocarpal portal to visualize the SLIOL. However, the dorsal portion of the SLIOL can be best seen with the scope in the 6 R portal. A probe is used to assess the nature of the SL ligament injury. In cases where the ligament is ruptured in the center, with two ligament stumps remaining attached to the scaphoid and lunate, the original Mathoulin SL suture technique to suture the ligament arthroscopically is performed.

An absorbable monofilament suture (3–0 or 4–0) is passed through a needle. This needle is inserted through the 3–4 portal, and then shifted slightly distally so as to cross the joint capsule. The needle is localized inside the joint through the scope and then pushed through the SLIOL stump on the scaphoid side. The needle is then oriented dorsal to volar and angled proximal to distal, allowing it to enter the midcarpal joint. A second needle and suture are then inserted parallel to the first into the SLIOL stump attached to the lunate (▶ Fig. 14.2a). The scope is returned to the midcarpal ulnar portal. The two tips of the needles are now found inside the midcarpal joint, after they have passed between the scaphoid and lunate. The two sutures can be caught through the midcarpal radial portal (▶ Fig. 14.2b). The needles are removed and both sutures are pulled outside. A knot is tied between the two sutures. Traction is applied to both sutures through the 3–4 portal to pull the first knot into the midcarpal joint so that it comes to lie between the scaphoid and lunate (▶ Fig. 14.2c) just volar to the remaining dorsal portions of the SLIOL. The degree of reduction in the SL gap is determined by maintaining tension on the sutures after releasing wrist traction. If reduction is satisfactory, the ligament is sutured to the dorsal capsule by the last knot, which is tied subcutaneously (▶ Fig. 14.2d). The wrist is immobilized in extension (45–60 degrees) with an anterior splint for 6 weeks.

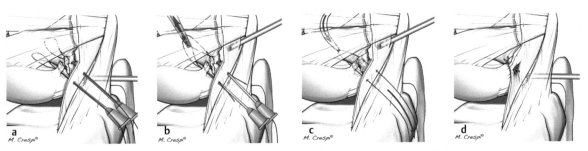

Fig. 14.2 (a–d) Illustration of the classic arthroscopic repair. (Courtesy of Christopher Mathoulin, MD, PhD.)

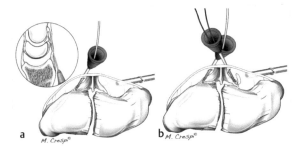

Fig. 14.3 (a,b) Insertion of the suture for capsulodesis with two cannulas in divergent course from radiocarpal to midcarpal level. (Courtesy of Christopher Mathoulin, MD, PhD.)

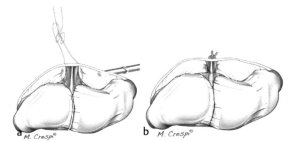

Fig. 14.4 (a,b) Final placement of the suture and completion of capsulodesis. (Courtesy of Christopher Mathoulin, MD, PhD.)

Arthroscopic Scapholunate Capsulodesis (Haerle)

In frequent situations where the remnants of the SL ligament are already degenerated or avulsed from one of the bones, a direct suture is not feasible. For those cases, a dorsal capsuloligamentous repair has been described by Haerle. The setup and approach are the same as for the conventional technique. In chronic cases, aggressive shaving provides a good visualization and converts the chronic into an acute lesion with better healing potential. In addition, it has been found that the scaphoid is still reducible after cleaning up the local fibrosis using an extended synovectomy, thus extending the indications of this technique to the stage where the scaphoid is so-called "fixed."[21,25] Under arthroscopic control via the 6R-Portal, a first cannula loaded with a 2–0 suture is inserted into the radiocarpal joint radially to the 3–4 portal, then it is slightly retracted and routed through the dorsal capsule into the midcarpal joint (▶ Fig. 14.3a). Noteworthy, the route of the suture is not aiming toward any possible ligament remnants in order to reunify them, but to grasp a considerable fraction of the dorsal capsule. Therefore, the second cannula with a 2–0 FibreWire is inserted ulnarly to the SL ligament on the radiocarpal level and then passed in a diverging direction to the midcarpal joint (▶ Fig. 14.3b). Thereupon, the arthroscope is changed to the MCU portal. After visualizing the cannulas, the

sutures are pulled out through the MCR portal. A single suture limb of the FiberWire is conducted through the PDS loop and pulled back through the capsule to the radiocarpal level, thus creating a U-shaped intracapsular course of the suture. After making sure that no extensor tendon is caught in the suture, traction on the wrist is released and the capsulodesis is completed with a tight suture knot, whereby the SL interval is realigned and stabilized (▶ Fig. 14.4a,b).

Postoperatively, the wrist is immobilized in a removable splint for a period of 8 weeks. In the following period of 6 weeks, free range of motion is allowed, but the patients are still dissuaded from bearing load or having physiotherapy so as not to impair the formation of a stable scar of the dorsal capsule. On further maturation and incorporation of elastic proteins, the scar might biomechanically emulate the properties of the former ligament.

Large Arthroscopic Repair (Mathoulin)

Another modification of this technique is described by C. Mathoulin. The setup and approach of this technique are the same as that of the conventional technique. In chronic cases, aggressive shaving debrides the fibrous ligament stumps and creates optimal conditions for effective suturing of the ligament to the capsule. In addition, it has been found that the scaphoid is still reducible after cleaning up the local fibrosis using an extended synovectomy, thus extending the indications of this technique to the stage where the

14

III

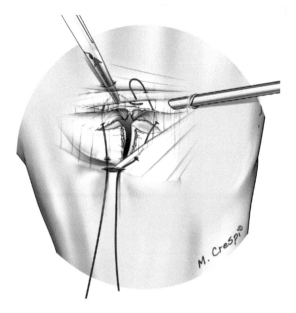

Fig. 14.5 The wires are recovered in the midcarpal region through two different orifices. (Courtesy of Christopher Mathoulin, MD, PhD.)

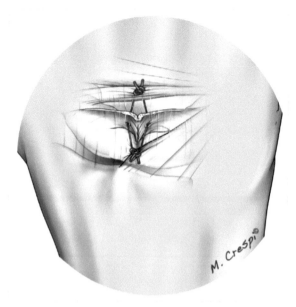

Fig. 14.6 The nodes are made and positioned extracapsularly at the midcarpal and radiocarpal levels. (Courtesy of Christopher Mathoulin, MD, PhD.)

scaphoid is so-called "fixed."[21,25] The first needle is introduced through the 3–4 cutaneous route but crosses the capsule in an offset manner at the standard capsular entry port. A second needle must be introduced using the same procedure but on the ulnar side of the SL joint, through the ligament stump attached to the lunate. Two different entry points are made on either side of the MCR capsular port to retrieve the PDS wire ends with hemostasis forceps, each through one of the two passages created (▶ Fig. 14.5).

An enlargement of the 3–4 and MCR tract can be performed to avoid trapping an extensor tendon in the suture. The distal end of the recovered PDS sutures will be tied in an extracapsular knot (as opposed to the classic dorsal capsuloligamentous repair, which is intracapsular). The second knot, also extracapsular, will be made after release of traction, allowing effective constriction of the dorsal capsule and thus reduction of the SL space while avoiding the use of pins (▶ Fig. 14.6).

The approaches will then be closed with a simple skin suture, but with the progression curve, the incisions become smaller and smaller, requiring no closure. The wrist is then immobilized at 45-degree extension for 6 weeks. Active and passive rehabilitation is started after a period of immobilization.

14.4 Results

14.4.1 Classic Arthroscopic Repair

In the Mathoulin series, there were 139 males and 82 females with a mean age of 38.11 (range: 17–63 y).

The mean time since injury was 7.13 (range: 3–26 mo) and the mean follow-up was 39.43 months (range: 12–83 mo). The mean range of motion improved in all directions. The mean difference between the preoperative and postoperative extension was 14.03 degrees ($p < 0.001$), while the mean difference between the preoperative and postoperative flexion was 11.14 degrees ($p < 0.0001$). The mean difference in the visual analog scale (VAS) score was 5.46 ($p < 0.0001$). The mean postoperative grip strength on the affected side was 38.42 ± 10.27 kg (range: 20–60 kg) as compared with the mean preoperative grip strength of 24.07 kg (range: 8–40 kg; $p < 0.0001$). The mean postoperative grip strength of the operated side was 93.4% of that on the unaffected side. In 19% of cases, the dorsal intercalated segment instability (DISI) was uncorrected on postoperative radiographs. The mean difference between the preoperative and postoperative SL angles was 9.45 degrees ($p < 0.0001$). The mean postoperative disabilities of the arm, shoulder, and hand (DASH) score was 9.4 as compared with the mean preoperative DASH score of 47.04 ($p < 0.0001$). There was a negative correlation between the overall DASH score and the postoperative correction of the DISI deformity with a lower DASH score associated with increasing SL angles. All patients returned to work in an average of 9 weeks (range: 1–12 wk) and all the professional athletes resumed their sporting activities at their preinjury levels. Two hundred and fifteen patients (95.7%) were very satisfied or satisfied with their result. Five patients had a fair result and one was unsatisfied, mainly due to postoperative wrist stiffness and nonreduction of the SL gap. All failures were cases of Garcia-Elias stage 5 dissociation (5 cases/7). Some of the cases with high-grade injuries were clear failures. This surgical technique was found to be quite ineffective when a lunotriquetral ligament injury was present. The authors do not currently recommend this technique in cases of Geissler stage 4 or in association with lunotriquetral instabilities.

14.4.2 Arthroscopic Scapholunate Capsulodesis

A cohort consisted of a prospective study conducted in the Institute de la Main, Paris (France), from 05/2020 to 05/2022 involving 112 patients (70 men and 42 women) with an average age of 31.63 years. The mean time to surgery was 5.11 months and in the associated lesions the authors found 22 lesions of the triangular fibrocartilage complex (TFCC) and 5 lunotriquetral ligament lesions, all of which were treated surgically. No patient was excluded from the study during its course.

A total of 3 EWAS stage 3A, 12 stage 3B, 29 stage 3C, 56 stage 4, and 12 stage 5 were included. Postoperatively, all joint ranges were significantly improved (p < 0.0001) except for flexion, probably due to greater folding of the back capsule. An improvement in pain, strength, and qDASH was recorded, with a mean difference of 2.86 (p < 0.0001), 13.25 (p < 0.0001), and 25.91 (p < 0.0001), respectively. There was a significant reduction in the SL angle from 74.64 to 55.09 degrees on average (p < 0.0001) and in the radiolunate angle from −7.37 to 4.34 (p < 0.0001). Moreover, when faced with a very large SL angle (more than 85 degrees in nine patients), the authors' technique was effective at reducing radiological signs and functional signs. Only one complication was reported in 112 patients: a tendon rupture of the extensor digitorum communis of the fourth compartment, which was detected intraoperatively and sutured. This is the first prospective cohort of this technique and therefore results can be considered as preliminary. The authors' technique effectively reduced radiological and functional signs in the face of a very large SL angle (more than 85 degrees in nine patients). However, it will be interesting to compare this technique in very large flexions of the lunate with the addition or not of a repair/attachment of the palmar extrinsic system and of the palmar part under arthroscopy as described by del Piñal.[22]

14.5 Discussion

SL lesions and their treatment remain controversial and also depend on the surgeon's habits, particularly whether or not he or she likes wrist arthroscopy. In the authors' opinion, the strong point of the arthroscopic techniques is "simplicity." The difficulty of current arthroscopic techniques such as Corella's[23] and Ho's[24] techniques can be a hindrance, particularly because of the difficulty of making

bone tunnels with the passage of tendons through the tunnel, and the non-negligible but pejorative risk of avascular necrosis of one of the two bones. Open techniques such as ScaphoLunate Intercarpal ligamentoplasty (SLIC)[26] and Anatomical Front And Back ligamentoplasty (ANAFAB)[27] with the need for a capsulotomy may also be a hindrance to their use. Concerning the three-ligament tenodesis, Blackbrun et al reported results at 1 year (in 203 patients) that are certainly significant in terms of pain and functional scores as well as joint amplitudes, but that were much poorer than those reported by the authors' cohort, particularly in terms of joint amplitudes. Moreover, in a study with 9 years of follow-up, three-ligament tenodesis (TLT) demonstrated a success rate of 63% and a high number of complications.[28] The question of scaphoid reducibility can be criticized because very often, in advanced stages of SL instability, the scaphoid remains flexed in dynamic and static maneuvers, and the extension of the lunate. As Garcia-Elias proposes in his classification, stages 4 and 5 are differentiated by the reducibility of the carpal instability. However, as proposed by Mathoulin et al, irreducible lesions may become reducible by a major periscaphoid arthrolysis, allowing scaphoid flexion to be overcome under arthroscopy.[21] In severe cases, a scaphotrapezoid arthrolysis would be recommended. In addition, this aggressive shaving would make it possible to transform a chronic lesion into a fresh lesion.[29] Although some authors report the use of SL and scaphocapitate pins in chronic cases,[30,34] the authors of this text have never used pins to maintain the reduction of the scaphoid and lunate.

14.6 Conclusion

Dorsal capsuloligament repair or capsulodesis thus offers an effective therapeutic solution in the most common and the most advanced SL instabilities, while remaining minimally invasive and conservative, relatively easy and with few complications, offering not only a clear improvement in functional signs (especially joint amplitudes) but also a reduction in the radiological deformation of the instability.

Acknowledgment

Thanks to Prof. C. Mathoulin for his loan of illustrations and for his help in writing this chapter.

References

[1] Camus EJ, Millot F, Lariviere J, Raoult S, Rtaimate M. Kinematics of the wrist using 2D and 3D analysis: biomechanical and clinical deductions. Surg Radiol Anat. 2004; 26(5):399–410

[2] Berger RA, Imeada T, Berglund L, An KN. Constraint and material properties of the subregions of the scapholunate interosseous ligament. J Hand Surg Am. 1999; 24(5):953–962

[3] Sokolow C, Saffar P. Anatomy and histology of the scapholunate ligament. Hand Clin. 2001; 17(1):77–81

14

[4] Short WH, Werner FW, Green JK, Sutton LG, Brutus JP. Biomechanical evaluation of the ligamentous stabilizers of the scaphoid and lunate: part III. J Hand Surg Am. 2007; 32(3):297–309

[5] Meade TD, Schneider LH, Cherry K. Radiographic analysis of selective ligament sectioning at the carpal scaphoid: a cadaver study. J Hand Surg Am. 1990; 15(6):855–862

[6] Mitsuyasu H, Patterson RM, Shah MA, Buford WL, Iwamoto Y, Viegas SF. The role of the dorsal intercarpal ligament in dynamic and static scapholunate instability. J Hand Surg Am. 2004; 29(2):279–288

[7] Pérez AJ, Jethanandani RG, Vutescu ES, Meyers KN, Lee SK, Wolfe SW. Role of ligament stabilizers of the proximal carpal row in preventing dorsal intercalated segment instability: a cadaveric study. J Bone Joint Surg Am. 2019; 101(15):1388–1396

[8] Lee SK, Desai H, Silver B, Dhaliwal G, Paksima N. Comparison of radiographic stress views for scapholunate dynamic instability in a cadaver model. J Hand Surg Am. 2011; 36(7):1149–1157

[9] Ruby LK, An KN, Linscheid RL, Cooney WP, III, Chao EYS. The effect of scapholunate ligament section on scapholunate motion. J Hand Surg Am. 1987; 12(5 Pt 1):767–771

[10] Van Overstraeten L, Camus EJ. Arthroscopic classification of the lesions of the dorsal capsulo-scapholunate septum (DCSS) of the wrist. Tech Hand Up Extrem Surg. 2016; 20(3):125–128

[11] Overstraeten LV, Camus EJ, Wahegaonkar A, et al. Anatomical description of the dorsal capsulo-scapholunate septum (DCSS): arthroscopic staging of scapholunate instability after DCSS sectioning. J Wrist Surg. 2013; 2(2):149–154

[12] Elsaidi GA, Ruch DS, Kuzma GR, Smith BP. Dorsal wrist ligament insertions stabilize the scapholunate interval: cadaver study. Clin Orthop Relat Res. 2004(425):152–157

[13] Binder AC, Kerfant N, Wahegaonkar AL, Tandara AA, Mathoulin CL. Dorsal wrist capsular tears in association with scapholunate instability: results of an arthroscopic dorsal capsuloplasty. J Wrist Surg. 2013; 2(2):160–167

[14] Daly LT, Daly MC, Mohamadi A, Chen N. Chronic scapholunate interosseous ligament disruption: a systematic review and meta-analysis of surgical treatments. Hand (N Y). 2020; 15(1):27–34

[15] Rohman EM, Agel J, Putnam MD, Adams JE. Scapholunate interosseous ligament injuries: a retrospective review of treatment and outcomes in 82 wrists. J Hand Surg Am. 2014; 39(10):2020–2026

[16] Loisel F, Orr S, Ross M, Couzens G, Leo AJ, Wolfe S. Traumatic nondissociative carpal instability: a case series. J Hand Surg Am. 2022; 47(3):285.e1–285.e11

[17] Raja S, Williams D, Wolfe SW, Couzens G, Ross M. New concepts in carpal instability. In: Geissler WB, ed. Wrist and elbow arthroscopy with selected open procedures. Springer International Publishing; 2022:173–185. doi:10.1007/978-3-030-78881-0_14

[18] Kuo CE, Wolfe SW. Scapholunate instability: current concepts in diagnosis and management. J Hand Surg Am. 2008; 33(6):998–1013

[19] Wolfe SW, Katz LD, Crisco JJ. Radiographic progression to dorsal intercalated segment instability. Orthopedics. 1996; 19(8):691–695

[20] Messina JC, Van Overstraeten L, Luchetti R, Fairplay T, Mathoulin CL. The EWAS classification of scapholunate tears: an anatomical arthroscopic study. J Wrist Surg. 2013; 2(2):105–109

[21] Mathoulin CL, Dauphin N, Wahegaonkar AL. Arthroscopic dorsal capsuloligamentous repair in chronic scapholunate ligament tears. Hand Clin. 2011; 27(4):563–572, xi

[22] del Piñal F. Arthroscopic volar capsuloligamentous repair. J Wrist Surg. 2013; 2(2):126–128

[23] Corella F, Del Cerro M, Ocampos M, Simon de Blas C, Larrainzar-Garijo R. Arthroscopic scapholunate ligament reconstruction, volar and dorsal reconstruction. Hand Clin. 2017; 33(4):687–707

[24] Ho PC, Wong C, Tse WL. Arthroscopic-assisted combined dorsal and volar scapholunate ligament reconstruction with tendon graft for chronic SL instability. J Wrist Surg. 2015; 4(4):252–263

[25] Wahegaonkar AL, Mathoulin CL. Arthroscopic dorsal capsulo-ligamentous repair in the treatment of chronic scapho-lunate ligament tears. J Wrist Surg. 2013; 2(2):141–148

[26] Athlani L, Pauchard N, Dautel G. Outcomes of scapholunate intercarpal ligamentoplasty for chronic scapholunate dissociation: a prospective study in 26 patients. J Hand Surg Eur Vol. 2018; 43(7):700–707

[27] Sandow M, Fisher T. Anatomical anterior and posterior reconstruction for scapholunate dissociation: preliminary outcome in ten patients. J Hand Surg Eur Vol. 2020; 45(4):389–395

[28] Goeminne S, Borgers A, van Beek N, De Smet L, Degreef I. Long-term follow-up of the three-ligament tenodesis for scapholunate ligament lesions: 9-year results. Hand Surg Rehabil. 2021; 40(4):448–452

[29] del Piñal F, Haerle M, Krimmer H, eds. Distal radius fractures and carpal instabilities: FESSH IFSSH 2019 instructional book. Georg Thieme Verlag; 2019:b-006–163731. doi:10.1055/b-006–163731

[30] Busse F, Felderhoff J, Krimmer H, Lanz U. Die skapholunäre Bandverletzung. Therapie durch dorsale Kapsulodese. Handchir Mikrochir Plast Chir. 2002; 34(3):173–181

[31] Deshmukh SC, Givissis P, Belloso D, Stanley JK, Trail IA. Blatt's capsulodesis for chronic scapholunate dissociation. J Hand Surg Am. 1999; 24(2):215–220

[32] Slater RR, Jr, Szabo RM, Bay BK, Laubach J. Dorsal intercarpal ligament capsulodesis for scapholunate dissociation: biomechanical analysis in a cadaver model. J Hand Surg Am. 1999; 24(2):232–239

[33] Szabo RM, Slater RR, Jr, Palumbo CF, Gerlach T. Dorsal intercarpal ligament capsulodesis for chronic, static scapholunate dissociation: clinical results. J Hand Surg Am. 2002; 27(6):978–984

[34] Wintman BI, Gelberman RH, Katz JN. Dynamic scapholunate instability: results of operative treatment with dorsal capsulodesis. J Hand Surg Am. 1995; 20(6):971–979

15 Chronic "R"econstruction (Ligamentoplasties): Open Treatment

Rupert Wharton and Mike Hayton

Abstract

Chronic scapholunate (SL) ligament injuries are widely considered to lead to a predictable pattern of wrist arthritis (scapholunate advanced collapse [SLAC]). Prior to the development of arthritis they may present with a painful clunking wrist, a sense of instability, and a reduced movement in wrist extension particularly. In such chronic cases the SL ligament atrophies with little or no healing potential. The SL and scaphotrapeziotrapezoid (STT) joints fill with scar tissue which can block reduction, and at this stage a direct repair does not address failure of the STT ligaments which lead to a dorsal-intercalated segment instability (DISI) pattern.

Ligament reconstruction using a distally based flexor carpi radialis (FCR) tendon graft was described by Brunelli in 1995 and was the first technique to address these failures. This technique was modified by the authors to avoid crossing the radiocarpal joint by using the dorsal radiotriquetral (RTq) ligament to act as a pulley around which the FCR graft was passed and sutured back down onto itself over a lunate anchor. This was later termed the three-ligament tenodesis, and good results with this technique have been reported both in the general population and in athletes. Cadaveric studies have shown the dorsal component of the SL ligament to have the greatest strength, and this was traditionally targeted by reconstruction. More recently interest has returned to the possibility of volar reconstruction in addition to dorsal reconstruction. The use of a palmaris graft with suture tape and interference screws has been suggested, and this has been termed "the Scapholunate Ligament Internal Brace 360-degree Tenodesis (SLITT)."

From a tertiary unit involved in technique development in the United Kingdom, the authors describe their experience with using open techniques and suggestions for pitfall avoidance.

Keywords: three-ligament tenodesis, Brunelli, ligamentoplasty, reconstruction, SLITT

15.1 Introduction

Garcia-Elias has defined a spectrum of injuries to the scapholunate interosseous ligament (SLIL) via a series of questions indicating progression of severity of injury.[1,2] Stage III represents a complete SLIL injury which is non-repairable, with a normally aligned scaphoid and lunate, and Stage IV describes this with reducible rotary subluxation of the scaphoid leading to the characteristic dorsal-intercalated segment instability (DISI) deformity.

The time point at which the ruptured ligament atrophies, shortens, and becomes nonviable is not clear, but most authors define acute repair as occurring within 6 weeks of injury.[3,4] After that time point, primary repair becomes increasingly difficult and a reconstruction is preferred. The maintenance of a normal scapholunate (SL) angle suggests integrity of the anterolateral scaphotrapeziotrapezoid (STT) ligament, volar capsule, and dorsal intercarpal ligaments,[5] while scaphoid flexion suggests attenuation of these (Stage IV). SL diastasis may only be present with dynamic stress, and the patient may be symptomatic only on loading the wrist.[6] Although it is now accepted that untreated SLIL injuries will progress to radiological degenerative arthritis,[6,7] surgical intervention is not without risk, and asymptomatic patients should be assessed and counselled carefully before deciding on optimal treatment.[8]

15.2 Ligamentoplasties

15.2.1 The Brunelli Procedure

For symptomatic Stage III and IV SLIL injury in the absence of arthritis, most surgeons favor variants of the now eponymous procedure described in 1995 by Brunelli and Brunelli. The authors' unit opted this technique following disappointing results with the Blatt capsulodesis[9] compared with published reports in the literature.[10] The Brunelli procedure was derived following the concern that ligamentoplasties available until that time addressed only the SL ligament, while cadaveric mechanical studies sectioning that ligament did not result in scaphoid flexion.[11] Scaphoid flexion, Brunelli postulated, occurred only after failure of the STT ligaments. Of these the more important is the palmar ligament complex comprising the floor of the sheath of the flexor carpi radialis (FCR) in the prevention of rotatory subluxation (flexion) of the scaphoid. They sought a technique that would address this problem without resorting to arthrodesis which had yielded poor midterm results despite initial encouragement.[12]

The goal instead was to find a technique to reduce the scaphoid, correct the dissociation, re-establish carpal height, and maintain the correction. In their description of the technique initially, a Berger flap is made to open the dorsum of the wrist and scar tissue is removed from the SL joint and STT joint, sparing the cartilage surfaces. A 7-cm slip of the FCR tendon is harvested with preservation of the distal attachment (▶ Fig. 15.1). This is passed retrograde through a 2.5-mm drill hole in the palmar scaphoid tubercle exiting dorsally. The tendon slip is then

15

III

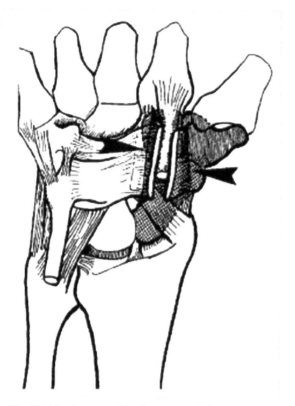

Fig. 15.1 The deep part of the flexor carpi radialis (FCR) sheath (*arrow*) is the most important element of the ligamentous complex that ties the scaphoid to the trapezium and trapezoid. (Reproduced with permission from Brunelli GA, Brunelli GR. A new technique to correct carpal instability with scaphoid rotary subluxation: a preliminary report. J Hand Surg. 1995;20A(3):S82–S85.)

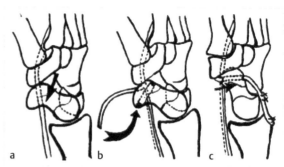

Fig. 15.2 Surgical procedure (lateral view). (a) Rotary subluxation of the scaphoid; (b) prepared flexor carpi radialis (FCR) tendon slip ready to be passed through a tunnel made in the distal pole of the scaphoid, parallel to its distal articular surface; (c) FCR tendon slip is passed through the tunnel, pulled dorsally to reduce rotary subluxation, and sutured to fibrous elements of the lunate ligament and radius. (Reproduced with permission from Brunelli GA, Brunelli GR. A new technique to correct carpal instability with scaphoid rotary subluxation: a preliminary report. J Hand Surg. 1995;20A(3):S82–S85.)

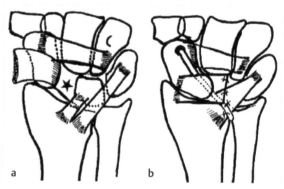

Fig. 15.3 Surgical procedure (sagittal view). (a) Incision and reflection of the capsuloligamentous tissues between the scaphoid and lunate to expose the dissociation (*star*) and remove the interarticular dorsal scar tissue; (b) after reduction of the scaphoid, the flexor carpi radialis (FCR) tendon slip is sutured to the dorsoulnar edge of the radius and the capsule is sutured back in place. (Reproduced with permission from Brunelli GA, Brunelli GR. A new technique to correct carpal instability with scaphoid rotary subluxation: a preliminary report. J Hand Surg. 1995;20A(3):S82–S85.)

pulled dorsally, reducing the scaphoid which is then held in extension via a K-wire into the capitate (▶ Fig. 15.2). The graft is inserted into fibrous tissue on the dorsoulnar side of the radius (▶ Fig. 15.3). The original description reported 13 cases with follow-up from 6 months to 2 years, at which point 11 of the 13 cases were pain free. There was a reduction in flexion of 30 to 60% compared with the contralateral wrist. Grip strength was 35% of the noninjured side and all patients returned to work after an average of 100 days, although it is not clear whether this was to original employment.

15.2.2 The Three-Ligament Tenodesis (3LT)

In 1998, authors from the tertiary unit described outcomes using a modification of the original Brunelli technique.[13] Instead of suturing the FCR tendon slip to the distal radius it was passed under and around the obliquely orientated dorsal radiolunotriquetral ligament, and then sutured back on itself using a 3–0 Prolene suture

(▶ Fig. 15.4). Rotatory subluxation of the scaphoid can be reduced using "joystick" K-wires prior to tensioning. One surgeon from the unit additionally sutured the same graft onto the lunate using an anchor. Encouraging short-term outcomes were reported in 22 patients with a mean of 9 months (range 6–16).[13]

Subsequently, outcomes were reported in 162 patients operated on in the unit, over a range of 7 years. Of these 162 patients, 117 were contactable for review at the time of publication.[14] Mean follow-up was 4.1 years for the

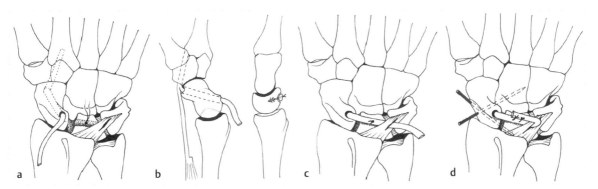

Fig. 15.4 The 3LT technique. **(a)** A strip of flexor carpi radialis (FCR) tendon is passed obliquely from the palmar scaphoid tuberosity to the dorsal ridge of the scaphoid where the dorsal scapholunate (SL) ligament normally inserts. **(b)** The tendon graft is set across the SL joint to be buried in a trough created on the dorsum of the lunate by means of an anchor suture. **(c)** To obtain adequate graft tension a slit at the distal portion of the dorsal radiotriquetral (RTq) ligament is made, through which the tendon is passed. **(d)** The graft finally is sutured onto itself while two K-wires neutralize both the SL and scaphocapitate (SC) joints. Unlike Brunelli's tenodesis the tendon graft does not cross the radiocarpal joint. (Reproduced with permission from Garcia-Elias M, Lluch AL, Stanley JK. Three-ligament tenodesis for the treatment of scapholunate dissociation: indications and surgical technique. J Hand Surg. 2006;31A:125–134.)

dynamic instability group, and 3.7 years for the reducible static instability group. Out of these, 62% were pain free, 28% had moderate pain, and 6% had severe pain. Mean pain score was 3.7. There was a 33-degree (26%) loss of flexion-extension and 13-degree (12%) loss of radial-ulnar deviation compared with the nonoperated side, and the grip strength was 80% of the nonoperated side. Those with legal claims scored more poorly on patient-reported outcome measures (PROMS). Four patients had tender palmar scars and of those three required exploration and neuroma excision. Two had gone on to have scaphocapitate fusion, and two to total wrist fusion, all for persistent mechanical pain.

In 2013, the senior author (M.H.) reported outcomes of the modified Brunelli procedure in 14 professional athletes operated on over a 3-year period.[15] Eleven were rugby players, two were boxers, and one was a golfer. Eleven returned to play within 4 months of the procedure. Three did not return to professional sport partly due to symptoms and partly for unrelated reasons. Nine had returned to preinjury levels, two had not, on account of knee injuries. The senior author continues to map these early results.

Further evolutions of this technique were described by the senior hand surgeon of our unit together with surgeons from the Institut Kaplan, Barcelona.[2] In view of the technique's ability to reconstruct the function of the STT, dorsal SL, and dorsal radiotriquetral (RTq) ligaments, it became known as the 3LT. The original Wrightington approach preserved the posterior interosseous nerve (PIN) but it evolved to recommend a proximal sectioning of the nerve to avoid a painful neuroma in the wrist capsule. The importance of leaving enough dorsal RTq ligament is emphasized to prevent failure of the ulnar portion of

the ligament which acts as a pulley. The joint is inspected according to Garcia-Elias' five factors guiding treatment: dorsal SL integrity, dorsal SL healing potential, resting alignment of the scaphoid (indicating status of STT capsule and ligaments), reducibility of carpal alignment, and cartilage status of both the radiocarpal and midcarpal joints. A 3.2-mm drill hole is used to pass the tendon graft. The connections of the FCR to the trapezium are left intact, allowing the obliquity of the tendon strip as it passes through the scaphoid tubercle to mimic the scaphocapitate ligament. The graft is secured to the lunate with a bone anchor before it is passed through the RTq ligament. The scaphoid, lunate, and capitate are reduced and held with 1.6-mm K-wires prior to tensioning of the sutures anchoring the graft in position. The capsule and the extensor retinaculum are repaired, and the wires are buried subcutaneously, with anticipated removal at 8 weeks postoperatively. Garcia-Elias reported the results in 38 patients and noted pain relief at rest in 28 of those at an average follow-up of 46 months (range 7–98). Eight patients experienced mild discomfort on strenuous activity and two had pain in most activities of daily living. Twenty-nine out of 38 returned to their original occupation, 7 had to reduced strength activities, and 2 retired. Patients achieved 74% of flexion and 77% of extension of the noninjured side (range of movement [ROM]: 52–0–52 degrees); 78% of radial and 28% of ulnar inclination (ROM: 15–0–28 degrees). Grip strength recorded was 65% of the contralateral side. Two wrists collapsed into DISI, and one was overcorrected into a flexed lunate position. Seven wrists demonstrated mild degenerative change on radiographs, and two showed global osteoarthritis, although none required analgesia.

15

15.2.3 Volar Scapholunate Ligament Reconstruction

Surgical practice to date has traditionally focused on dorsal reconstruction, in view of Berger's original work on cadavers with sectioned ligaments, and Short's subsequent insights into failure strengths.[5,16] These suggested failure strengths in the order of 300 N for the dorsal SLIL, and 120 N for the volar ligament. Published literature does not yet allow comparison of dorsal-only versus dorsal-plus volar ligament reconstruction for isolated SLIL pathology or Mayfield Stage I injury,[17] although a number of modifications of the 3LT have been described to provide volar stability. Postoperative radiographs following a Brunelli-type procedure often suggest the presence of persistent SL diastasis following dorsal-only techniques, although when present this correlates poorly with symptoms or satisfaction.[18] An early advocate of open volar and dorsal reconstruction was the Policlinico of Modena, Italy group who described a combined open approach but then suture anchor repair rather than reconstruction. Six patients were reported with average 32 months follow-up[19] in patients presenting up to 6 months post injury. Two had no pain at final follow-up, three had pain after work, and one had pain with daily activities. However, the dual approach with release of the dorsal capsule for exposure carries greater concern where bone tunnels are also being placed in poorly vascularized bone, which led to the evolution of arthroscopic capsular-sparing techniques discussed in the following chapter.[20,22]

The majority of described volar approaches aim to address multidirectional instability in a Mayfield 2–4 injury. Chee and colleagues, together with Garcia-Elias, recommended an open approach for volar and dorsal fixation of instability following perilunate dislocation.[23] They termed this procedure "the Antipronation Spiral Tenodesis." A strip of FCR is passed through the scaphoid as in the Brunelli technique, and is then passed dorsal to volar through the triquetrum, retrieved through the carpal tunnel and passed under the flexor tendons, and sutured to the volar aspect of the radial styloid using an anchor. Their description included a review of five patients treated in this way, of whom three had follow-up of over 1 year. Three had sustained a perilunate injury, and two had an SLIL injury with ulnar translocation of the lunate. They lost 15% of range of motion and had 70% of contralateral grip strength, but all were reported to have returned to previous activities, but two had pain at extremes of motion or performing strenuous tasks.

In 2013, Henry[24] suggested an alternative open volar and dorsal reconstruction for multidirectional instability confirmed arthroscopically after SLIL injury. In this technique the FCR graft is passed volar to dorsal through the lunate, and then dorsal to volar through the lunate, and sutured to the distal residual FCR attachment. A single case in which the technique was employed is described.

The author recognizes the possibility of avascular necrosis or iatrogenic fracture with this method, and currently a large series data is not available to support routine use.

15.2.4 The 360 Tenodesis (SLITT)

In 2019, authors from the Mayo Clinic, Rochester, USA described an alternative to the 3LT, borne out of concerns regarding the need for prolonged immobilization, the risk of retained broken wires, and the focus on dorsal reconstruction, with no consideration for the palmar SLIL which provides in the order of 120 N of failure strength.[16] They named their technique "the Scapholunate Ligament Internal Brace 360-degree Tenodesis (SLITT)" procedure.[25] They described a case using a palmaris longus autograft anchored dorsally using biotenodesis screws, and the reconstruction was reinforced with suture-tape passed through the biotenodesis screws and tied volarly. Their subsequent biomechanical study compared 360-degree reconstructions via palmaris longus graft only, and 360-degree tenodesis using an internal brace (suture-tape) in 24 fresh frozen cadavers.[26] The SLILs were sectioned and the wrist was disarticulated for testing. The grafts were passed dorsal to volar through the lunate, volar to dorsal through the scaphoid, and dorsal to volar through the lunate to achieve 360-degree stability, and were then held with biotenodesis screws. In the suture-tape arm these were passed through the biotenodesis screws to prevent cut-out through cortical bone. The suture-tape group failed at 283.47 +/- 100 N, compared with the internal brace group which failed at 143.61 +/- 90.54 N. The authors suggest that consideration of this technique in a clinical setting may allow more rapid return of active movement. They also suggest that an extension of the technique could be considered to reconstruct the long radiolunate ligament in cases of ulnar translocation of the lunate described by Taleisnik.[27,28]

15.3 The Author's Preferred Technique and Pitfalls

The senior author's experience with modified Brunelli has been reported historically,[14] and it remains his preferred technique today. This is done via dorsal approach to the wrist with an incision no more proximal than Lister's tubercle, retaining extensor pollicis longus (EPL) in its subsheath. A distally based capsular flap is made (▶ Fig. 15.5), with retention of the full thickness of the RTq to act as a pulley.[29] The drill hole in the scaphoid is made dorsal to volar prior to graft harvest, to avoid the risk of wrapping the graft around the K-wire or cannulated drill. The pitfall is aiming pole to pole in the scaphoid as a surgeon might do for scaphoid fixation, as this will not allow enough extension on the scaphoid. Instead, the dorsal entry point for the guidewire is at the sweet spot of the proximal pole just next to the dorsal SL

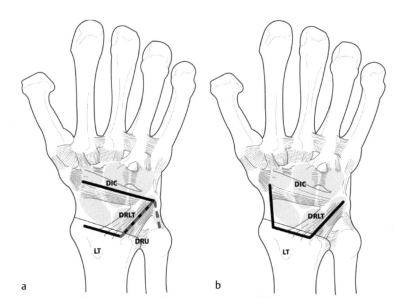

Fig. 15.5 The modified capsulotomy. **(a)** Line drawing of Berger's dorsal capsulotomy showing standard incisions for radiocarpal access marked by a *solid line* and an additional capsulotomy for ulnar-sided access using a *dotted line*. DIC, dorsal intercarpal ligament; DRLT, dorsal radiolunotriquetral ligament; DRU, dorsal radioulnar ligament; LT, Lister's tubercle. **(b)** Line drawing of modified distally based capsulotomy. DIC, dorsal intercarpal ligament; DRLT, dorsal radiolunotriquetral ligament; LT, Lister's tubercle. (Reproduced with permission Anakwe RE, Middleton SD, Hayton MJ. A modified dorsal capsulotomy for improved radiocarpal exposure. J Hand Surg Eur Vol. 2013;38(7):805–806.)

footprint, and the exit point slightly more proximal to the ST joint, such that when the graft pulls, the scaphoid tubercle is brought into extension. This must be tempered with the risk of fracture if the entry is too distal, and not enough cortical bone is left to support a 3.2-mm drill hole. The scaphoid tubercle is exposed through a small J-shaped incision retracting the FCR tendon prior to harvest of the volar third. This incision should be made carefully using blunt dissection retracting branches of the palmar cutaneous branch of the median nerve to avoid a painful postoperative neuroma. The K-wire and drill is brought out volarly and radially in the scaphoid under direct vision and checked on X-ray image intensifier.

The volar ulnar one-third of the FCR tendon is harvested and the spiraling nature of the fibers of the tendon ensure they are radiodorsal at their insertion. A blunt Carroll tendon passer is passed along the FCR sheath at the level of the scaphoid tubercle incision, and is used to retrieve the graft distally via a separate 1-cm transverse incision approximately 10 cm from the tubercle. The graft should be sized carefully—an oversized graft will not pass through the drill hole or will bunch preventing appropriate extension of the scaphoid. A 0.8-mm cerclage wire loop is fashioned to act as tendon passer through the bone tunnel and passed from dorsal to volar through the scaphoid drill hole. Only the very end of the FCR graft should be placed into the wire loop to avoid bunching. The graft is brought carefully into the hole under direct vision at the tubercle, and then delivered dorsally. An appropriate bone anchor is placed in the reduced neutral lunate. The graft is brought through and around the RTq ligament and passed back onto itself. This is then all tied down to the lunate with the anchor sutures.

A video demonstrating the senior author's technique is available at https://www.vumedi.com/video/brunelli-triligament-tenodesis-for-scapholunate-instability/.

15.4 Conclusion

Open reconstruction for chronic SL deficiency remains a challenging diagnosis for wrist surgeons to manage. Multiple procedures have been described; all of these procedures aim to restore pain-free stability, but most of them will sacrifice ROM to achieve this. The tertiary unit remains advocates of the modified Brunelli on account of the satisfactory published outcomes achieved with this technique in both the general and athletic populations. This is a technically demanding operation with a resultant learning curve, and the tips described in this chapter have evolved with the authors' experience. The authors appreciate that the prolonged immobilization period remains challenging for patients, and they look forward to seeing case series data from the Mayo clinic's SLITT procedure when it is available in the future.

References

[1] Garcia-Elias M. The non-dissociative clunking wrist: a personal view. J Hand Surg Eur Vol. 2008; 33(6):698–711

[2] Garcia-Elias M, Lluch AL, Stanley JK. Three-ligament tenodesis for the treatment of scapholunate dissociation: indications and surgical technique. J Hand Surg Am. 2006; 31(1):125–134

[3] Chen RE, Calfee RP, Stepan JG, Osei DA. Outcomes of acute versus subacute scapholunate ligament repair. J Hand Surg Glob Online. 2021; 4(2):103–110

[4] Zarkadas PC, Gropper PT, White NJ, Perey BH. A survey of the surgical management of acute and chronic scapholunate instability. J Hand Surg Am. 2004; 29(5):848–857

15

[5] Short WH, Werner FW, Green JK, Sutton LG, Brutus JP. Biomechanical evaluation of the ligamentous stabilizers of the scaphoid and lunate: part III. J Hand Surg Am. 2007; 32(3):297–309

[6] Watson HK, Weinzweig J, Zeppieri J. The natural progression of scaphoid instability. Hand Clin. 1997; 13(1):39–49

[7] Watson HK, Ballet FL. The SLAC wrist: scapholunate advanced collapse pattern of degenerative arthritis. J Hand Surg Am. 1984; 9 (3):358–365

[8] Trail IA, Stanley JK, Hayton MJ. Twenty questions on carpal instability. J Hand Surg Eur Vol. 2007; 32(3):240–255

[9] Deshmukh SC, Givissis P, Belloso D, Stanley JK, Trail IA. Blatt's capsulodesis for chronic scapholunate dissociation. J Hand Surg [Br]. 1999; 24(2):215–220

[10] Blatt G. Capsulodesis in reconstructive hand surgery. Dorsal capsulodesis for the unstable scaphoid and volar capsulodesis following excision of the distal ulna. Hand Clin. 1987; 3(1):81–102

[11] Brunelli G, Libassi G, Stafani G. La instabilita del polso (wrist instability). Riv Chir Mano. 1981; 18:27–46

[12] Kleinman WB. Long-term study of chronic scapho-lunate instability treated by scapho-trapezio-trapezoid arthrodesis. J Hand Surg Am. 1989; 14(3):429–445

[13] Van Den Abbeele KLS, Loh YC, Stanley JK, Trail IA. Early results of a modified Brunelli procedure for scapholunate instability. J Hand Surg [Br]. 1998; 23(2):258–261

[14] Talwalkar SC, Edwards ATJ, Hayton MJ, Stilwell JH, Trail IA, Stanley JK. Results of tri-ligament tenodesis: a modified Brunelli procedure in the management of scapholunate instability. J Hand Surg [Br]. 2006; 31(1):110–117

[15] Williams A, Ng CY, Hayton MJ. When can a professional athlete return to play following scapholunate ligament delayed reconstruction? Br J Sports Med. 2013; 47(17):1071–1074

[16] Berger RA. The gross and histologic anatomy of the scapholunate interosseous ligament. J Hand Surg Am. 1996; 21(2):170–178

[17] Mayfield JK, Johnson RP, Kilcoyne RK. Carpal dislocations: pathomechanics and progressive perilunar instability. J Hand Surg Am. 1980; 5(3):226–241

[18] Viegas S. Ligamentous repair following acute scapholunate dissociation. In: Gelberman RH, ed. The Wrist. New York: Raven Press; 1994:135–146

[19] Marcuzzi A, Leti Acciaro A, Caserta G, Landi A. Ligamentous reconstruction of scapholunate dislocation through a double dorsal and palmar approach. J Hand Surg [Br]. 2006; 31(4):445–449

[20] Corella F, Del Cerro M, Ocampos M, Simon de Blas C, Larrainzar-Garijo R. Arthroscopic scapholunate ligament reconstruction, volar and dorsal reconstruction. Hand Clin. 2017; 33(4):687–707

[21] Ho PC, Wong CW, Tse WL. Arthroscopic-assisted combined dorsal and volar scapholunate ligament reconstruction with tendon graft for chronic SL instability. J Wrist Surg. 2015; 4(4):252–263

[22] Mathoulin C, Merlini L, Taleb C. Scapholunate injuries: challenging existing dogmas in anatomy and surgical techniques. J Hand Surg Eur Vol. 2021; 46(1):5–13

[23] Chee KG, Chin AYH, Chew EM, Garcia-Elias M. Antipronation spiral tenodesis: a surgical technique for the treatment of perilunate instability. J Hand Surg Am. 2012; 37(12):2611–2618

[24] Henry M. Reconstruction of both volar and dorsal limbs of the scapholunate interosseous ligament. J Hand Surg Am. 2013;38(8):1625–1634

[25] Kakar S, Greene RM. Scapholunate ligament internal brace 360-degree tenodesis (SLITT) procedure. J Wrist Surg. 2018; 7(4):336–340

[26] Kakar S, Greene RM, Denbeigh J, Van Wijnen A. Scapholunate ligament internal brace 360 tenodesis (SLITT) procedure: a biomechanical study. J Wrist Surg. 2019; 8(3):250–254

[27] Taleisnik J. The ligaments of the wrist. J Hand Surg Am. 1976; 1(2):110–118

[28] Taleisnik J. The wrist. New York: Churchill Livingstone; 1985

[29] Anakwe RE, Middleton SD, Hayton MJ. A modified dorsal capsulotomy for improved radiocarpal exposure. J Hand Surg Eur Vol. 2013; 38(7):805–806

III

16 Chronic "R"econstruction (Ligamentoplasties): Arthroscopic Treatment

Pak Cheong Ho and Jeffrey Justin Siu Cheong Koo

Abstract

Both the dorsal and the volar portion of the scapholunate interosseous ligament (SLIL) are major stabilizers of the scapholunate (SL) joint. Most reconstruction methods to restore SL stability do not address the volar constraints and frequently fail to reduce the SL gapping. With the assistance of arthroscopy and intraoperative imaging as a guide, a combined limited dorsal and volar incision exposed the dorsal and palmar SL interval without violating the wrist joint capsule. Bone tunnels were made on the proximal scaphoid and lunate. A palmaris longus tendon graft was delivered through the wrist capsule and the bone tunnels to reduce and connect the two bones in a boxlike fashion. Once the joint diastasis is reduced and any dorsal intercalated segment instability (DISI) malrotation corrected, the tendon graft was knotted and sutured on the dorsal surface of the SL joint extracapsularly in a shoe-lacing manner. The scaphocapitate joint could be transfixed with Kirschner wires (K-wires) to protect the reconstruction for 6 to 8 weeks. The authors have satisfactory results in their 17 patients regarding pain, range of motion, and grip strength. Recurrence of a DISI deformity was noted in four patients without symptoms. Ischemic change of proximal scaphoid was noted in one case without symptoms or progression. There were no major complications. All patients were satisfied with the procedure and outcome.

Keywords: wrist arthroscopy, scapholunate ligament, scapholunate instability, tendon graft

16.1 Introduction and Historical Perspective

Scapholunate interosseous ligament (SLIL) instability is the most common form of carpal instability. Falling onto an extended wrist is the usual injury mechanism to the SLIL. Mayfield et al described a sequential failure of carpal osteoligamentous architecture. Starting radially, the force is transmitted through either the scaphoid body (transscaphoid) or SLIL (SL dissociation) into the midcarpal joint and then to the ulnar aspect of the wrist. The SL joint stability depends on two systems of ligaments: the intrinsic SLIL and secondary extrinsic stabilizers such as dorsal radiocarpal (DRC) ligament, dorsal intercarpal (DIC) ligament, scaphotrapezial (ST) ligament, and radioscaphocapitate (RSC) ligament. Each has a distinct role; however, they work in concert to form the scapholunate ligament complex (SLLC).[1]

Different stages in SL instability have been described by Watson et al, which resulted from the rotary subluxation of scaphoid. Based on the findings on static X-ray and cineradiography, the instability can be categorized into predynamic, dynamic, static with or without dorsal intercalated segment instability (DISI), and finally with degeneration as seen in scapholunate advanced collapse (SLAC)[2] (▶ Table 16.1). The degree of malalignment seen is due to gradual loss of stabilizing structures during primary injury or attenuation after trauma. Therefore, SL diastasis would only occur in a combined intrinsic and extrinsic ligament injury or a primary SLIL injury with gradual attenuation of the extrinsic ligaments. Permanent malalignment occurs when SLIL and secondary stabilizers are disrupted, and the proximal row will progress to the typical deformity: lunate and triquetrum will go into extension. At the same time, the scaphoid flexes and pronates around the RSC ligament leading to the typical DISI deformity.[3] The proximal pole of the scaphoid subluxes dorsoradially, causing increased compressive and shear stresses on the dorsolateral aspect of the radioscaphoid fossa and producing characteristic dorsal wrist pain and degenerative changes over there. The extended lunate remains stable with the radius since both opposing articulating surfaces have the same radius of curvature. This can

Table 16.1 Severity of scapholunate instability classified by radiograph[2]

Group	Description
Predynamic instability	Radiographs not showing any abnormality but physical examination is positive with pain on wrist movement. There is only tear in palmar and proximal portion of SLIL. Pain is only due to synovitis.
Dynamic stability	Radiographs reveal the injury under stressed or dynamic loading. The secondary stabilizers of the scapholunate joint maintain the scapholunate alignment when no stress is applied.
Static scapholunate dissociation	Static radiographs show scaphoid displacement without stressed or dynamic loading. The SLL and secondary stabilizers are completely torn and malalignment exists.
Scapholunate advanced collapse	Radiographs show static scapholunate dissociation with wrist arthritis changes

Abbreviations: SLIL, scapholunate interosseous ligament; SLL, scapholunate ligament.

Table 16.2 Five Questions set by Garcia-Elias for developing stage-based treatment algorithms

Scapholunate dissociation stage	1	2	3	4	5	6
Is there a partial rupture with a normal dorsal SL ligament?	Yes	No	No	No	No	No
If ruptured, can the dorsal SL ligament be repaired?	Yes	Yes	No	No	No	No
Is the scaphoid normally aligned (radioscaphoid angle ≤ 45 degrees)?	Yes	Yes	Yes	No	No	No
Is the carpal malalignment easily reducible?	Yes	Yes	Yes	Yes	No	No
Are the cartilages at both RC and MC joints normal?	Yes	Yes	Yes	Yes	Yes	No

Abbreviations: MC, midcarpal; RC, radiocarpal; SL, scapholunate.
Reproduced with permission from Garcia-Elias M, Lluch AL, Stanley JK. Three-ligament tenodesis for the treatment of scapholunate dissociation: indications and surgical technique. J Hand Surg Am. 2006; 31(1):125–134.[5]

explain why the radiolunate (EL) joint seldom shows degeneration in the SLAC wrist unless very advanced.[4]

A set of questions have been proposed by Garcia-Elias et al, helping to determine the severity of SLIL injury and providing a framework to develop stage-based treatment[5] (▶ Table 16.2). Combining with Geissler's arthroscopic classification for SLIL injuries[6] (▶ Table 16.3), a treatment algorithm can be devised to guide decision-making based on the chronicity of injury, presence of dynamic or static radiographic changes, and presence of arthritic changes (▶ Fig. 16.1). Newer classification such as European Wrist Arthroscopy Society (EWAS) arthroscopic classification further defines which portion of SLIL has been injured[7] (▶ Table 16.4).

Choosing the optimal treatment requires consideration of several factors: the amount of instability (static vs dynamic), the elapsed time between injury and treatment (acute vs chronic), and the presence of associated injury or degenerative changes. Timing of the injury is crucial as the healing potential of the disrupted ligament is better in the acute setting and has a significantly better surgical outcome.[8]

16.2 Literature Review and Different Surgical Techniques

In chronic SLIL injuries (> 6 weeks), ligament reconstruction results are superior to repair.[9] Reconstruction can change the deteriorating pattern of instability, but the function is restored in a limited fashion with wrist mobility sacrificed in return.[10] Salvage procedures will be considered in the presence of degenerative arthritis.

Planning of SLIL reconstruction needs careful assessment. The diagnostic wrist arthroscopy findings provide important information for decision-making in the

Table 16.3 Geissler arthroscopic classification of scapholunate interosseous ligament tear[6]

Grade	Description
I	Hemorrhage and attenuation of the interosseous ligament viewed from the radiocarpal joint and no step-off at the midcarpal joint
II	Hemorrhage and attenuation of the interosseous ligament at the radiocarpal joint. Step-off can be viewed at the midcarpal joint and the probe can be placed between the scaphoid and lunate
III	Step-off between the scaphoid and lunate is viewed at both the radiocarpal and midcarpal joints. The probe can be easily placed and rotated between the scaphoid and lunate gap
IV	Gross instability is noted at the scapholunate interval and a 2.7-mm arthroscope can be placed in the scapholunate diastasis

management plan. Not only the degree of SLIL tear can be assessed, it also helps to discover any associated intra-articular soft tissue lesions and the extent of articular degeneration in the chronic situation.

Traditionally, Open reconstruction is considered for tears beyond acute grade IV and Chronic grade III. Numerous surgical techniques, including bone-ligament-bone graft, three-ligament tenodesis, dorsal and volar capsulodesis, and scapholunate axis method (SLAM), have been described to restore or improve the stability of the SL joint and retard or prevent the progression to arthritis.[5,11,29] However, there is no consensus on the optimal treatment of chronic SLIL ligament tears. Among those focused on SLIL reconstruction, most methods provide only dorsal and uniplanar reconstructions, and

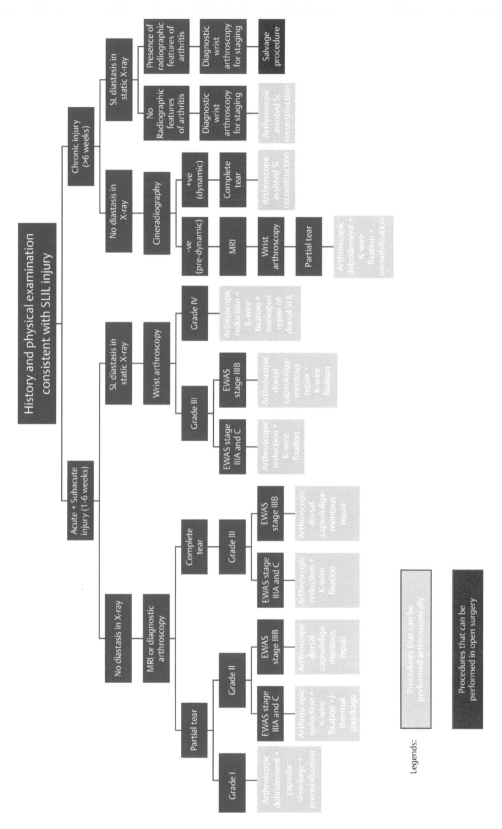

Fig. 16.1 Flowchart showing the treatment algorithm based on the chronicity of injury, presence of dynamic or static radiographic changes, and presence of arthritic changes.

Table 16.4 Arthroscopic EWAS classification and relative anatomical findings in cadaver specimens

EWAS arthroscopic stage	Arthroscopic findings of SLIL from midcarpal joint	Anatomical findings
I	The tip of the probe cannot enter SL space, only synovitis	Not found in cadaver specimens
II lesion of membranous portion of SLIL	The passage of the tip can go through the SL space without widening (stable)	Lesion of proximal portion of SLIL
IIIA partial lesion involving volar portion of SLIL	Volar SL widening on dynamic testing from midcarpal joint (volar laxity)	Lesion of volar and proximal portion of SLIL with or without lesion of RSC
IIIB partial lesion involving dorsal portion of SLIL	Dorsal SL widening on dynamic testing from midcarpal joint (dorsal laxity)	Lesion of proximal and dorsal portion of SLIL with partial lesion of DIC
IIIC complete SLIL tear, reducible SL joint	Complete widening of SL space on dynamic testing, SL joint reducible upon removal of probe	Complete lesion of SLIL (volar, proximal, and dorsal), complete lesion of one extrinsic ligament (DIC or RSC)
IV complete SLIL with SL gap	SL gap with passage of arthroscope through SL joint No radiological abnormalities	Complete lesion of SLIL (volar, proximal, and dorsal), complete lesion of extrinsic ligaments (DIC and RSC)
V	Wide SL gap with passage of arthroscope through SL joint with X-ray abnormalities	Complete lesion of SLIL (volar, proximal, and dorsal), extrinsic ligaments (DIC and RSC) and one or more ligaments (TH, STT, DRC)

Abbreviations: DIC, dorsal intercarpal; DRC, dorsal radiocarpal; RSC, radioscaphocapitate; SL, scapholunate; SLIL, scapholunate interosseous ligament; STT, scapho-trapezial-trapezoidal; TH, triquetro-hamate.
Adapted from Messina JC, Van Overstraeten L, Luchetti R, Fairplay T, Mathoulin CL. The EWAS classification of scapholunate tears: an anatomical arthroscopic study. J Wrist Surg. 2013;2(2):105–109.[7]

the importance of the SLIL volar component is often underrated.[14,15,21,22,25] Volar component has an important role in the rotational constraint of the SL joint and will create shear stress between the scaphoid and lunate when sectioned.[30,31] Yi et al used a palmaris longus (PL) tendon to pass through drill holes in the anteroposterior plane of the scaphoid and the lunate. As a result, the SL diastasis was effectively reduced to normal, and the scaphoid and lunate contact pressure on the radius and the scaphoid-to-lunate contact ratio were significantly improved after the reconstruction.[32] Zdero et al used bovine tendons passing through double bone tunnels of the scaphoid and lunate in 19 cadaveric wrists and found no difference in the mechanical property from the normal wrists.[33] Based on the result of biomechanical studies, restoring both the dorsal and volar components of the SLIL ligament is more logical and ideal.

Apart from biomechanical factors, there are concerns on open surgery about the extensive soft tissue dissection required for reconstruction which can lead to soft tissue and vascularity damage. Dobyns used a portion of the tendon to pass through anteroposterior bone tunnels in the proximal pole of the scaphoid and lunate to reconstruct the SL linkage. Stability was obtained by tightly looping the tendon graft across the scaphoid and lunate.[34] However, creating drill holes across poorly vascularized areas of bone in an open fashion severely compromised their blood supply and resulted in fractures and avascular necrosis. The joint capsule is often opened up, and important structures that are crucial for wrist stability are cut for exposure during surgery, especially the DIC ligament, which is a crucial secondary extrinsic stabilizer, and the posterior interosseous nerve (PIN) has an important role in proprioception and neuromuscular control on wrist stability.[35,41] Range of motion (ROM), especially wrist flexion, has decreased due to scarring and stiffness after open surgery.[5]

The recent development of arthroscopic-assisted reconstruction techniques for chronic SL dissociation showed promising results.[42,43] Corella et al created two bone tunnels: one on the scaphoid for dorsal SLIL ligament origin to scaphoid tubercle and the other on lunate perpendicular to the distal articular surface as seen in lateral view. Using a strip of flexor carpi radialis (FCR) harvested from distal to proximal with approximately 10 cm in length and 3 mm width, retrieved from distal harvesting wound close to the volar scaphoid tunnel entrance site. The FCR tendon graft is passed from the volar side of the scaphoid tunnel and exits through the dorsal end of the bone tunnel. The tendon graft is fixed to the scaphoid bone tunnel with a 3 × 8 mm tenodesis screw (Arthrex, Naples, NL). Through intra-articular passage with the help of a curved suture lasso (Arthrex, Naples, NL), the tendon

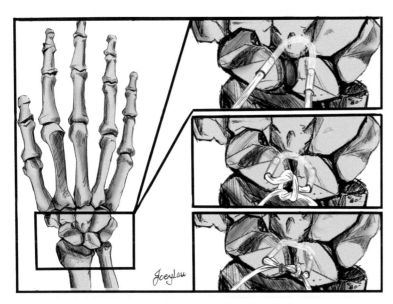

Fig. 16.2 Simultaneous reconstruction of the dorsal and palmar SL ligaments anatomically with the use of tendon graft in a boxlike manner. (Courtesy of Joey Lau Chun Yin.)

graft exits through the dorsal central wound, which is communicated with the dorsal entrance of the lunate bone tunnel. The tendon graft then passes through the lunate bone tunnel and leaves the volar bone tunnel exit. Finally, the graft passes extra-articularly over the volar joint capsule and is directly fixed to the SLIL ligament footprint over the scaphoid by Micro-Corkscrew 2/0 (Arthrex, Naples, NL). In their review of 27 patients (20 males and 7 females) performed between 2011 and 2016, 14 patients had EWAS Grade IIIC, and 13 had Grade IV lesions. The preoperative and 6 months postoperative ROM is the same, with significant improvement in grip strength and DASH score. Both dynamic and static instability groups (16 dynamic vs 11 static) have a significant decrease in average SL gap and average SL angle after surgery.[42]

In 2002, the senior author (PC Ho) developed an arthroscopic-assisted technique to reconstruct the dorsal and volar SL ligament simultaneously using a free tendon graft in a boxlike structure without violating the major blood supply to the scaphoid and soft tissue envelope (▶ Fig. 16.2).[43]

16.3 Indications and Contraindications for Surgery

The technique is indicated in subacute or chronic SL dissociation of 6 weeks or beyond with reducible SL diastasis and dorsal intercalated segmental instability (DISI) deformity confirmed arthroscopically and radiologically.

Contraindications include SLAC wrist beyond Watson stage I and chronic nonreducible SL dissociation after adequate intra-articular fibrosis and capsular contracture release.

16.4 Authors' Preferred Technique

The authors advise performing diagnostic wrist arthroscopy under portal site local anesthesia before the definitive surgery for complete diagnostic purposes, especially if the SL dissociation cannot be fully accounted for the wrist pain.[44] This helps to evaluate the cause of the chronic wrist pain, confirm the status of the SL ligaments, evaluate the reducibility of the SL diastasis and rotation malalignment, and assess any cartilage or SLAC changes. Also, arthroscopic lysis at this stage can help improve the SL joint reducibility. If not, alternative treatment methods need to be considered.

16.5 Patient Preparation and Positioning

After anesthesia and before the patient is subjected to surgery, a thorough fluoroscopic assessment of the SL joint stability and reducibility is conducted. The amount of SL joint diastasis, DISI deformity, and dorsal scaphoid translation are noted. Reducibility can be evaluated by doing a passive radial deviation of the wrist to observe for apposition of the SL gap (▶ Fig. 16.3). Reduction of the DISI deformity can be assessed by applying a volarly directed pushing force to the dorsal scaphoid (▶ Fig. 16.4). Easily reducible SL dissociation will constitute a good indication for the captioned technique.

The surgery is performed under general anesthesia or regional block with the patient in the supine position and the operated arm resting on a hand table in 90-degree shoulder abduction. The elbow joint is flexed to 90 degrees, and the affected hand is subjected to 10 to 13 lb of traction force through the plastic finger traps applied to

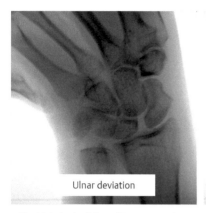
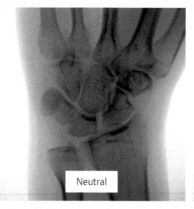
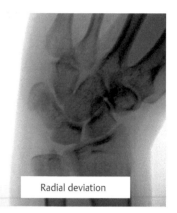

Ulnar deviation

Neutral

Radial deviation

Fig. 16.3 Reducibility of SL joint can be assessed under fluoroscopy, where radial deviation reduces the SL gap while ulnar deviation widens the gap.

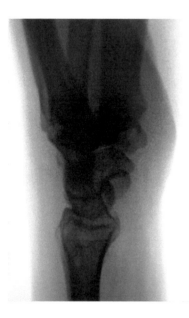
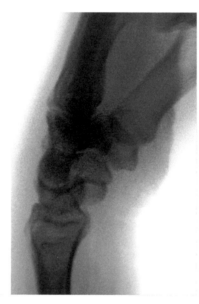

Fig. 16.4 By applying wrist flexion force, reducibility of lunate in DISI deformity can be seen under fluoroscope.

the middle three digits using a sterilizable Wrist Traction Tower (ConMed Linvatec Corp., Goleta, CA). The well-padded arm is strapped to the base plate of the tower to provide countertraction.

The arm tourniquet is not inflated initially. 2% ligno-caine with 1:200,000 adrenaline is injected into the portal sites over the skin and joint capsule to reduce bleeding. Continuous saline irrigation of the joint is achieved with a bag of 3 L of normal saline hung up at about 1.5 m instilled under gravity.

16.6 Exploration of Radiocarpal Joint and Midcarpal Joint

A 1.9-mm or 2.7-mm arthroscope is used. Small transverse skin crease incisions are made on the portal sites. Radiocarpal joint arthroscopy is performed initially

through the 3–4 and 4–5 portals with 6 U as the outflow portal, followed by midcarpal joint arthroscopy through the midcarpal radial (MCR) and midcarpal ulnar (MCU) portals. SL joint gapping, drive-through sign, articular step-off, the torn SL ligament remnant status, associated chondral lesions, and changes in the extrinsic ligaments can be observed. Synovectomy and radial styloidectomy can be performed simultaneously if necessary using a 2-mm shaver, small radiofrequency ablation probe, and 2.9-mm bur.

16.7 Taking-Down of Intra-Articular Fibrosis

In chronic SL dissociation with significant diastasis and DISI deformity, intra-articular fibrosis and capsular contracture are often found. In addition, a bundle of scar tissue interposed at the SL joint interval can prevent its adequate reduction (▶ Fig. 16.5). Fibrosis and scar tissue are resected with a shaver to improve the capsular elasticity and to facilitate subsequent reduction of the SL gap, malalignment, and DISI deformity. The carpal bones in the proximal carpal row can be squeezed manually under a reduced traction force to assess the reduction of the SL gap (▶ Fig. 16.6). Reducibility of scaphoid and lunate should also be confirmed by fluoroscopy before proceeding to the next stage.

16.8 Identification of Scaphoid and Lunate Bone Tunnel Sites

The operated arm is taken off the traction tower and put on the hand table. The arm tourniquet is then inflated after the hand and forearm are exsanguinated. A 2-cm transverse incision is centered at the 3–4 portal and extended 1 cm radially and 1 cm ulnarly toward the 4–5 portal (▶ Fig. 16.7). The extensor retinaculum is split along its oblique fibers. The extensor digitorum communis (EDC), extensor carpi radialis brevis (ECRB), and the extensor carpi radialis longus (ECRL) tendons are identified. Lunate can be exposed by retracting the EDC

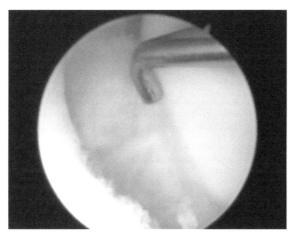

Fig. 16.5 A view from MCR portal looking into the midcarpal joint showing the dense scar tissue interposed between SL interval, which would hinder subsequent reduction.

tendons ulnarward or, more preferably, by passing between the EDC tendons. The ideal scaphoid tunnel position can be spotted between ECRB and ECRL tendons (▶ Fig. 16.8). The tendons are being slung with cotton tapes for protection and retraction.

Volarly, a transverse incision is made along the proximal wrist crease from the radial border of the palmaris longus (PL) to the ulnar border of the FCR tendon (▶ Fig. 16.9). Palmar cutaneous branch of the median nerve should be dissected out and safeguarded (▶ Fig. 16.10). PL-free graft is harvested with a tendon stripper. The volar forearm fascia is incised. The interval between the FCR tendon, the finger flexor tendons, and the median nerve is entered to reach the volar wrist joint capsule (▶ Fig. 16.11). The volar and dorsal wrist joint capsules contain the important extrinsic ligaments. Hence secondary stabilizers of the SL joint are carefully preserved without violation. The soft tissue dissection is kept to minimal.

16.9 Correction of DISI Deformity

DISI deformity needs to be corrected before drilling the bone tunnel. The hand is examined under the fluoroscope. The Linscheid maneuver can correct the extended lunate with wrist flexion to realign the lunate with radius. The lunate position can be maintained by transfixing the RL joint with a 1.6-mm K-wire inserted percutaneously through the dorsum of distal radius. The RL pin should be aimed at the ulnar half of the lunate to avoid conflict with the lunate bone tunnel (▶ Fig. 16.12). The wrist is now ready for bone tunnel preparation.

16.10 Preparation of Lunate Bone Tunnel

A lunate bone tunnel is created through the dorsal incision. Either by retracting the tendons ulnarly, or more preferably, passing through the EDC tendons, the dorsal portion of the lunate can be reached. A 1.1-mm guide pin is inserted into the lunate perpendicular to the long axis of the lunate, i.e., parallel to the line joining the tip of the volar and dorsal lips of the lunate, through the capsule under fluoroscopic guidance. The guide pin should aim at the center of the lunate to avoid an iatrogenic blow-out

Before reduction   After reduction

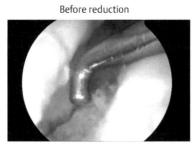 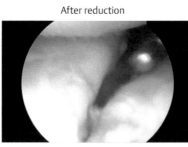

Fig. 16.6 By removing the scar tissue in between SL interval, the gap can be reduced with squeezing proximal carpal bone externally.

III

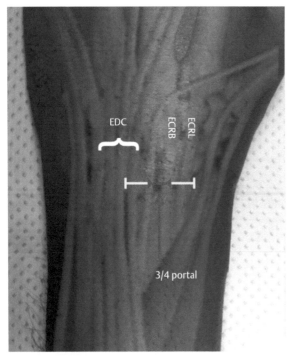

Fig. 16.7 Planning of dorsal skin incision. Using the 3-4 portal as the center, skin incision is extended 1 cm radially and 1 cm ulnarly.

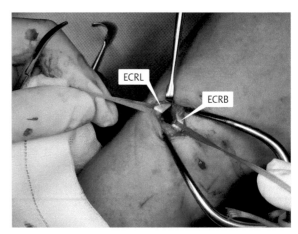

Fig. 16.8 By retracting the ECRB and ECRL, the "sweet" spot for placing the scaphoid bone tunnel can be located.

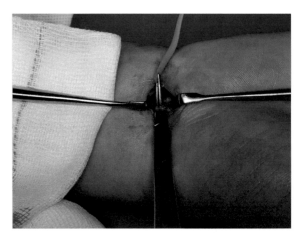

Fig. 16.10 The palmar cutaneous branch of median nerve should be dissected out and safeguarded, which is often found on radial side of skin incision.

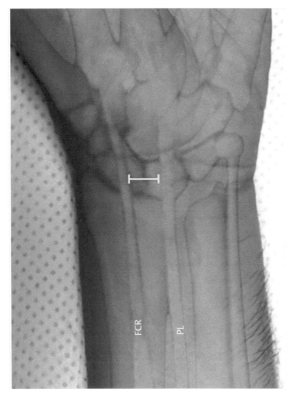

Fig. 16.9 Placement of volar skin incision. Transverse incision is made along the proximal wrist crease from the radial border of the palmaris longus (PL) to the ulnar border of the flexor carpi radialis (FCR) tendon.

fracture. For cases with mild DISI deformity, RL pinning may not be necessary. If the lunate is not being transfixed to the radius, manual traction of the wrist can help bring the lunate to a more distal position to uncover the lunate from the distal radius's dorsal rim facilitating the pinning process. Over the volar side, an assistant helps to gently retract and protect the flexor tendons and median nerve ulnarward. The surgeon advances the lunate tunnel guide pin to perforate the volar cortex of the lunate, volar joint capsule, and exit through the volar wound (▶ Fig. 16.13).

16.11 Preparation of Scaphoid Bone Tunnel

Another guide pin is inserted through the dorsal wound onto the scaphoid in the interval between the ECRB and

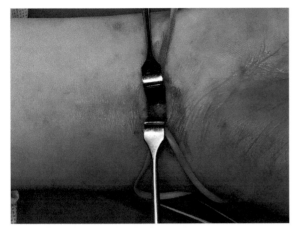

Fig. 16.11 Photo showing the volar joint capsule can be visualized by retracting FCR and palmar cutaneous branch of median nerve radially while median nerve and finger flexor tendons retract ulnarly.

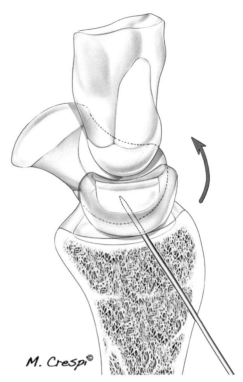

M. Crespi©

Fig. 16.12 Drawing showing the lunate reduction by the Linscheid maneuver. The radiolunate joint is transfixed with a 1.6-mm K-wire with the lunate in a neutral position. (Reproduced from Mathoulin C. Wrist Arthroscopy Techniques; Copyright © 2021 Thieme. All rights reserved.)

ECRL tendons. The guide pin aims at the proximal scaphoid at least 2 to 3 mm from the surrounding articular margin to avoid iatrogenic fracture both in coronal and sagittal planes. It provides a counter-rotational force on the scaphoid to correct the flexion pronation deformity when the guide pin trajectory is slightly directed proximally and volarly (▶ Fig. 16.14, ▶ Fig. 16.15). When the FCR tendon retracts radially, the scaphoid guide pin exits through the volar wound. Both the lunate and scaphoid bone tunnels are subsequently enlarged using 2.0-mm and 2.4-mm cannulated drill bits. We must bear in mind that the bone tunnels should not be too large as there is a risk of iatrogenic fracture or inducing bone ischemia. Too small the tunnel size may cause jamming of tendon graft inside the tunnel, causing graft attrition or even avulsion when being pulled through the tunnel. It is mandatory to use protection sheaths of adequate size on both the dorsal and volar side to protect the soft tissue during the pinning and drilling processes under fluoroscopic control.

16.12 Passing the Palmaris Longus Tendon Graft Through the Scaphoid and Lunate Bone Tunnel

The free PL tendon graft is delivered through the capsular vents and the bone tunnels with a 2-mm arthroscopic grasper, from the volar side of the scaphoid to the dorsal (▶ Fig. 16.16). It is critically important to be sure that the grasper is passing through inside the tunnels instead of slipping through the surface of the carpal bones. The grasper is then passed through the lunate bone tunnel from the dorsal to the volar side to grab onto the volar limb of the tendon graft. It is then brought to the dorsal side again through the lunate bone tunnel. Thus the tendon graft is passed outside the capsule to cross the SL

interval so that the reconstruction also helps to tighten the capsule and the extrinsic ligaments, which confer added stability to the SL joint (▶ Fig. 16.17). It is mandatory to check that the volar loop of the tendon graft does not trap on any of the flexor tendons and the median nerve before tying the tendon.

16.13 Assessment Through Midcarpal Joint Arthroscopy and Scapholunate Interval Reduction with Palmaris Longus Tendon Graft

The hand is put on the traction tower again. The midcarpal Joint is inspected through the MCR portal. The RL pin is then withdrawn from the lunate so that the lunate becomes mobile to facilitate reduction of the diastasis. Traction should be reduced to the minimum. When the two ends of the tendon graft are pulled manually, any SL gapping and step-off are corrected and can be visualized under arthroscopic and fluoroscopic surveillance. Any interposing soft tissue at the SL joint can be removed arthroscopically. Quality of reduction can be reassessed. If necessary, a large bone reduction clamp placed between

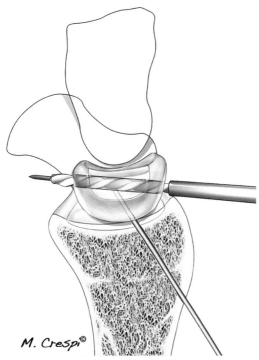

Fig. 16.13 Drawing showing preparation of lunate bone tunnel. 1.1-mm guide pin is inserted into the lunate perpendicular to the long axis of the lunate under fluoroscopic guidance. The guide pin should aim at the center of lunate and not too close to the articular margin to avoid iatrogenic blow-out fracture. Then the bone tunnel is prepared with cannulated drill from dorsal to volar direction. Using a 4.5-mm drill sleeve to protect the soft tissue from the K-wire and cannulated drill is often useful to avoid iatrogenic damage to flexors and median nerve. (Reproduced from Mathoulin C. Wrist Arthroscopy Techniques; Copyright © 2021 Thieme. All rights reserved.)

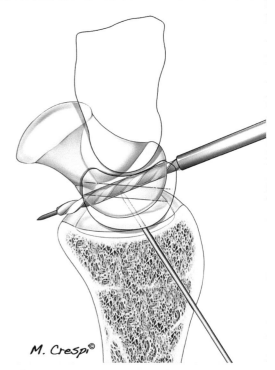

Fig. 16.14 Drawing showing preparation of scaphoid bone tunnel. Again, guide pin should be 2 to 3 mm away from articular margin to avoid blow-out. Guide pin trajectory is preferably slightly directed proximally and volarly to correct the flexion pronation deformity when the tendon graft is tightened. (Reproduced from Mathoulin C. Wrist Arthroscopy Techniques; Copyright © 2021 Thieme. All rights reserved.)

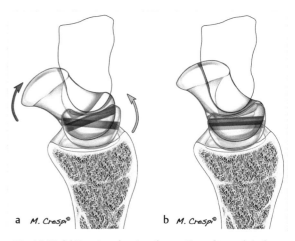

Fig. 16.15 **(a)** Drawing showing the position of tunnels before passage of tendon graft and before reduction. **(b)** Drawing showing the reduction of both tunnels after tensioning of the PL graft. (Reproduced from Mathoulin C. Wrist Arthroscopy Techniques; Copyright © 2021 Thieme. All rights reserved.)

the scaphoid and triquetrum percutaneously can facilitate the reduction. Once adequate reduction is confirmed by tensioning the tendon graft, the hand is put back on the hand table. The two ends of the tendon graft are passed underneath all the extensor tendons to meet each other at the SL joint. The tendon graft is maximally tensioned and tied in a shoelace manner over the dorsal capsule and secured with 2–0 nonabsorbable braided sutures on a noncutting needle (▶ Fig. 16.18). Additional sutures can be stitched through the adjacent capsular structure to augment the repair strength. SL reduction and stability are confirmed arthroscopically and fluoroscopically. If the reduction and stability are suboptimal, the suturing can be revised after further tensioning until the reduction is satisfactory. The tendon graft is then tied once more and sutured securely. Two knots of the tendon graft suffice as further knotting may produce an unacceptable bump at the back of the wrist. In case of chronic instability

with wide diastasis and difficult reduction, two 1.1-mm K-wires can be inserted through a small incision in the

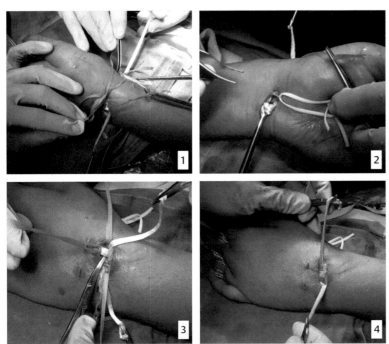

Fig. 16.16 Operative view of PL tendon graft is delivered through the wrist capsule and the bone tunnels. (1) Passing the 2-mm arthroscopic grasper from dorsal side to volar side to grab the PL tendon graft end and deliver through the bone tunnel to dorsal side. (2) Careful retraction helps prevent unnecessary trapping of flexor tendons and median nerve by the tendon graft. (3) Passing of PL tendon graft underneath the extensors to avoid iatrogenic entrapment of extensors. (4) After checking no soft tissue entrapment, it is ready for reduction and tightening of tendon graft.

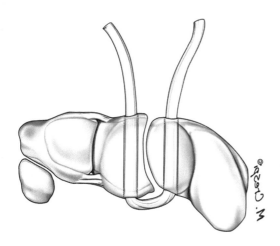

Fig. 16.17 Drawing showing the passage of PL tendon graft from scaphoid, volar to the volar capsule and through the lunate before final tightening and suture. (Reproduced from Mathoulin C. Wrist Arthroscopy Techniques; Copyright © 2021 Thieme. All rights reserved.)

additional repair strength. The RL pin is then advanced to maintain the lunate reduction if necessary. The protective pinning can be omitted if the reconstruction is considered solid and stable. The extensor tendons are repositioned, and the extensor retinaculum is repaired.

16.14 Closure and Postoperative Care

The wound is closed with absorbable subcuticular sutures. Bulky dressing and scaphoid plaster slab are applied with the wrist in a neutral position and the thumb in neutral palmar abduction.

The wrist is immobilized in a short arm thumb spica cast for 6 weeks. The RL pin is removed at the beginning of the third week. The cast is then changed to a thumb spica splint for an additional 2 weeks, at which time gentle active wrist mobilization exercise is allowed out of the splint. The SC pins are removed at the beginning of the ninth week under local anesthesia. The splint is worn at nighttime for another 4 to 6 weeks. Gradual wrist ROM exercise under physiotherapist supervision is started after the pin removal. Passive ROM exercise can be commenced at the beginning of the 11th week and gradual strengthening exercises in the 13th week after surgery. The SL reduction should be monitored at intervals with the radiological examination.

16.15 Clinical Outcome

In the first 17 patients with chronic SL instability operated between October 2002 and June 2012, there were three Geissler Grade 3 and fourteen Grade 4 instability cases. The average preoperative SL interval was 4.9 mm (range

anatomic snuffbox region to transfix the scaphocapitate (SC) joint to unload the SL joint and hence protect the reconstructed ligament during the healing process (▶ Fig. 16.19). The pins are cut short and buried underneath the skin for later removal. The authors advise against pinning the SL joint as this may risk injury and weakening of the tendon graft at the bone tunnels. Additional suture anchors can be placed next to the dorsal bone tunnels over the scaphoid and lunate and tied for

III

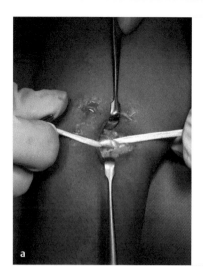
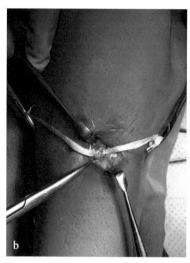

Fig. 16.18 (a) The tendon graft is knotted and **(b)** sutured under maximal tension on the dorsal surface of the SL joint extra-capsularly in shoelace manner.

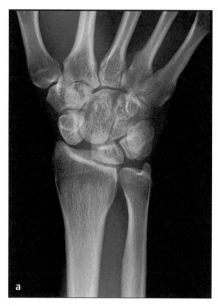
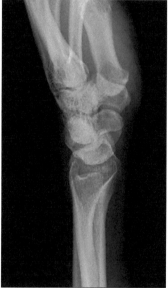
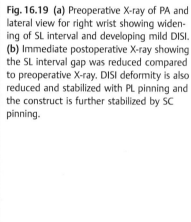

Fig. 16.19 (a) Preoperative X-ray of PA and lateral view for right wrist showing widening of SL interval and developing mild DISI. **(b)** Immediate postoperative X-ray showing the SL interval gap was reduced compared to preoperative X-ray. DISI deformity is also reduced and stabilized with PL pinning and the construct is further stabilized by SC pinning.

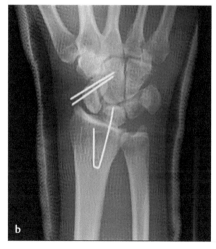
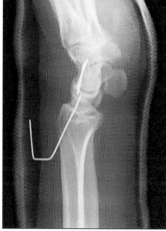

39 mm). DISI deformity was present in 13 patients. Six patients had Stage 1 SLAC wrist change radiologically. Concomitant procedures were performed on four patients.

The average follow-up was 48.3 months (range 11–132 mo). Thirteen returned to their preinjury job level. Eleven patients had no wrist pain, and 6 had some pain on either maximum exertion or at the extreme of motion. The average extension range compared to pre-op improved by 13%, flexion range by 16%, radial deviation by 13%, and ulnar deviation by 27%. Mean grip strength was 32.8 kg (120% of the preoperative status, 84% of the contralateral side). The average SL interval after reconstruction was 2.9 mm (range 1.6–5.5 mm). Recurrence of a DISI deformity was noted in four patients but remained asymptomatic. No case reported progressive SLAC wrist change. Ischemic change of proximal scaphoid was noted in one case without symptom or progression. It is likely due to the large 3.5-mm bone tunnel creation. There was no neurovascular or tendon complication. All patients were satisfied with the procedure and outcome.

Naqui et al reviewed the 1191 papers on managing chronic nonarthritic SL dissociation, of which 17 papers were valid for analysis. The study concluded that the authors' current technique had better pain reduction than others (63% in authors' study vs 50% in capsulodesis vs 52% in tenodesis). This would be attributed to the soft tissue preservation as the authors' technique was performed with minimal soft tissue dissection under arthroscopic guidance. Flexion-extension arc improved by 15%, while the tenodesis and capsulodesis decreased in flexion-extension range by 32% and 22%, respectively. The greater loss of motion in tenodesis and capsulodesis can be explained by tenodesis crossing radiocarpal and midcarpal joint. In contrast, capsulodesis reinforce the dorsal SLIL repair through the capsular flap, which limited the radiocarpal joint motion.[45] The authors' technique involves tendon graft spanning over scaphoid and lunate only, which minimizes the restraining effect on other carpal bones motion. Also, tendon graft is placed at the extracapsular level, which helps tighten the extrinsic secondary stabilizers within the joint capsule when the graft is tied at its maximum tension. Moreover, another potential advantage is that the joint capsule does not need to be opened to expose the SL interval. This leaves innervation pathways intact, thus improving the SL stabilizing effect further.[38,46]

The following case illustrates the clinical result of one of the cases with chronic SL dissociation. The patient had a right wrist injury one year earlier while playing tennis. He felt pain in the right wrist during the backhand serve and had persistent weakness of grip and painful clicks during movement for one year. Physical examination showed tenderness at the anatomical snuffbox, proximal scaphoid, and SL interval region. Watson test was positive with a painful clunk. Radiologically, widely open SL interval, marked DISI deformity, and mild dorsal scaphoid translation were noted (▶ Fig. 16.19). With the SL ligament complex reconstructed by PL graft, SL interval, DISI deformity, and dorsal translation were well reduced. The construct was stabilized by the RL pin and SC joint pinning. The reconstruction remained stable with a well-maintained SL angle and SL interval after 9.5 years (▶ Fig. 16.20). He had no pain (VAS 0) with a reasonable range of wrist motion (extension 77.8%, flexion 60%), grip strength (107% compared with contralateral side), and good outcome in the functional score (DASH score 0.83/100, PWRE 5/100).

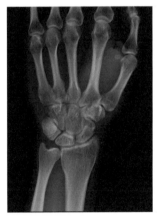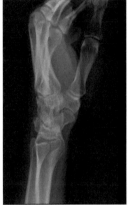

Fig. 16.20 X-ray of PA view and lateral view of the same patient taken 9.5 years after the SL reconstruction. There is no reopening up of the SL interval and corrected scapholunate angle maintained.

16.16 Tips and Tricks

Reducibility of scaphoid and lunate	Intra-articular fibrosis is often found in radiocarpal joint interposed at the region between dorsal joint capsule and the region of previous ligament. These fibrosis and scar tissue need to be shaved away to restore the reducibility of scaphoid and lunate which facilitates subsequent reduction of SL malalignment. Fluoroscopic assessment is required to assess whether DISI deformity can be reduced or not before proceeding to tendon harvesting and bone tunnel creation.
Protecting the palmar cutaneous branch of median nerve during creation of volar skin incision	When making skin incision for volar incision, palmar cutaneous branch of median nerve should be identified and protected; otherwise, the nerve will be injured in subsequent procedure.

RL joint K-wire pinning should be aimed at ulnar half of lunate	When transfixing the RL joint, the 1.6-mm K-wire is inserted percutaneously through the dorsum of distal radius. Blunt dissection is required to avoid iatrogenic injury to the extensor tendons. The RL pin should be aimed at the ulnar half of the lunate to avoid conflict with the lunate bone tunnel.
Precise bone tunnel position should be confirmed with fluoroscopy to avoid blow-out fracture	The lunate bone tunnel should be perpendicular to the long axis of the lunate, i.e., parallel to the line joining the tip of the volar and dorsal lips of the lunate. The pin should aim at the center of lunate to avoid iatrogenic blow-out fracture.
	In more severe case of DISI deformity, using Linscheid maneuver helps reduce the deformity. Whereas in mild case of DISI, the lunate pin can be inserted slightly obliquely from dorsal proximal to volar distal direction to increase the correction force on the dorsal rotation of the lunate.
	The scaphoid bone tunnel aims at the proximal scaphoid at least 2 to 3 mm from the surrounding articular margin to avoid iatrogenic fracture. The guide pin trajectory is slightly directed proximally and volarly so that it provides counter-rotational force on the scaphoid to correct the flexion pronation deformity when tendon graft is passed and tightened.
	Under fluoroscopic guidance, we can assess guide pin placement inside scaphoid and lunate before proceeding with bone tunnel drilling.
Pay attention to bone tunnel size, and soft tissue protection is needed when passing K-wire and cannulated drill	The bone tunnels should not be too large as there is risk of iatrogenic fracture or inducing bone ischemia. Tunnel size of about 2.5 mm is appropriate. If the tunnel size is too small it may cause jamming of tendon graft inside the tunnel, causing graft attrition or even avulsion when pulled through the tunnel. The tunnels should not be close to the articular surfaces.
	The flexor tendons and median nerve have to be gently retracted and protected when the guide pins and cannulated drills are passing out from the volar side of scaphoid and lunate. A large soft tissue protection sheath is essential when using the cannulated drills.
	The assistant surgeon working on the volar side should preferably be a knowledgeable and reliable partner as it is hard for the arthroscopic surgeon to visualize both dorsal and palmar side at the same time. There should be good lighting and loupe magnification to avoid complications.
Use nonabsorbable round-bodied suture when securing the tied tendon graft	Make sure the suture is equipped with round-bodied suture needle; otherwise, it can create iatrogenic injury and lacerate the tendon graft.
Avoid to insert K-wire for pinning the SL joint	It may injure and weaken the tendon graft inside the scaphoid and lunate bone tunnels.

16.17 Conclusion

Different methods have been described to reconstruct the SL ligament in chronic SL dissociation over the past 50 years. It is logical and preferable to reconstruct the dorsal and volar components and augment the extrinsic ligaments. The authors' study demonstrated that it could be performed in an arthroscopic-assisted manner. The ideal indication for this technique is a non-reparable but easily reducible complete SL ligament injury with dissociation. The presence of DISI deformity does not preclude this method. While arthroscopic shaving of intra-articular fibrosis and lysis of capsular scar may help to convert a nonreducible DISI into a reducible one, the DISI deformity can be corrected and stabilized using Linscheid maneuver with the RL pinning.

References

[1] Short WH, Werner FW, Green JK, Sutton LG, Brutus JP. Biomechanical evaluation of the ligamentous stabilizers of the scaphoid and lunate: part III. J Hand Surg Am. 2007; 32(3):297–309

[2] Watson H, Ottoni L, Pitts EC, Handal AG. Rotary subluxation of the scaphoid: a spectrum of instability. J Hand Surg [Br]. 1993; 18(1):62–64

[3] Andersson JK, Garcia-Elias M. Dorsal scapholunate ligament injury: a classification of clinical forms. J Hand Surg Eur Vol. 2013; 38(2):165–169

[4] Watson HK, Weinzweig J, Zeppieri J. The natural progression of scaphoid instability. Hand Clin. 1997; 13(1):39–49

[5] Garcia-Elias M, Lluch AL, Stanley JK. Three-ligament tenodesis for the treatment of scapholunate dissociation: indications and surgical technique. J Hand Surg Am. 2006; 31(1):125–134

[6] Geissler WB, Freeland AE, Savoie FH, McIntyre LW, Whipple TL. Intracarpal soft-tissue lesions associated with an intra-articular fracture of the distal end of the radius. J Bone Joint Surg Am. 1996; 78(3):357–365

[7] Messina JC, Van Overstraeten L, Luchetti R, Fairplay T, Mathoulin CL. The EWAS classification of scapholunate tears: an anatomical arthroscopic study. J Wrist Surg. 2013; 2(2):105–109

[8] Whipple TL. The role of arthroscopy in the treatment of scapholunate instability. Hand Clin. 1995; 11(1):37–40

[9] Rohman EM, Agel J, Putnam MD, Adams JE. Scapholunate interosseous ligament injuries: a retrospective review of treatment and outcomes in 82 wrists. J Hand Surg Am. 2014; 39(10):2020–2026

[10] Melone CP, Jr, Polatsch DB, Flink G, Horak B, Beldner S. Scapholunate interosseous ligament disruption in professional basketball players: treatment by direct repair and dorsal ligamentoplasty. Hand Clin. 2012; 28(3):253–260, vii

[11] Palmer AK, Dobyns JH, Linscheid RL. Management of post-traumatic instability of the wrist secondary to ligament rupture. J Hand Surg Am. 1978; 3(6):507–532

[12] Glickel SZ, Millender LH. Ligamentous reconstruction for chronic intercarpal instability. J Hand Surg Am. 1984; 9(4):514–527

[13] Blatt G. Capsulodesis in reconstructive hand surgery. Dorsal capsulodesis for the unstable scaphoid and volar capsulodesis following excision of the distal ulna. Hand Clin. 1987; 3(1):81–102

[14] Conyers DJ. Scapholunate interosseous reconstruction and imbrication of palmar ligaments. J Hand Surg Am. 1990; 15(5):690–700

[15] Almquist EE, Bach AW, Sack JT, Fuhs SE, Newman DM. Four-bone ligament reconstruction for treatment of chronic complete scapholunate separation. J Hand Surg Am. 1991; 16(2):322–327

[16] Brunelli GA, Brunelli GR. A new surgical technique for carpal instability with scapholunate dissociation. Surg Technol Int. 1996; 5: 370–374

[17] Wintman BI, Gelberman RH, Katz JN. Dynamic scapholunate instability: results of operative treatment with dorsal capsulodesis. J Hand Surg Am. 1995; 20(6):971–979

[18] Rosenwasser MP, Miyasajsa KC, Strauch RJ. The RASL procedure: reduction and association of the scaphoid and lunate using the Herbert screw. Tech Hand Up Extrem Surg. 1997; 1(4):263–272

[19] Uhl RL, Williamson SC, Bowman MW, Sotereanos DG, Osterman AL. Dorsal capsulodesis using suture anchors. Am J Orthop. 1997; 26(8): 547–548

[20] Van Den Abbeele KL, Loh YC, Stanley JK, Trail IA. Early results of a modified Brunelli procedure for scapholunate instability. J Hand Surg [Br]. 1998; 23(2):258–261

[21] Weiss AP. Scapholunate ligament reconstruction using a bone-retinaculum-bone autograft. J Hand Surg Am. 1998; 23(2):205–215

[22] Harvey EJ, Hanel DP. Bone-ligament-bone reconstruction for scapholunate disruption. Tech Hand Up Extrem Surg. 2002; 6(1):2–5

[23] Moran SL, Ford KS, Wulf CA, Cooney WP. Outcomes of dorsal capsulodesis and tenodesis for treatment of scapholunate instability. J Hand Surg Am. 2006; 31(9):1438–1446

[24] Darlis NA, Kaufmann RA, Giannoulis F, Sotereanos DG. Arthroscopic debridement and closed pinning for chronic dynamic scapholunate instability. J Hand Surg Am. 2006; 31(3):418–424

[25] Papadogeorgou E, Mathoulin C. Extensor carpi radialis brevis ligamentoplasty and dorsal capsulodesis for the treatment of chronic post-traumatic scapholunate instability. Chir Main. 2010; 29(3):172–179

[26] Mathoulin CL, Dauphin N, Wahegaonkar AL. Arthroscopic dorsal capsuloligamentous repair in chronic scapholunate ligament tears. Hand Clin. 2011; 27(4):563–572, xi

[27] Camus EJ, Van Overstraeten L. Dorsal scapholunate stabilization using Viegas' capsulodesis: 25 cases with 26 months-follow-up. Chir Main. 2013; 32(6):393–402

[28] Ross M, Couzens G. A new technique for scapholunate ligament reconstruction utilizing FCR and interference screw fixation: level 4 evidence. J Hand Surg Am. 2013; 38(10):e51

[29] Yao J, Zlotolow DA, Lee SK. Scapholunate axis method. J Wrist Surg. 2016; 5(1):59–66

[30] Berger RA, Imeada T, Berglund L, An KN. Constraint and material properties of the subregions of the scapholunate interosseous ligament. J Hand Surg Am. 1999; 24(5):953–962

[31] Berger RA. The ligaments of the wrist. A current overview of anatomy with considerations of their potential functions. Hand Clin. 1997; 13 (1):63–82

[32] Yi IS, Firoozbakhsh K, Racca J, Umeda Y, Moneim MS. Treatment of scapholunate dissociation with palmaris longus tendon graft: a biomechanical study. Univ Pa Orthop J. 2000; 13:53–59

[33] Zdero R, Olsen M, Elfatori S, et al. Linear and torsional mechanical characteristics of intact and reconstructed scapholunate ligaments. J Biomech Eng. 2009; 131(4):041009

[34] Dobyns H. Traumatic instability of the wrist. AAOS Instr Course Lect. 1975; 24:182–199

[35] Elsaidi GA, Ruch DS, Kuzma GR, Smith BP. Dorsal wrist ligament insertions stabilize the scapholunate interval: cadaver study. Clin Orthop Relat Res. 2004(425):152–157

[36] Mitsuyasu H, Patterson RM, Shah MA, Buford WL, Iwamoto Y, Viegas SF. The role of the dorsal intercarpal ligament in dynamic and static scapholunate instability. J Hand Surg Am. 2004; 29(2):279–288

[37] Esplugas M, Garcia-Elias M, Lluch A, Llusá Pérez M. Role of muscles in the stabilization of ligament-deficient wrists. J Hand Ther. 2016; 29 (2):166–174

[38] Hagert E, Lluch A, Rein S. The role of proprioception and neuromuscular stability in carpal instabilities. J Hand Surg Eur Vol. 2016; 41(1):94–101

[39] Hagert E. Proprioception of the wrist joint: a review of current concepts and possible implications on the rehabilitation of the wrist. J Hand Ther. 2010; 23(1):2–17

[40] Hagert E, Ljung BO, Forsgren S. General innervation pattern and sensory corpuscles in the scapholunate interosseous ligament. Cells Tissues Organs. 2004; 177(1):47–54

[41] Hagert E, Persson JK, Werner M, Ljung BO. Evidence of wrist proprioceptive reflexes elicited after stimulation of the scapholunate interosseous ligament. J Hand Surg Am. 2009; 34(4):642–651

[42] Corella F, Del Cerro M, Ocampos M, Simon de Blas C, Larrainzar-Garijo R. Arthroscopic scapholunate ligament reconstruction, volar and dorsal reconstruction. Hand Clin. 2017; 33(4):687–707

[43] Ho PC, Wong CW, Tse WL. Arthroscopic-assisted combined dorsal and volar scapholunate ligament reconstruction with tendon graft for chronic SL instability. J Wrist Surg. 2015; 4(4):252–263

[44] Koo SJJ, Ho PC. Wrist arthroscopy under portal site local anesthesia without tourniquet and sedation. Hand Clin. 2017; 33(4):585–591

[45] Naqui Z, Khor WS, Mishra A, Lees V, Muir L. The management of chronic non-arthritic scapholunate dissociation: a systematic review. J Hand Surg Eur Vol. 2018; 43(4):394–401

[46] Salva-Coll G, Garcia-Elias M, Hagert E. Scapholunate instability: proprioception and neuromuscular control. J Wrist Surg. 2013; 2(2): 136–140

17 Chronic "R"esection (Palliative): Open Salvage Surgery after SL Degeneration

Hermann Krimmer

Abstract

Longstanding scapholunate (SL) lesion leads to degenerative changes with carpal collapse. These degenerative changes are seen in different stages starting at the proximal pole of the scaphoid (Stage I), spreading over the whole radio scaphoid joint (Stage II), and finally entering the midcarpal joint (Stage III). Usually the radiolunate joint is preserved and only in rare cases (Stage IV) it is damaged. Indication for treatment depends not only on the stage but also on the complaints of the patient. Wrist denervation in case of still good mobility, PRC (proximal row carpectomy) for Stage II, and four-corner fusion mainly for Stage III represent the most frequent procedures whereas total wrist fusion and wrist replacement stay for the rare Stage IV and for failed surgeries.

Keywords: SLAC-wrist, SL degeneration, Denervation, Proximal row carpectomy, four-corner fusion

17.1 Introduction

17.1.1 Carpal Collapse—SLAC Pattern

Longstanding scapholunate (SL) dissociation leads to significant degenerative changes of the wrist. This pattern first was described by Watson and Ballet[1] as SLAC-wrist (scapholunate advanced collapse), which is caused by palmar flexion of the scaphoid and dorsal extension of the lunate (dorsal intercalated segment instability [DISI]-position) due to the damaged scapholunate complex. These changes reduce load-bearing areas in the radiocarpal as well the midcarpal joint significantly and lead to damage of the cartilage with time. The occurrence of these degenerative changes shows different stages where the time period is unpredictable depending mainly on the amount of instability and loading.

The damage starts at the proximal pole of the scaphoid (*Stage I*) because of impingement to the dorsal rim of the radius (▶ Fig. 17.1). This is different to the similar pattern of carpal collapse due to longstanding scaphoid nonunion (SNAC-wrist) where the degenerative changes start at the radial styloid. This occurrence of the proximal pole frequently is missed, and the majority of the patients are seen in *Stage II* when the arthritic changes already involve the whole radioscaphoid joint (▶ Fig. 17.2). Finally, the degenerative changes enter the midcarpal joint between head of the capitate and lunate and later on include hamate and triquetrum (*Stage III* ▶ Fig. 17.3). In all these stages the radiolunate joint remains preserved as by the DISI position of the lunate load bearing is changed but

not reduced due to the spheric configuration of this joint. In rare cases even the radiolunate joint shows degenerative changes according to *Stage IV*.

17.2 Indication for Treatment

Indication for treatment mainly depends on the complaints of the patient, function of the wrist, and stage based on radiograph and arthroscopy.[2] *Stage I* usually is found when in chronic SL damage arthroscopy is performed to decide if ligament reconstruction still makes sense. If the damage of the cartilage is limited reconstruction still might be possible; however in more severe degenerative changes of the proximal pole denervation for reducing pain is of good alternative as the usually preserved motion of the wrist is not reduced.

In *Stage II* where the whole radioscaphoid joint is damaged, indication depends on the complaints and function. If movement and grip strength is not significantly reduced arthroscopy with synovectomy and denervation is preferred as it does not lead to alteration of the movement in contrast to invasive procedures such as proximal row carpectomy (PRC) or four-corner fusion where the patient would lose function. However, if severe restriction of mobility in combination with obvious swelling is found, salvage of the carpus by PRC or four-corner is indicated. For Stage II where PRC and four-corner are competitive,

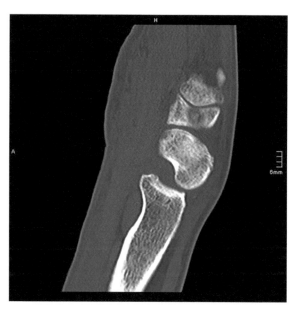

Fig. 17.1 Scapholunate advanced collapse (SLAC) wrist Stage I.

most of the surgeons tend to prefer PRC due to similar outcome, less morbidity, and complications (▸ Fig. 17.4).[3] However under special conditions where previous ligament reconstruction has failed and significant ulnar translocation

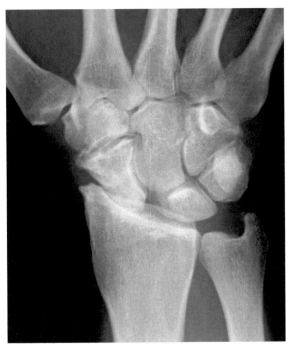

Fig. 17.2 Scapholunate advanced collapse (SLAC) wrist Stage II.

of the carpus is found, both procedures have a high risk of failure, and therefore radioscapholunate (RSL fusion) as motion-preserving procedure should be preferred as it allows stable correction of the ulnar translocation and similar movement in the preserved midcarpal joint (▸ Fig. 17.5).

In *Stage III* where the midcarpal joint is involved four-corner fusion is indicated (▸ Fig. 17.6).

The preserved radiolunate joint should not be sacrificed with interposing a capsular flap to force a PRC and the authors don't see any indication for total wrist replacement in Stage III.

Finally, in *Stage IV* total wrist fusion represents the last line of defense; alternatively depending on patients' profile total wrist replacement might be done. Replacement of the head of the capitate by a pyrocarbon implant to make PRC possible seems to be an attractive option[4]; however, the outcome was not predictable, and the authors gave it up.

17.3 Operative Procedures

17.3.1 Denervation

For denervation the authors don't perform a complete procedure as described by Wilhelm.[5] The dorsal and palmar interosseous nerve are just included as main pain branches of the wrist. A 3-cm longitudinal straight dorsal incision is made just 2 cm proximal to the wrist and the extensor retinaculum is exposed and opened over the ulnar border of the radius. The extensor tendons are

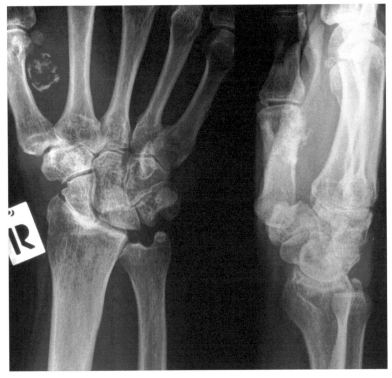

Fig. 17.3 Scapholunate advanced collapse (SLAC) wrist Stage III advanced flexion of the scaphoid and DISI position of the lunate.

III

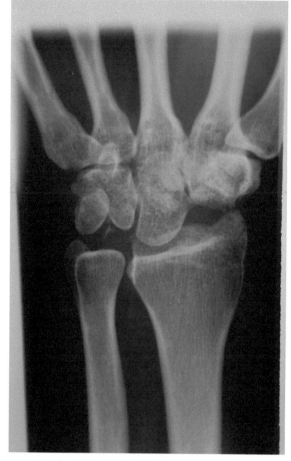

Fig. 17.4 Proximal row carpectomy.

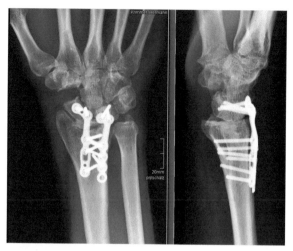

Fig. 17.5 Radioscapholunate (RSL) fusion for Stage II in case of ulnar translocation.

retracted ulnarly and at the bottom the interosseous nerve is mobilized taking care of the accompanying vessels (▶ Fig. 17.7). After coagulation proximal and distal at a distance of 2 cm this part is resected. Next the interosseous membrane is opened and the same is done with the palmar interosseous nerve.

17.3.2 Proximal Row Carpectomy (PRC)

PRC is done in a standard manner via dorsal incision opening the capsule over the radiocarpal joint. Key point means avoiding any damage to the cartilage of the head of the capitate by cautious mobilizing scaphoid, lunate, and triquetrum from the attached ligaments, especially palmar at the distal part of the scaphoid and palmar at the lunate. After resection of the carpal row the head of the capitate moves smoothly in the lunate fossa. Concerning the debate with the radial styloid, the authors perform only partial resection if it is felt that there might be risk for impingement. Alternatively, PRC can be done through a palmar approach as described by Luchetti et al

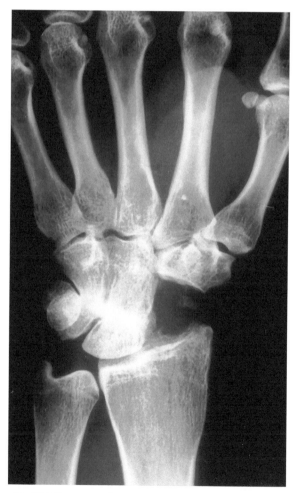

Fig. 17.6 Four-corner fusion.

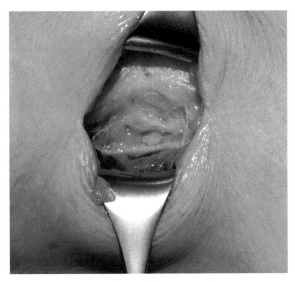

Fig. 17.7 Denervation through dorsal incision.

pointing out that resection of the proximal row is easier by direct visualization of the attached palmar carpal ligaments.[6]

17.3.3 Four-Corner Fusion (Video 17.1)

The authors prefer a slight oblique dorsal incision where the extensor retinaculum is exposed taking care of the sensitive nerve branches. The third extensor compartment is opened and the second and fourth compartment are opened like a window. The dorsal interosseous nerve is resected and the wrist capsule is opened by mobilizing a radial-based flap. Intensive synovectomy is performed to get good overview of the proximal and distal carpal row and the radiolunate joint is checked. Complete removal of the scaphoid in one piece can be facilitated by detaching the carpal ligaments with a curved chisel; alternatively, the scaphoid is separated in the middle and removed step by step which, however, is more time consuming. Under traction the midcarpal joint is exposed and the cartilage is removed using luer forceps and chisel. It is important to remove the sclerotic bone till cancellous bone area is visible; to facilitate this maneuver the authors use a 2.0-mm drill to open the sclerotic area by numerous drill holes. Interposing cancellous bone is mandatory, which in the majority of cases can be harvested from the radial styloid. In addition, the resected scaphoid can be used as a source. Only in case of cystic changes with larger defects cancellous bone from the iliac crest is necessary.

Key point of this procedure is based on realignment of the carpus by restoring the lunate from its dorsal position up to neutral (▶ Fig. 17.8). This is a prerequisite to get regular extension and flexion. Pressing the head of the capitate to the palmar lip of the lunate bimanually

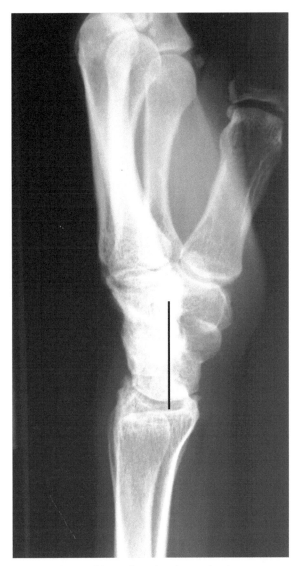

Fig. 17.8 Restored lunate from dorsal intercalated segment instability (DISI) position.

restores the lunate. If this maneuver is not sufficient the joystick procedure is used in which a K-wire is drilled dorsally into the lunate as a lever to restore the lunate. One should take care that the head of the capitate is positioned central into the lunate and not remain dorsally displaced as this results in painful dorsal impingement at the dorsal rim of the radius. In addition, by reducing capitate and lunate in one line, the palmar carpal ligaments are tightened to stabilize the remaining carpus.

In case of using K-wires for fixation two of them should be placed into capitate and lunate and one into hamate and triquetrum (▶ Fig. 17.9). At first the K-wires are predrilled till visible at the midcarpal joint, next the cancellous bone is interposed at the bottom, and finally after realignment of the carpus the K-wire are further drilled till

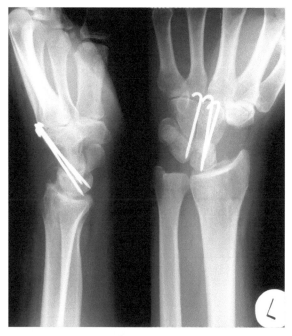

Fig. 17.9 Four-corner with K-wires.

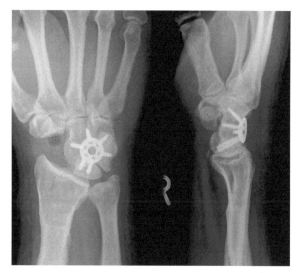

Fig. 17.10 Four-corner with circular plate.

they catch safely lunate and triquetrum. Precise X-ray control is needed to make sure that the wires are not penetrating the radiocarpal joint. Positioning of the wires often is difficult as frequently they run steep and catch the proximal bones only partially. In the end the remaining spaces are filled with cancellous bone. Using cannulated headless screws instead of K-wires follows the same principles.[7]

For circular plates at first after interposing the cancellous bone at the bottom the carpus is realigned as described and temporarily stabilized. The authors prefer one K-wire running proximally into the radius, with lunate and capitate at the radial side. In addition, if not stable a second wire can be placed from ulnar into triquetrum and lunate. Stable conditions are needed for reaming the bed for the circular plate with the tip of the reamer in the center of the four bones. Reaming should be performed not too deep but exactly such that the rim of the circular plate can be placed slightly under the bone area to avoid impingement at the radius. First two nonlocking screws, one into the lunate and one into the capitate, are placed to reduce the plate against the bones and after X-ray control the K-wire is removed and the remaining holes are filled with locking screws and finally the gaps are filled with cancellous bone (▶ Fig. 17.10).

17.4 Results

The success rate for denervation resulting in significant pain relief differs from 50 to 70%, but it leaves the door open for invasive open procedures with the advantage that it does not worsen function.[8]

PRC as well as four-corner show similar outcome and if properly done both treatments lead to significant pain relief and preserve motion of about 30 degrees for extension and 30 degrees for flexion with grip strength of 60 to 80% compared to the opposite site.

17.5 Conclusion

Degenerative changes after SL lesion are seen in different stages. Treatment depends not only on the stage but also on the complaints of the patient. In case of good function denervation might be the first choice. If swelling and significant limitation of function is dominant in Stage II, PRC is preferred due to similar results and a lower complication rate in comparison to four-corner. However, in Stage III four-corner fusion represents the adequate treatment. For Stage IV or failed previous PRC or four-corner, total wrist fusion is a reliable option where total wrist replacement might be the alternative if mobility is required.

References

[1] Watson HK, Ballet FL. The SLAC wrist: scapholunate advanced collapse pattern of degenerative arthritis. J Hand Surg Am. 1984; 9 (3):358–365

[2] Krimmer H, Lanz U. [Post-traumatic carpal collapse. Follow-up and therapeutic concept]. Unfallchirurg. 2000; 103(4):260–266

[3] Ahmadi AR, Duraku LS, van der Oest MJW, Hundepool CA, Selles RW, Zuidam JM. The never-ending battle between proximal row carpectomy and four corner arthrodesis: a systematic review and meta-analysis for the final verdict. J Plast Reconstr Aesthet Surg. 2022; 75(2):711–721

[4] Fulchignoni C, Caviglia D, Rocchi L. Resurfacing capitate pyrocarbon implant after proximal row carpectomy: a literature review. Orthop Rev (Pavia). 2020; 12 Suppl 1:8679

[5] Wilhelm A. Anatomical aspects of wrist denervation. J Hand Surg [Br]. 1996; 21(6):834

[6] Luchetti R, Soragni O, Fairplay T. Proximal row carpectomy through a palmar approach. J Hand Surg [Br]. 1998; 23(3):406–409

[7] Hayes E, Cheng Y, Sauder D, Sims L. Four-corner arthrodesis with differing methods of osteosynthesis: a systematic review. J Hand Surg Am. 2022; 47(5):477.e1–477.e9

[8] Fuchsberger T, Boesch CE, Tonagel F, Fischborn T, Schaller HE, Gonser P. Patient-rated long-term results after complete denervation of the wrist. J Plast Reconstr Aesthet Surg. 2018; 71(1):57–61

17

18 Chronic "R"esection (Palliative): Arthroscopic Salvage Surgery after Scapholunate Degeneration

Eva-Maria Baur and Jean-Baptiste de Villeneuve Bargemon

Abstract

The management of wrist osteoarthritis has been studied for many decades. The etiologies of wrist osteoarthritis are multiple, including scapholunate instability, but the appearance of osteochondral lesions changes the prognosis as well as the dimension of the management. Reconstruction is no longer possible, so treatment becomes palliative. Although some techniques have proven to be effective, the appearance of new technologies, such as wrist arthroscopy, has made it possible to modernize the traditional treatment methods and to propose new ones. In this chapter, we will detail the different arthroscopic possibilities in the treatment of wrist osteoarthritis according to the different stages of osteoarthritis after scapholunate instability.

Keywords: carpus, wrist, arthroscopy, bone fusion, joint

Table 18.1 Possible palliative arthroscopic techniques according to the different scapholunate degenerative disorders

SLAC 1	Styloidectomy +/− scaphocapitate fusion
SLAC 2	Arthroscopic radiocarpal tendinous interposition or arthroscopic-assisted PRC Two-, three-, or four-corner fusion (with scaphoidectomy)
SLAC 3	Two-, three-, or four-corner fusion (with scaphoidectomy)
SLAC 4	No indication for arthroscopy (limited to synovectomy)

Note: Other open indications (denervation and others) can also be used.

18.1 Introduction

The range of possible lesions of the scapholunate capsulo-ligamentous complex is very wide, from a simple ligament sprain to osteoarthritis of all the articular surfaces of the wrist. Initially, when this complex is repairable, multiple arthroscopic or open solutions are proposed.[1,3] However, when a lesion of this complex is neglected, the disorganization of the carpal biomechanics leads to pathological friction on the articular surfaces of the wrist, resulting in an irreversible loss of cartilage. Depending on the arthritic evolution, these lesions can lead to *scapholunate advanced collapse* (SLAC), which is described by Weiss and Rodner in four stages[4]:

- SLAC 1 = styloscaphoid arthrosis.
- SLAC 2 = radioscaphoid arthrosis.
- SLAC 3 = SLAC 2 + lunocapitate osteoarthritis (then more or less scaphocapitate, depending on Type 1 or 2 of lunate).
- SLAC 4 = SLAC 3 + radioulnar osteoarthritis.

As soon as a lesion appears, the indications for repair or reconstruction are no longer relevant, and more palliative solutions must be proposed. For this situation, open techniques have been described and will be presented in another chapter. With the advent of arthroscopy, these methods could be applied in a minimally invasive manner. In this chapter, the authors will present the possible arthroscopic techniques and their indications (▶ Table 18.1).

18.2 Styloidectomy

This minimally invasive technique can be performed alone for early forms of SLAC and in combination with other surgical techniques for more advanced forms. Initially described using two approaches (3–4 or 4–5 for the camera and 1–2 for the instrumentation) (▶ Fig. 18.1), Herzberg and Burnier developed this technique with an additional palmar approach (radial portal volar) without more complications than with two dorsal approaches, allowing better visualization of degenerative lesions, particularly dorsal ones.[5] Noback et al even reported its use in association with partial denervation of the wrist in SLAC 2 and 3, with encouraging results at 5 years, particularly in terms of joint amplitude maintenance and pain reduction.[6]

18.2.1 Tips and Tricks

- The resection must be vertical and must not exceed 3 to 4 mm from the original radius or the radial insertion of the radioscaphocapitate ligament; otherwise, ulnar translation of the carpus may occur.[7]
- To avoid overlay generous resections, the diameter of the bur (usually 3 or 3.5) can be used as a marker, thus avoiding the need for perioperative fluoroscopic control, although this is useful at the end of the procedure.
- Some laboratories allow the removal of the bur's cannula resulting in a more complete and faster resection.

18.3 Radiocarpal Interposition

Few reports exist on radiocarpal interposition,[8,9] and few solutions have been developed that conserve the first row. These procedures are performed openly with the risk of stiffness counterbalanced by the maintenance of

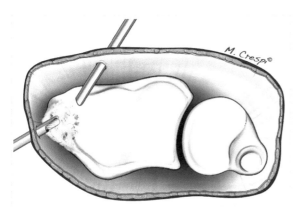

Fig. 18.1 Drawing showing a classic two-portal styloidectomy. The scope through the radial palmar radiocarpal portal and the bur through the 1–2 portal. (Reproduced from Mathoulin C. Wrist Arthroscopy Techniques; Copyright © 2021 Thieme. All rights reserved.)

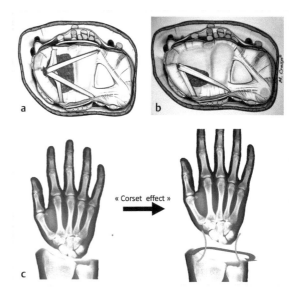

« Corset effect »

Fig. 18.2 Arthroscopic radiocarpal tendinous interposition (ARTI). **(a)** ARTI according to Mathoulin. **(b)** ARTI according to Levadoux. **(c)** Illustration of the "corset effect" by applying tension to the tendon on the capsule. (Reproduced from Mathoulin C. Wrist Arthroscopy Techniques; Copyright © 2021 Thieme. All rights reserved.)

joint range of motion during resection of the first row of the carpus. The only known interposition under arthroscopy was initially reported by Levadoux and Mathoulin, who performed radiocarpal tendon interposition while preserving the bony structures.[10] In 2018, Mathoulin and Arianni, using a four-strand interposition in combination with a conventional dorsal capsuloligamentous repair, reported significant improvements in strength, pain, and DASH scores as well as improvement in joint ranges[11] (▶ Fig. 18.2a). However, this technique remains technically demanding with potential intraoperative failures, notably due to the graft length, and requires significant skill in wrist arthroscopy.

18.3.1 Tips and Tricks

- In a personal series,[12] Levadoux et al reported identical results according to the same criteria with an average follow-up of 42 months while greatly simplifying the technique to a single dorsal loop (two strands) (▶ Fig. 18.2b). According to the authors, coverage of the entire radiocarpal surface by tendon interposition is not necessary because the radioscaphoid friction phenomena are concentrated on the posterior region of the radius.
- In addition, the authors believe that suturing the graft in traction leads to a "corset effect," which increases the radiocarpal spacing of this procedure by "retensioning" of the dorsal capsule (▶ Fig. 18.2c).

18.4 Scaphocapitate Arthrodesis (▶ Fig. 18.3)

In chronic scapholunate instability, scaphocapitate fusion produces good functional results, significantly decreasing flexion and extension ranges and slightly decreasing

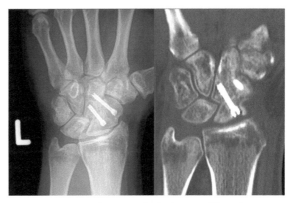

Fig. 18.3 Computed tomography (CT) image of frontal sections of scaphocapitate arthrodesis performed arthroscopically with bone grafting from the iliac crest.

ulnar and radial tilts; however, strength and pain seem to improve.[13,15] Scaphocapitate arthrodesis does not stop the arthrosis phenomenon but slows it down, with a rate of 16% of radioscaphoid arthrosis at 60-month follow-up according to Delétang et al and of 30% at 122-month follow-up according to Luegmair and Saffar.[13,15] The rate of nonunion was 23% in a cohort of 13 patients according to Chantelot et al.[14]

These series of scaphocapitate arthrodesis were all performed by open surgery. More recently, the advent of arthroscopy has led to a miniaturization of the technique and to the development of an entirely arthroscopic technique,[16,17] which preserves the surrounding structures and thus theoretically reduces the risk of nonunion and postoperative stiffness. Its indication will be limited to SLAC 0 to 1.

18.4.1 Tips and Tricks

- Scaphocapitate arthrodesis should be performed only in the absence of radioscaphoid arthritic lesions (or limited to the radial styloid) as well as in the absence of midcarpal arthrosis.
- It is advisable to perform a resection of the distal scaphoid so as not to interfere with the biomechanics of the thumb at the scaphotrapezoidal joint. This can be performed by open (osteotome) or arthroscopic surgery.
- The rotation of the scaphoid should be reduced, and it should be fixed slightly in extension.

18.5 Partial Arthrodesis

18.5.1 Radioscapholunate Arthrodesis

Some authors report a satisfaction rate of 88% for radioscapholunate (RSL) arthrodesis over a minimum of 10 years with a "test" period of the first 2 years.[18] This seems to be an effective technique but does not prevent the appearance of midcarpal arthrosis in the long term.[19,21] In addition, the nonunion rate is high, up to 30%.[19] The development of arthroscopic techniques has made it possible to perform RSL arthrodesis in a minimally invasive manner (▶ Fig. 18.4)[16,22] and theoretically reduces the risk of nonunion, although no comparative series exists. However, the question remains: Is RSL arthrodesis ultimately an effective solution for the management of SLAC 2? A randomized, blinded study comparing RSL arthrodesis with bicolumnar arthrodesis reported improved wrist function and a lower rate of reintervention in favor of bicolumnar arthrodesis.[23] According to the authors, in SLAC II arthritis, the expected benefit of preserving the midcarpal joint is not observed, and this procedure should be reserved for cases of posttraumatic radiocarpal arthrosis because the scaphoid and lunate form a biomechanical monoblock, ensuring coronal congruence of the midcarpal joint.

Whether open or arthroscopic, the technique is demanding.

Tips and Tricks

- Resection of the distal pole of the scaphoid seems to be an essential step, avoiding conflict of an immobile scaphoid with the scaphotrapezoid joint. Moreover, it appears that the rate of nonunion is less important when the distal pole of the scaphoid is removed,[20] and there is a significant improvement in radial

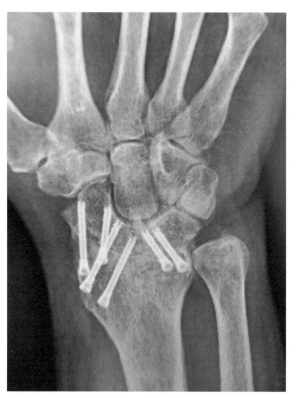

Fig. 18.4 Front wrist radiograph with radioscapholunate arthrodesis performed arthroscopically.

inclination.[24] This excision can be performed arthroscopically (STT approach) or through a mini-open approach.

- Special attention should be paid to the triquetrum and its excision. The decrease in carpal height may lead to ulnocarpal impingement if the triquetrum is retained. Though the technique is classically performed to increase joint amplitudes,[25,26] more recent studies do not seem to find this effect and find no difference in the appearance of mediocarpal osteoarthritis, proposing instead that distal radioulnar joint arthroplasty be performed to combat ulnocarpal impingement if necessary.[20,21] In addition, a recent biomechanical study reported that excision of the triquetrum is likely to induce midcarpal instability.[24]
- During screw fixation, when the pins are well positioned on the scan, removal of all but one pin allows for better compression. These pins will be reintroduced once the first set of screws is fixed (▶ Fig. 18.5).

18.5.2 Intracarpal Arthrodesis

In the more advanced stages (SLAC 2 or 3), two possible solutions are the most widely used: intracarpal arthrodesis or proximal row carpectomy (with more or less resurfacing of the capitatum in SLAC 3).[27,28] The

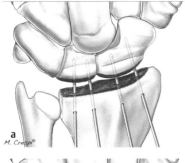
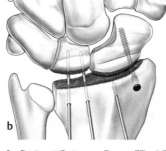

Fig. 18.5 Screw fixation technique to optimize compression in radioscapholunate arthrodesis. (a) Correct positioning of the pins. (b) Removal of all pins but one for each bone. Note that a pin remains in the lunate to block its extension. This pin could be triquetrolunar. (c) Screw fixation completed with maximum compression on the arthrodesis surfaces. (d) Poor compression when holding the pins during screw fixation.

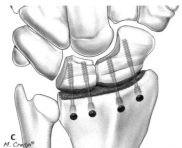
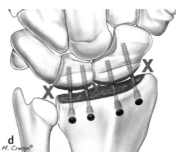

main disadvantage of intracarpal arthrodesis is the inevitable loss of joint range of motion. Initially, four-corner arthrodesis was the first to be described, but the most recent studies attempt to limit the number of bones to be fused.[29,31] This tendency to reduce the number of fused joints is probably due to the operative difficulty of four-corner arthrodesis. Excision of the scaphoid with capitolunate arthrodesis results in better amplitude, especially in flexion, than the three- (▶ Fig. 18.6) or four-corner method.[32,33] To counter this loss of mobility caused by capsulotomy and intracarpal arthrodesis, arthroscopy represents a definite advantage.[34] These techniques have already been published under arthroscopy.[16,35]

Tips and Tricks

- *Lunate anatomy:* Special attention should be paid to the anatomy of the lunate,[36] which can be a source of conflict when performing a bicolumnar arthrodesis and a Viegas 2 lunate.[30]
- *Reduction:* The authors recommend a slight overcorrection of the dorsal intercalated segment instability (DISI) deformity to achieve more wrist extension than flexion, but no overcorrection of the ulnar translation. Therefore, we need to pay attention on the type 1 or 2 of the lunate.
- *Wet or dry arthroscopy:* There is no proven difference, and the use of wet or dry arthroscopy varies according to the surgeon's habits. However, the authors recommend alternating the two modes, with dry milling (to avoid a "snowstorm effect") accompanied by

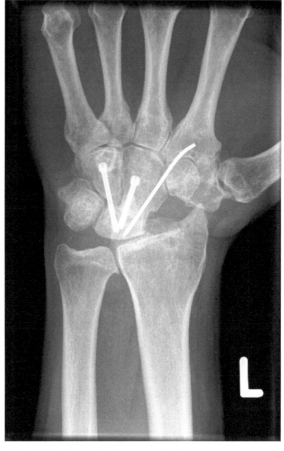

Fig. 18.6 Arthroscopic three-corner fusion.

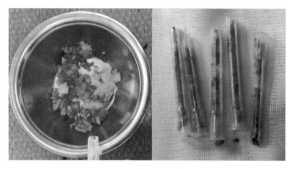

Fig. 18.7 The "Gun Barrel Trick." **Left:** Bone graft taken from the radius. **Right:** Twenty-gauge syringe cut at a bevel and filled with bone graft material. The caps can be filled using an operating aid, which saves operating time. The caps are then introduced via the arthroscopic portal. The metal introducer of the arthroscope is used as a pusher to introduce the graft into the joint. (Reproduced from Levadoux M. How to optimize a bone graft in arthroscopy of the wrist: the "Gun Barrel Trick." J Wrist Surg. Copyright © 2022 Thieme. All rights reserved.)

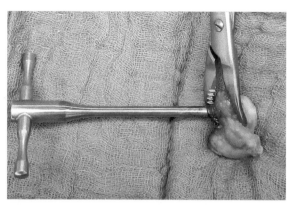

Fig. 18.8 Carpal stick. (Courtesy of KLS Martin.)

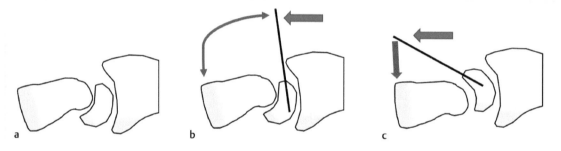

a   b   c

Fig. 18.9 (a–c) Reduction of the lunate with a threaded pin.

washouts to eliminate debris and avoid thermal burns on the bone. It should be noted that any humid environment should be avoided when the bone graft is in the intra-articular area. And while burring we need to prevent too much heating and "burning" of the bone.

- *Harvesting the graft:* This can require a long operating time. However, simple tricks such as the "Gun Barrel Trick" can be used to optimize the operating time[37] (▶ Fig. 18.7).
- *Useful instrument:* The presence of a "carpal stick" (type KLS Martin) with a threaded tip allows for a good grip on the scaphoid and greatly simplifies its excision (▶ Fig. 18.8). In the absence of this instrument, in the ancillary equipment, a threaded pin with a large diameter can help.
- *Lunate reduction:* Very often in advanced cases of scapholunate instability, wrist flexion is not sufficient for good lunate reduction. A practical tip is to use 1- or 1.2-mm threaded pins as joysticks introduced dorsally (▶ Fig. 18.9). Another option that may be useful is the

Linscheid maneuver by inserting a radiolunate pin during flexion and ulnar tilt of the wrist (▶ Fig. 18.10).

- *Crossing cartilage to optimize fixation:* The perfect fixation would avoid crossing a cartilage zone that is still mobile after arthrodesis (▶ Fig. 18.11). Although possible, retrograde screw fixation is sometimes difficult, particularly regarding the orientation of the screws, which can lead to poor positioning and failure. As with scaphoid screw fixation, the authors propose the trick of fixing the screws from proximal to distal through the "healthy" cartilage. Sometimes, the reduction of the lunate is good but does not leave a satisfactory screw-fixation angle. A trick can be to make a bone tunnel in the radius to allow optimal positioning of the screws (▶ Fig. 18.12).
- *Intracarpal urinary catheter:* To prevent leakage of the bone graft into the empty space after scaphoidectomy, a balloon catheter (e.g., a urinary catheter) can be inserted and inflated intra-articularly to prevent the graft from spreading.

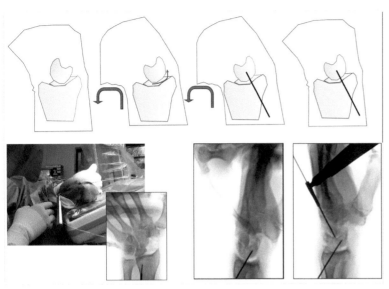

Fig. 18.10 Lunate deformity reduction according to Linscheid.

18

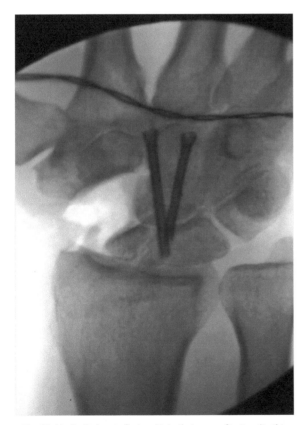

Fig. 18.11 Capitolunate fusion. Note that screw fixation (in this case, retrograde) is performed under optimal conditions, without crossing healthy cartilage. However, anterograde screw fixation is possible. In addition, the authors did not perform a total scaphoidectomy, leaving the proximal pole intact.

18.6 First-Row Carpal Bone Resection

This procedure has already proven its effectiveness in the long term[38,40] as well as for young patients (< 45 years).[41] Its indication in SLAC 2 remains a solution of choice when compared to intracarpal arthrodesis.[42] Under arthroscopy, Weiss et al describe their technique on a cohort of 16 patients with an average operating time of 70 minutes.[43] With their series, the authors report a flexion-extension rotation arc of 94 degrees compared to 79 degrees with the open techniques presented in their publication, as well as preservation of overall strength. Although the results are encouraging, there are too few series to draw a conclusion on the real benefit of arthroscopy in the resection of the first row of carpal bones.

18.6.1 Tips and Tricks

- Ocampos Hernandez et al report an interesting trick using a central palmar route.[44] The addition of this extra channel allows the surgeon to use two instruments at the same time while the operating assistant maintains the camera, with the aim of facilitating the procedure and reducing the operating time.
- To allow proper mobilization, the intrinsic and extrinsic ligaments must be cut with a 20-gauge needle bevel or with suitable knives.
- The carpal bones will then be removed by mini-approaches: an ulnodorsal approach for the lunate and triquetrum and a radiopalmar approach for the scaphoid.

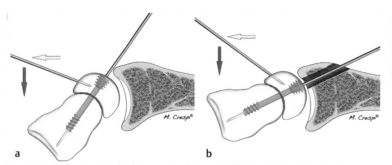

a   b

Fig. 18.12 Screw fixation for intracarpal arthrodesis. **(a)** Positioning of the screw through the healthy cartilage of the lunate. **(b)** Creation of a bone tunnel in the radius for optimal positioning of the screw.

III

- The authors recommend starting with a dorsal release of the carpal bones to avoid their collapse, which makes the excision more difficult.
- The "carpal stick" is also very useful.

18.7 Total Arthrodesis under Arthroscopy (SLAC 4)

In cases of advanced osteoarthritis (SLAC 4), the choice will be between a total wrist arthrodesis and a prosthetic arthroplasty. Total wrist arthrodesis under arthroscopy has been reported only once in the literature, for spastic patients, in 2019.[45] In the authors' opinion, arthroscopic total wrist arthrodesis is not a recommended procedure because it is difficult to perform, and the only theoretical advantage is better consolidation. At present, the literature is too sparse to draw a conclusion on the advantage of arthroscopy in this instance.

18.8 Authors' Preferred Technique

Arthroscopy can therefore be used for all stages of scapholunate degeneration. ▶ Table 18.1 describes the indications the authors prefer according to the different stages of degeneration. This list is exhaustive, and only the arthroscopic solutions are proposed herewith.

18.9 Conclusion

In the degenerative setting, palliative arthroscopic surgery is demanding. However, it remains particularly suitable for the management of these pathologies, in particular by checking for cartilage damage and thus confirming the indication. The advantage of minimally invasive surgery, particularly regarding the preservation of joint amplitudes and vascularization, is the undeniable advantage of arthroscopy. Some procedures are generally lengthy, and an operating timeslot should be reserved accordingly with a prepared team.

References

[1] Corella F, Del Cerro M, Ocampos M, Simon de Blas C, Larrainzar-Garijo R. Arthroscopic scapholunate ligament reconstruction, volar and dorsal reconstruction. Hand Clin. 2017; 33(4):687–707

[2] Mathoulin CL, Dauphin N, Wahegaonkar AL. Arthroscopic dorsal capsuloligamentous repair in chronic scapholunate ligament tears. Hand Clin. 2011; 27(4):563–572, xi

[3] Wahegaonkar AL, Mathoulin CL. Arthroscopic dorsal capsuloligamentous repair in the treatment of chronic scapho-lunate ligament tears. J Wrist Surg. 2013; 2(2):141–148

[4] Patel N, Russo G, Rodner C. Osteoarthritis of the wrist. In: Chen Q, ed. Osteoarthritis: diagnosis, treatment and surgery. InTech; 2012. doi:10.5772/28113

[5] Herzberg G, Burnier M. Isolated arthroscopic radial styloidectomy: the three-portal approach. J Wrist Surg. 2020; 9(4):353–356

[6] Noback PC, Seetharaman M, Danoff JR, Birman M, Rosenwasser MP. Arthroscopic wrist debridement and radial styloidectomy for advanced scapholunate advanced collapse wrist: long-term follow-up. Hand (N Y). 2018; 13(6):659–665

[7] Nakamura T, Cooney WP, III, Lui WH, et al. Radial styloidectomy: a biomechanical study on stability of the wrist joint. J Hand Surg Am. 2001; 26(1):85–93

[8] Rabinovich RV, Lee SJ. Proximal row carpectomy using decellularized dermal allograft. J Hand Surg Am. 2018; 43(4):392.e1–392.e9

[9] Gaspar MP, Pham PP, Pankiw CD, et al. Mid-term outcomes of routine proximal row carpectomy compared with proximal row carpectomy with dorsal capsular interposition arthroplasty for the treatment of late-stage arthropathy of the wrist. Bone Joint J. 2018; 100-B(2):197–204

[10] Levadoux M, Mathoulin C. Traitement arthroscopique du SLAC wrist stade I et II par styloïdectomie élargie et ligamentoplastie d'interposition tendue en Hamac, technique et résultats préliminaires. Chir Main. 2012; 31(6):390–391

[11] Arianni M, Mathoulin C. Arthroscopic interposition tendon arthroplasty for Stage 2 scapholunate advanced collapse. Arthroscopy. 2019; 35(2): 392–402

[12] Bargemon JBDV, Levadoux M, Mathoulin C, Merlini L. Arthroscopic radiocarpal tendinous interpositions (ARTI) for SLAC I and 2: "a new conservative solution" technique. Hand Surg Rehabil. 2021; 40(6):859

[13] Luegmair M, Saffar P. Scaphocapitate arthrodesis for treatment of scapholunate instability in manual workers. J Hand Surg Am. 2013; 38(5):878–886

[14] Chantelot C, Becquet E, Leconte F, Lahoude-Chantelot S, Prodomme G, Fontaine C. Etude rétrospective de 13 arthrodèses scaphocapitatum pour instabilité scapholunaire chronique. Chir Main. 2005; 24(2):79–83

[15] Delétang F, Segret J, Dap F, Dautel G. Chronic scapholunate instability treated by scaphocapitate fusion: a midterm outcome perspective. Orthop Traumatol Surg Res. 2011; 97(2):164–171

[16] Baur EM. Arthroscopic-assisted partial wrist arthrodesis. Hand Clin. 2017; 33(4):735–753

[17] de Villeneuve Bargemon JB, Peras M, Hasegawa H, Levadoux M. Arthroscopic scaphocapitate fusion: surgical technique. Arthrosc Tech. 2022; 11(7):e1289–e1294

[18] Ha NB, Phadnis J, MacLean SBM, Bain GI. Radioscapholunate fusion with triquetrum and distal pole of scaphoid excision: long-term follow-up. J Hand Surg Eur Vol. 2018; 43(2):168–173

[19] Montoya-Faivre D, Pomares G, Calafat V, Dap F, Dautel G. Clinical and radiological outcomes following radioscapholunate fusion. Orthop Traumatol Surg Res. 2017; 103(7):1093–1098

[20] Degeorge B, Dagneaux L, Montoya-Faivre D, et al. Radioscapholunate fusion for posttraumatic osteoarthritis with consecutive excision of the distal scaphoid and the triquetrum: a comparative study. Hand Surg Rehabil. 2020; 39(5):375–382

[21] Degeorge B, Montoya-Faivre D, Dap F, Dautel G, Coulet B, Chammas M. Radioscapholunate fusion for radiocarpal osteoarthritis: prognostic factors of clinical and radiographic outcomes. J Wrist Surg. 2019; 8(6):456–462

[22] de Villeneuve Bargemon JB, Ben Hadid N, Hasegawa H, Levadoux M. Arthroscopic radioscapholunate fusion: surgical technique. Arthrosc Tech. 2022; 11(6):e1081–e1085

[23] Chan SSM, Sikora S, Harvey JN, Tham SKY. A blinded, randomized trial comparing bicolumnar arthrodesis to radioscapholunate arthrodesis in scapholunate advanced collapse II arthritis: a pilot study. J Hand Surg Eur Vol. 2018; 43(8):813–819

[24] Suzuki D, Omokawa S, Iida A, et al. Biomechanical effects of radioscapholunate fusion with distal scaphoidectomy and triquetrum excision on dart-throwing and wrist circumduction motions. J Hand Surg Am. 2021; 46(1):71.e1–71.e7

[25] Berkhout MJ, Shaw MN, Berglund LJ, An KN, Berger RA, Ritt MJPF. The effect of radioscapholunate fusion on wrist movement and the subsequent effects of distal scaphoidectomy and triquetrectomy. J Hand Surg Eur Vol. 2010; 35(9):740–745

[26] Bain GI, Ondimu P, Hallam P, Ashwood N. Radioscapholunate arthrodesis: a prospective study. Hand Surg. 2009; 14(2–3):73–82

[27] De Vitis R, Passiatore M, Cilli V, et al. Secondary wrist arthritis in active workers: does capitate pyrocarbon resurfacing (RCPI) improve proximal row carpectomy? A retrospective cohort study. J Hand Surg Asian Pac Vol. 2021; 26(4):625–634

[28] Fulchignoni C, Caviglia D, Rocchi L. Resurfacing capitate pyrocarbon implant after proximal row carpectomy: a literature review. Orthop Rev (Pavia). 2020; 12 Suppl 1:8679

[29] Undurraga S, Au K, Dobransky J, Gammon B. Scaphoid excision and bicolumnar carpal fusion with retrograde headless screws. J Wrist Surg. 2021; 10(3):201–207

[30] Gauci MO, Waitzenegger T, Chammas PE, Coulet B, Lazerges C, Chammas M. Comparison of clinical outcomes of three-corner arthrodesis and bicolumnar arthrodesis for advanced wrist osteoarthritis. J Hand Surg Eur Vol. 2020; 45(7):679–686

[31] Dunn JC, Polmear MM, Scanaliato JP, Orr JD, Nesti LJ. Capitolunate arthrodesis: a systematic review. J Hand Surg Am. 2020; 45(4):365.e1–365.e10

[32] Duraku LS, Hundepool CA, Hoogendam L, et al. Hand-Wrist Study Group. Two-corner fusion or four-corner fusion of the wrist for midcarpal osteoarthritis? A multicenter prospective comparative cohort study. Plast Reconstr Surg. 2022; 149(6):1130e–1139e

[33] Gaston RG, Greenberg JA, Baltera RM, Mih A, Hastings H. Clinical outcomes of scaphoid and triquetral excision with capitolunate arthrodesis versus four-corner arthrodesis. J Hand Surg Am. 2009; 34(8):1407–1412

[34] Azócar C, Lecaros JJ, Bernal N, Sanhueza M, Liendo R, Cifras JL. Four-corner arthrodesis: comparative analysis of open technique versus percutaneous technique with arthroscopic assistance. J Wrist Surg. 2021; 11(2):127–133

[35] Ho PC. Arthroscopic partial wrist fusion. Tech Hand Up Extrem Surg. 2008; 12(4):242–265

[36] Viegas SF, Wagner K, Patterson R, Peterson P. Medial (hamate) facet of the lunate. J Hand Surg Am. 1990; 15(4):564–571

[37] de Villeneuve Bargemon JB, Peras M, Hasegawa H, Baur EM, Levadoux M. How to optimize a bone graft in arthroscopy of the wrist: the "gun barrel trick". J Wrist Surg. 2022; 11(6):561–562

[38] Green DP, Perreira AC, Longhofer LK. Proximal row carpectomy. J Hand Surg Am. 2015; 40(8):1672–1676

[39] Chim H, Moran SL. Long-term outcomes of proximal row carpectomy: a systematic review of the literature. J Wrist Surg. 2012; 1(2):141–148

[40] Zeidan M, Garcia BN, Lu CC, et al. Risk of total wrist arthrodesis following proximal row carpectomy: an analysis of 1,070 patients. J Hand Surg Am. 2023; 48(2):195.e1–195.e10

[41] Wagner ER, Barras LA, Harstad C, Elhassan BT, Moran SL. Proximal row carpectomy in young patients. JBJS Essential Surg Tech. 2021; 11(1):54–54

[42] Garcia BN, Lu CC, Stephens AR, et al. Risk of total wrist arthrodesis or reoperation following 4-corner arthrodesis or proximal row carpectomy for Stage-II SLAC/SNAC arthritis: a propensity score analysis of 502 wrists. J Bone Joint Surg Am. 2020; 102(12):1050–1058

[43] Weiss ND, Molina RA, Gwin S. Arthroscopic proximal row carpectomy. J Hand Surg Am. 2011; 36(4):577–582

[44] Ocampos Hernandez M, Corella Montoya F, Del Cerro Gutierrez M, Larrainzar Garijo R. Arthroscopic proximal row carpectomy using the volar central portal. Arthrosc Tech. 2017; 6(4):e1427–e1430

[45] Nazerani S, Nazerani T, Molayem A, Keramati MR. A modified surgical technique for minimally invasive arthroscopic total wrist fusion. J Wrist Surg. 2019; 8(1):84–88

18

Section IV

Lunotriquetral Injury and Instability

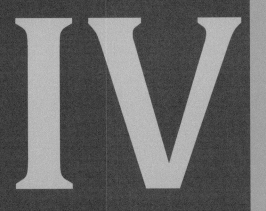

19 Isolated Lunotriquetral Interosseous Ligament Ruptures

Teun Teunis, David Ring, Liron Duraku, and Marco J.P.F. Ritt

Abstract

Traumatic lunotriquetral interosseous ligament (LTIL) rupture is obvious in perilunate, reverse perilunate, and axial carpal dislocations. In these settings, when the lunate and triquetrum are realigned the LTIL likely heals without direct repair, or at least it does not seem associated with carpal malalignment.[1,3] While insufficiency of the scapholunate interosseous ligament can result in progressive arthritis (scapholunate advanced collapse [SLAC]), there is no established equivalent for LTIL pathology. The idea that isolated LTIL pathology could account for persistent, troubling wrist pain seems related to the development of imaging techniques such as arthrogram, magnetic resonance imaging (MRI), and diagnostic wrist arthroscopy. For instance, contrast medium leaking through the LTIL on wrist arthrogram in people seeking care for wrist pain was assumed by some to indicate traumatic rupture and stabilization of the LTIL was proposed to reduce pain.[4] However, the link between variations in LTIL anatomy and wrist pain is not at all clear, given the evidence that such variations are common and increase with age in people with and without symptoms. There is limited evidence regarding (1) the reliability and accuracy of diagnosis of isolated LTIL pathology; (2) the ability to establish LTIL pathology as a source of wrist pain; (3) the natural history of isolated LTIL variations encountered on imaging and arthroscopy; and (4) the notion that surgery to address LTIL pathology alleviates symptoms better than surgery that simulates treatment of pathology (placebo). The latter is important, because subjective outcomes are always improved by nonspecific effects (regression to the mean, self-limiting course, placebo effect) in addition to any improvements that might be related to alterations in the pathology.[4]

Keywords: lunotriquetral interosseous ligament, perilunate injuries, base rate neglect, confirmation bias, natural history, volar-intercalated segment instability, hamate arthrosis lunotriquetral tear

19.1 Introduction

Survey-based experiments show substantial variation in how surgeons approach wrist pain, magnetic resonance imaging (MRI) signal changes, and wrist arthroscopy findings.[5] This supports our notion that lunotriquetral interosseous ligament (LTIL) variations are inconsistently diagnosed and treated. This variation in part might be related to common cognitive biases, prevalent in humans and in surgeons.[6] Common cognitive biases include base rate neglect, which results in overestimating the meaning of a positive test, like MRI signal changes, or wrist arthroscopy findings; confirmation bias, where confirmatory tests are emphasized, and disconfirmatory tests neglected; and anchoring and framing heuristics. Anchoring and framing might occur because most studies on LTIL variations discuss surgical stabilization, potentially creating an unconscious emphasis on surgical treatment without exploring the natural history and the potential self-limiting nature of wrist pain in structurally sound joints. As a debiasing strategy, the authors reviewed the experimental evidence regarding diagnosis and management of isolated LTIL variations.

19.2 Definition of the Key Concepts

The word "rupture" is used to describe complete traumatic disruption of the LTIL. The word "variation" is used to describe any findings that vary from the usual anatomy whether they are developmental deficiencies, expected anatomical variations, age-related variations (senescence), or possible damage from past trauma.

19.3 LTIL Rupture in Carpal Dislocations

Traumatic LTIL rupture is obvious in the setting of perilunate, reverse perilunate, and axial carpal dislocations. Studies of perilunate injuries and fracture dislocations show that when the lunate and triquetrum are aligned, the LTIL likely heals without direct repair—or at least it is not associated with carpal malalignment.[1,3] In the proposed stages of reverse perilunate dislocations, type 1 consists of an isolated partial or complete LTIL rupture (type 2: disruption of alignment between lunate and triquetrum [▶ Fig. 19.1]; type 3: progression of the injury through the midcarpal joint [▶ Fig. 19.2]).[7,8] Since the treatment of perilunate injuries shows that the LTIL heals to the extent that it does not cause problems if the lunate and triquetrum are aligned, it is probably safe to assume this applies to isolated LTIL ruptures without carpal malalignment.

19.3.1 Consequences of LTIL Rupture

Several studies noted that isolated sectioning of the LTIL in cadavers has little effect on carpal alignment and wrist biomechanics.[8,9] One study noting the potential limited role of the LTIL in maintaining LT joint alignment suggested the extensor carpi ulnaris tendon might play a role in LT joint stability.[10] Lunate flexion (or volar-intercalated segment instability [VISI]) is common in the absence of LTIL variations[4] and uncommon in their presence.[11]

IV

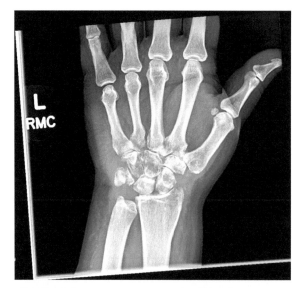

Fig. 19.1 Left posteroanterior wrist radiographs of a 57-year-old man with a type 2 reverse perilunate injury after a fall from wheel chair. Note the triquetral body fracture and disruption of the lunotriquetral interval and disruption of the normally smooth arc distal to the proximal carpal row. (Copyright Teun Teunis.)

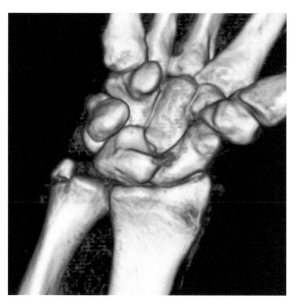

Fig. 19.2 A 27-year-old man injured his wrist in a fall. Volar view on the 3D computed tomography (CT) reconstruction shows a type 3 dorsal reverse perilunate dislocation with maintained scapholunate relationship, and dislocation of the triquetrum, capitate, and rest of the wrist. (Copyright David Ring.)

While insufficiency of the scapholunate interosseous ligament can result in progressive arthritis (scapholunate advanced collapse [SLAC]), there is no established equivalent for LTIL pathology. Others have proposed an association between wrist pain, LTIL variations, and hamate arthrosis (hamate arthrosis LTIL tear; HALT) and recommend proximal hamate pole excision.[12] But hamate tip arthrosis is common when there is a separate lunate articulation, 38% (108/285) of cadavers with articulation vs only 2% (2/108) without.[13] Since both hamate tip arthrosis and LTIL variations are common there is a high probability of coincidence.

19.4 Prevalence of Wrist Pain

Wrist pain is common, perhaps more so with age, and is generally nonspecific. A study from the Netherlands found that about 5 per 1000 people will consult their physician for wrist symptoms in a given year.[14] One study from the United Kingdom found that among 6038 people, 11% (694/6038) experienced wrist pain for 1 day or longer in the past 7 days. Upon physical examination, 60% (419/694) of those pains were judged to be nonspecific (not associated with discrete pathology).[15] The prevalence of nonspecific wrist pain increases with age in the general population (▶ Fig. 19.3). One study found that among 634 people initially diagnosed with nonspecific arm pain, only 7 people were diagnosed with a potentially discrete pathology later on (1.1%), and only 1 (0.16%) was confirmed and felt likely to be accurate.[16]

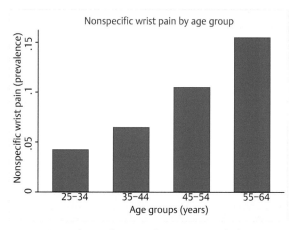

Fig. 19.3 Prevalence of nonspecific wrist pain in the last 7 days that lasted longer than 1 day in the general population between 25 and 64. (Based on Walker-Bone et al.[15] Copyright Teun Teunis.)

19.4.1 Prevalence of LTIL Variations

A scoping review of the prevalence of LTIL variations found that variations of the LTIL are common and increase with age both in people assumed to be without wrist pain (cadavers) and people with wrist pain (▶ Table 19.1). The authors found 5% (6/112) abnormalities in people < 20 years old, 14% (29/203) 20 to 39 years, 24% (37/154) 40 to 59 years, and 44% (177/402) in people over 60-year-old (▶ Fig. 19.4). The rate of developmental lack of LTIL is

Table 19.1 Study characteristics of reports on LTIL variations at different ages

Study	Method of identification	Wrist pain	Number of wrists per age group in each study				Total LTIL variations
			< 20	20–39	40–59	> 60	
Blair et al[18]	Arthrotomy	– (cadaver)	2	13	1	0	2
Cooney[19]	Arthroscopy	+	4	13	3	0	8
Dwek et al[20]	MRI	+	10	0	0	0	0
Levinsohn and Palmer[21]	Arthrography	+	26	83	0	0	11
Mahmood et al[22]	Arthroscopy	+	0	13	15	2	4
Mikic[23]	Arthrotomy	– (cadaver)	71	24	36	49	60
Viegas and Ballantyne[24]	Arthrotomy	– (cadaver)	2	4	18	76	21
Viegas et al.[13]	Arthrotomy	– (cadaver)	5	23	64	274	128
Weiss et al.[17]	Arthroscopy	+	2	30	17	1	15

Abbreviations: LTIL, lunotriquetral interosseous ligament; MRI, magnetic resonance imaging.

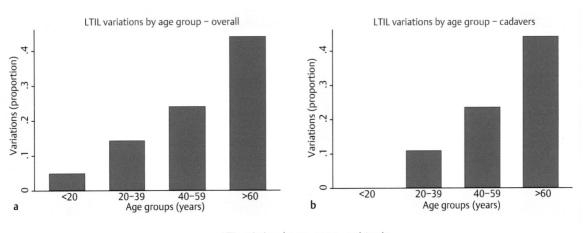

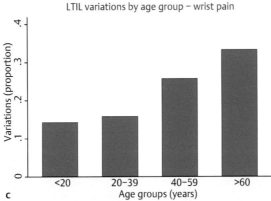

Fig. 19.4 **(a)** Lunotriquetral interosseous ligament (LTIL) variations by age group, including all studies. **(b)** LTIL variations by age group in assumed asymptomatic individuals. **(c)** LTIL variations by age group in people with wrist pain. There are only three people over 60 years of age, limiting the validity of this group. (Copyright Teun Teunis.)

unstudied and unknown. One study reported 20 LTIL variations in 62 cadavers (32%) with a mean age of 78 years (range 46–99) of which 12 were completely interrupted (60%, 12/20). One arthroscopy study reported 5 out of 15 (33%) of the LTIL variations were completely interrupted.[17]

19.4.2 The Association of LTIL Variations and Discomfort and Incapability

The high base rate of daily wrist pains in combination with the high base rate of LTIL variations makes coincidental overlap far more likely than a true association. We need a reliable and accurate diagnostic test for LTIL variations that cause a specific type of pain distinct from commonplace wrist pains. In the absence of such a test, there is a notable potential for overdiagnosis and overtreatment (Box 19.1).

Box 19.1 Testing with a low pretest probability of symptomatic LTIL rupture

Assume that 10% of people with LTIL variations have symptoms related to those variations (we expect this to be much lower), and assume we can diagnose LTIL variations with 90% sensitivity and specificity. If we test 1000 people with nonspecific wrist pain after interview, examination, and radiographs, 100 people will actually have a symptomatic LTIL variation. With a sensitivity of 90% our test will be positive in 90 people who have the symptomatic variation (100*90%), while we will miss 10 people—see the "symptomatic" column. There will be no LTIL variation, or it will be asymptomatic, in 900 people (1000 – 100). With a specificity of 90%, our test will accurately identify (900*90%) 810 people as such, and the test will be a false-positive in 90 people—see the absent/asymptomatic column. This means that 180 people will have a positive test, of which only 90 (50%) will actually have a symptomatic variation and our posttest probability is only 50%. If we treat everyone with a positive test, half of the people have unhelpful surgery, resulting in a number needed to harm of 2.

These numbers are hypothetical. Currently it is unclear if and when LTIL variations are painful, further increasing the probability of overdiagnosis and treatment (see ▶ Table 19.2).

19.5 Diagnosis and Treatment of LTIL Variations as the Cause of Wrist Pain

In 1984, Reagan et al described 24 people with wrist pain and normal radiographs. Thirteen (54%) had surgery, nine

Table 19.2 LTIL variation

		LTIL variation		
		Symptomatic	Absent/ Asymptomatic	Total
Test	Positive	90	90	180
	Negative	10	810	820
	Total	100	900	1000

Abbreviation: LTIL, lunotriquetral interosseous ligament.

(70%) based on passage of radiopaque injection material through the lunotriquetral interval. During surgery the authors encountered LTIL variations that they labeled as ruptures but did not otherwise describe. Surgery consisted of LT fusion, ligament repair, and ligament reconstruction. They noted satisfaction as "good" in 8, "fair" in 1, and "poor" in 4.[4]

Subsequent studies found that passage of radiopaque dye is often present in the asymptomatic contralateral side,[25] unrelated to the location of wrist pain,[26] and common in asymptomatic wrists.[27] Cadaver studies of presumed asymptomatic individuals showed LTIL variations are common and increase with age.[13]

A review published in 2016 found 7 studies reporting the results of arthroscopic LTIL debridement in 131 people; 8 studies of 184 people having LTIL reconstruction; and 12 studies of 232 people having LT joint fusion.[28] No report other than Reagan et al addressed nonoperative treatment (n=11),[4] reflecting notable publication bias in favor of operative treatment.

Most studies do not differentiate between LTIL ruptures and variations.[28,29,30,31] There is no evidence regarding the natural history of LTIL variations in people with and without wrist pain.

Steroid injections are often recommended as an initial treatment of presumed symptomatic LTIL variations.[29,30,31] There is no experimental evidence that steroid injections behave differently than placebo injections in this context. If LTIL variations are conceptualized as traumatic, the rationale for using a catabolic medication is a bit puzzling.

19.6 Potential Harms Associated with the Concept of LTIL Variations as a Cause of Wrist Pain

Mislabeling LTIL variations as damage or the source of wrist pains has potential for iatrogenic (unhelpful surgery), psychological (identity as damaged and vulnerable), social (job, housing, role security), and financial harms (out–of–pocket expenses, time off work). Referring to variations as "tears" can reenforce the common misconception that painful activity represents activity that will make the problem worse. The word "tear" may also reinforce the misconception that the problem can and should be repaired, generally through surgery. To avoid misleading clinicians and patients, the authors believe that LTIL variations should not be referred to as tears unless they can reliably and accurately be associated with recent trauma, which currently seems implausible.

Assuming one day we are able to reliably and accurately identify LTIL variations that cause symptoms (▶ Table 19.3, ▶ Fig. 19.5), we would still need evidence regarding the natural history of these variations. Do symptoms resolve

Table 19.3 Tests proposed to identify symptomatic LTIL variations and their limitations

Test	Description	Reliability, accuracy, reproducibility
Physical examination	Reagan et al proposed an LT ballottement test: fixing the lunate between thumb and index finger with one hand, and fixing the pisiform and triquetrum with the other hand, followed by displacing the triquetrum dorsal and volar.[4] Other authors report slight variations of this maneuver, such as the Kleinman shear test,[32] or a different ballottement test.[33]	One study found the tests to be positive <65% in people having LT stabilization surgery.[34] Another study found no association between positive tests in people with wrist pain and LTIL variations on arthrogram.[25]
Arthrogram	Contrast medium flowing from the radiocarpal joint, through the LT space, into the midcarpal joint, or the other way around. Can be a radiograph or MRI.	Passage of radiopaque dye is often present in the asymptomatic contralateral side,[25] unrelated to the location of wrist pain,[26] and common in asymptomatic people.[27]
Arthroscopy	Geissler proposed a classification of arthroscopic staging of ligament "tears."	There is no reference test to identify LTIL variations and to differentiate symptomatic and asymptomatic variations. There are no studies using latent class analysis. One study found interobserver agreement (kappa) between three surgeons to be 0.31 for LTIL pathology.[35] A study with a larger group of surgeons might find even lower agreement.[5]

Abbreviations: LT, lunotriquetral; LTIL, lunotriquetral interosseous ligament; MRI, magnetic resonance imaging.

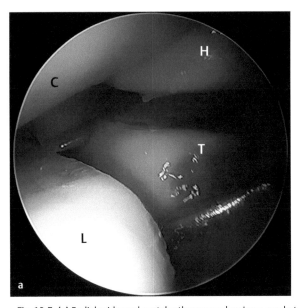
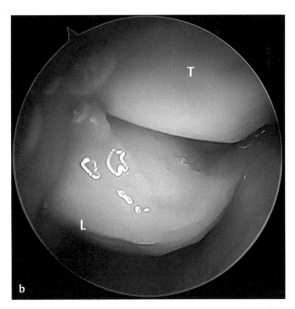

Fig. 19.5 (a) Radial midcarpal portal arthroscopy showing a gap between the lunate (L) and triquetrum (T), capitate (C), hamate (H). (b) Radiocarpal six-radial portal arthroscopy of the same patient showing a gap between the lunate (L) and triquetrum (T). It is important to keep in mind that the shown abnormalities are common in people with and without wrist pain. Currently there is no reference test to differentiate symptomatic and asymptomatic variations. It is not known if intervention to address lunotriquetral interosseous ligament (LTIL) pathology alleviates symptoms beyond nonspecific effects such as regression to the mean and the placebo effect. (Copyright Fernando Corella.)

19

over time? Will arthritis develop without treatment? Does an intervention to address LTIL pathology alleviate symptoms beyond nonspecific effects such as regression to the mean and the placebo effect?

Until these gaps in the evidence are filled, there seems to be relatively little potential for harm in managing the structurally sound, painful wrist supportively, limiting both diagnostic tests and reconstructive interventions.

References

[1] Capo JT, Corti SJ, Shamian B, et al. Treatment of dorsal perilunate dislocations and fracture-dislocations using a standardized protocol. Hand (N Y). 2012; 7(4):380–387

[2] Herzberg G, Burnier M, Marc A, Merlini L, Izem Y. The role of arthroscopy for treatment of perilunate injuries. J Wrist Surg. 2015; 4 (2):101–109

[3] Kim JP, Lee JS, Park MJ. Arthroscopic treatment of perilunate dislocations and fracture dislocations. J Wrist Surg. 2015; 4(2):81–87

[4] Reagan DS, Linscheid RL, Dobyns JH. Lunotriquetral sprains. J Hand Surg Am. 1984; 9(4):502–514

[5] Bakker D, Kortlever JTP, Kraan GA, Mathijssen N, Colaris JW, Ring D, Science of Variation Group. Treatment recommendations for suspected scapholunate ligament pathology. J Wrist Surg. 2021; 11 (1):62–68

[6] Janssen SJ, Teunis T, Ring D, Parisien RC. Cognitive biases in orthopaedic surgery. J Am Acad Orthop Surg. 2021; 29(14):624–633

[7] Murray PM, Palmer CG, Shin AY. The mechanism of ulnar-sided perilunate instability of the wrist: a cadaveric study and 6 clinical cases. J Hand Surg Am. 2012; 37(4):721–728

[8] Viegas SF, Patterson RM, Peterson PD, et al. Ulnar-sided perilunate instability: an anatomic and biomechanic study. J Hand Surg Am. 1990; 15(2):268–278

[9] Horii E, Garcia-Elias M, An KN, et al. A kinematic study of lunotriquetral dissociations. J Hand Surg Am. 1991; 16(2):355–362

[10] León-Lopez MM, Salvà-Coll G, Garcia-Elias M, Lluch-Bergadà A, Llusá-Pérez M. Role of the extensor carpi ulnaris in the stabilization of the lunotriquetral joint. An experimental study. J Hand Ther. 2013; 26(4): 312–317, quiz 317

[11] Wright TW, Del Charco M, Wheeler D. Incidence of ligament lesions and associated degenerative changes in the elderly wrist. J Hand Surg Am. 1994; 19(2):313–318

[12] Harley BJ, Werner FW, Boles SD, Palmer AK. Arthroscopic resection of arthrosis of the proximal hamate: a clinical and biomechanical study. J Hand Surg Am. 2004; 29(4):661–667

[13] Viegas SF, Patterson RM, Hokanson JA, Davis J. Wrist anatomy: incidence, distribution, and correlation of anatomic variations, tears, and arthrosis. J Hand Surg Am. 1993; 18(3):463–475

[14] Bot SD, van der Waal JM, Terwee CB, et al. Incidence and prevalence of complaints of the neck and upper extremity in general practice. Ann Rheum Dis. 2005; 64(1):118–123

[15] Walker-Bone K, Palmer KT, Reading I, Coggon D, Cooper C. Prevalence and impact of musculoskeletal disorders of the upper limb in the general population. Arthritis Rheum. 2004; 51(4):642–651

[16] Kortlever JT, Janssen SJ, Molleman J, Hageman MG, Ring D. Discrete pathophysiology is uncommon in patients with nonspecific arm pain. Arch Bone Jt Surg. 2016; 4(3):213–219

[17] Weiss AP, Akelman E, Lambiase R. Comparison of the findings of triple-injection cinearthrography of the wrist with those of arthroscopy. J Bone Joint Surg Am. 1996; 78(3):348–356

[18] Blair WF, Berger RA, el-Khoury GY. Arthrotomography of the wrist: an experimental and preliminary clinical study. J Hand Surg Am. 1985; 10(3):350–359

[19] Cooney WP. Evaluation of chronic wrist pain by arthrography, arthroscopy, and arthrotomy. J Hand Surg Am. 1993; 18(5):815–822

[20] Dwek JR, Cardoso F, Chung CB. MR imaging of overuse injuries in the skeletally immature gymnast: spectrum of soft-tissue and osseous lesions in the hand and wrist. Pediatr Radiol. 2009; 39 (12):1310–1316

[21] Levinsohn EM, Palmer AK. Arthrography of the traumatized wrist. Correlation with radiography and the carpal instability series. Radiology. 1983; 146(3):647–651

[22] Mahmood A, Fountain J, Vasireddy N, Waseem M. Wrist MRI arthrogram v wrist arthroscopy: what are we finding? Open Orthop J. 2012; 6:194–198

[23] Mikić ZD. Age changes in the triangular fibrocartilage of the wrist joint. J Anat. 1978; 126(Pt 2):367–384

[24] Viegas SF, Ballantyne G. Attritional lesions of the wrist joint. J Hand Surg Am. 1987; 12(6):1025–1029

[25] Cantor RM, Stern PJ, Wyrick JD, Michaels SE. The relevance of ligament tears or perforations in the diagnosis of wrist pain: an arthrographic study. J Hand Surg Am. 1994; 19(6):945–953

[26] Metz VM, Mann FA, Gilula LA. Lack of correlation between site of wrist pain and location of noncommunicating defects shown by three-compartment wrist arthrography. AJR Am J Roentgenol. 1993; 160(6):1239–1243

[27] Kirschenbaum D, Sieler S, Solonick D, Loeb DM, Cody RP. Arthrography of the wrist. Assessment of the integrity of the ligaments in young asymptomatic adults. J Bone Joint Surg Am. 1995; 77(8):1207–1209

[28] van de Grift TC, Ritt MJ. Management of lunotriquetral instability: a review of the literature. J Hand Surg Eur Vol. 2016; 41(1):72–85

[29] Shin AY, Battaglia MJ, Bishop AT. Lunotriquetral instability: diagnosis and treatment. J Am Acad Orthop Surg. 2000; 8(3):170–179

[30] Nicoson MC, Moran SL. Diagnosis and treatment of acute lunotriquetral ligament injuries. Hand Clin. 2015; 31(3):467–476

[31] Wagner ER, Elhassan BT, Rizzo M. Diagnosis and treatment of chronic lunotriquetral ligament injuries. Hand Clin. 2015; 31(3):477–486

[32] Kleinman WB. Diagnostic exams for ligamentous injuries. Am Soc Surg Hand, Correspondence Club Newsletter. 1985;51

[33] Beckenbaugh RD. Accurate evaluation and management of the painful wrist following injury. An approach to carpal instability. Orthop Clin North Am. 1984; 15(2):289–306

[34] Shin AY, Weinstein LP, Berger RA, Bishop AT. Treatment of isolated injuries of the lunotriquetral ligament. A comparison of arthrodesis, ligament reconstruction and ligament repair. J Bone Joint Surg Br. 2001; 83(7):1023–1028

[35] Löw S, Prommersberger KJ, Pillukat T, van Schoonhoven J. [Intra- and interobserver reliability of digitally photodocumented findings in wrist arthroscopy]. Handchir Mikrochir Plast Chir. 2010; 42(5):287–292

20 Acute Management: Open Treatment of LT Injury and Instability

Lauren E. Dittman and Alexander Y. Shin

Abstract

This chapter discusses open treatment options of acute lunotriquetral (LT) injuries, including surgical techniques of LT repair and reconstruction. Acute LT injuries often present with variable severity of ulnar-sided wrist pain after a trauma and can be elusive to diagnose. Accurate early diagnosis is key to successful treatment of acute injuries and in preventing the sequelae of missed LT instability, including development of volar intercalated segment instability (VISI) deformity and arthritis. Diagnosis is often made with a combination of a high index of suspicion together with history, physical examination, radiographs (advanced imaging as necessary), and/or diagnostic arthroscopy.

Once the diagnosis is made, a broad range of treatment options exist, based on patient factors, concomitant injuries, the reducibility of deformity, and the degree of cartilage injury. Nonoperative and arthroscopic treatment can be applied in some settings, particularly those with partial injuries to the LT ligament with residual remaining stability. However, open repair or reconstruction is often necessary. This chapter will focus on the open treatment of acute injuries, typically performed through a dorsal approach with a ligament-sparing capsulotomy. Direct repair is facilitated with the aid of suture anchors, while reconstruction commonly utilizes a distally based strip of the extensor carpi ulnaris (ECU) tendon. The authors' preferred techniques of repair and reconstruction will be highlighted in this chapter.

Keywords: lunotriquetral ligament, acute, instability, ligament repair, ligament reconstruction

20.1 Introduction and Historical Perspective

The first report of LT injury was purportedly in 1903, when William Hessert described multiple cases of carpal dislocations.[1] An additional report of LT dissociation was later noted by von Mayersbach in 1913, when he described "the cuneiform (triquetrum) is separated from the semilunar bone (lunate), but is not substantially changed in position."[2] During the same year, Chaput and Vaillant described a deformity where the lunate fell into flexion, later to be known as a volar intercalated segmental instability (VISI) pattern.[3] A few years later, Navarro reports a series of patients with VISI deformity and noted the triquetrum was extended.[4] Throughout the remainder of the mid-1900s, additional reports of LT dissociation were reported.[5,7] It was not until 1972, when Linscheid

et al identified how the position of the lunate affected wrist stability and introduced the terms "dorsal intercalated segment instability (DISI)" and "VISI deformity."[8] Over the next 10 years, the role of the LT ligament as it relates to wrist stability slowly became understood.[9,10]

Acute lunotriquetral (LT) injury can be difficult to diagnose as it rarely occurs in isolation and may present as part of a wrist injury. Patients typically present with ulnar-sided wrist pain and decreased grip strength; however, there are numerous etiologies with similar clinical presentations. Mechanism of injury can be variable as well, ranging from perilunate or reverse perilunate injury patterns, dorsally directed forces across the wrist, to ulnar positive variance with ulnocarpal impaction. The spectrum of injury to the LT ligament complex can vary from partial injuries of the dorsal, volar, or membranous portions of the ligament, dorsal complete tear with partial volar tear, complete volar tear with partial dorsal tear, to complete disruption/dissociation of the entire ligament complex.

Unless there is frank dissociation with injury to secondary restraints, radiographs are usually normal. Magnetic resonance imaging (MRI) or MR arthrography may be performed to help aid in diagnosis; however, the sensitivity is variable with respect to LT injury.[11,12] Wrist arthroscopy remains the gold standard for accurate diagnosis and staging of LT injury and instability.[12,13] Geissler et al proposed a classification system based on intraoperative arthroscopic ligament stability.[14] Low-grade or partial tears can often be managed nonoperatively, or with arthroscopic debridement and possible pinning. However high-grade tears, or Geissler Grade III and IV, typically require open surgical treatment (see Video 20.1).

20.2 Surgical Anatomy

The LT ligament is a C-shaped structure with three components: the volar, dorsal, and proximal portions. The volar LT ligament is the thickest and strongest, and acting as the main restraint to extension of the triquetrum. It also acts to transmit the force from the triquetrum to the lunate during wrist extension as the triquetrum engages the hamate. The dorsal portion of the ligament is much thinner and acts as a rotational restraint. The proximal region, also known as the membranous portion, is composed of fibrocartilage and is the weakest of the three. It provides little restraint and has no significant biomechanical role. The volar and dorsal portions of the ligament are intimately associated with extrinsic ligaments of the wrist. The volar portion is intertwined with the ulnocapitate ligament and the dorsal portion with the

20

177

dorsal radiotriquetral ligament.[15] This allows the ulnocapitate ligament and the dorsal radiotriquetral ligament to act as secondary stabilizers to the LT joint.

20.3 Indications and Contraindications for Surgery

The decision for the appropriate treatment of LT ligament injuries is multifactorial. Not only is it important to consider the extent of instability and chronicity of the injury, but surgeons must also account for patient-specific factors, including age and functional wrist demands.[16,17] Concomitant traumatic or degenerative changes to the wrist need to be considered in the decision-making process.

Nonoperative treatment should be the initial treatment strategy for dynamic acute and chronic LT ligament injuries without dissociation/VISI deformity.[10,17,20] This typically consists of 4 weeks of immobilization in a long-arm Muenster cast with pisiform lift followed by an additional 4 weeks in a short-arm cast. The pisiform lift is created by molding a pad in the splint below the pisiform palmarly to prevent ulnar sag of the wrist and allow optimal ligamentous healing. After this immobilization period, hand therapy is crucial to help strengthening the extensor carpi ulnaris (ECU) and improve proprioception to neutralize the deforming forces in LT ligament injuries.[21,23] A corticosteroid injection into the midcarpal joint can also be considered to help with pain control and provides diagnostic validation of the diagnosis.

Surgical intervention is indicated for those who fail conservative management, have a clinical exam consistent with ligament disruption, or have acute injury with acute VISI deformity. The goal of surgery is to restore the anatomical lunocapitate axis, thereby eliminating VISI deformity (when present) and restoring rotational stability to the proximal carpal row.[17,24,25] This can be done through a variety of surgical techniques. These include debridement, thermal shrinkage of the attenuated ligament, direct ligament repair, ligament reconstruction, and varying forms of arthrodesis. Many of these can be done through either an arthroscopic or an open approach. Arthroscopic treatment was discussed in a prior chapter; therefore, the remainder of this chapter will focus on open surgical techniques.

Direct LT ligament repair is indicated in acute injuries where there is adequate remaining dorsal ligament for a successful repair. In addition, it is important to inspect the volar LT ligament, as incompetence would be a contraindication to dorsal ligament repair. If the dorsal or volar LT ligament is incompetent or lacks tissue for repair, reconstruction is indicated. A relative contraindication to direct repair is high functional demand. Manual laborers and high-level athletes should be considered for ligament reconstruction, as they pose a high risk for rerupture and attenuation leading to late failure of a direct repair.[26] In general, LT ligament reconstruction should be considered in virtually all patients as prior studies have shown that reconstruction has the lowest rate of reoperation compared to both direct repair and arthrodesis.[26]

Arthritic changes in the wrist are an absolute contraindication to both LT repair and reconstruction. This may be appreciated via radiographs or CT scan; however, diagnostic arthroscopy is considered the gold standard in assessing the status of the articular cartilage. This may be done in a single setting, prior to open surgical intervention, or in a staged manner, often several weeks apart, based on surgeon and patient preferences. If significant degenerative changes are found, partial or total carpal arthrodesis or proximal row carpectomy (depending on cartilage status) is indicated. A static VISI deformity is an indication for some variation of carpal arthrodesis.

Ulnar variance should also be considered during the surgical decision-making process. Patients with significant ulnar positivity or those with signs of ulnocarpal impingement would likely benefit from an ulnar shortening osteotomy alone or in addition to LT ligament repair or reconstruction.[27] Radiographs should be examined for ulnar variance and further imaging pursued if there is high clinical concern for ulnocarpal impingement. This may consist of pronated grip radiograph views to examine dynamic ulnar variance or MRI to look for signal changes secondary to impingement in the ulnar aspect of the lunate.[28,29]

20.4 Literature Review and Different Surgical Techniques

20.4.1 Debridement

Open versus arthroscopic debridement is perhaps the most conservative operative approach to patients with LT tears. It is accomplished with a relatively quick surgery and allows faster rehabilitation and recovery. Many times, the LT joint is held reduced and temporary K-wire fixation is placed. A small dorsal incision may be utilized to visualize and aid in a direct reduction of the LT joint. Prior studies have shown acceptable results with debridement alone. Weiss et al found that 78% of patients who had complete LT tears and 100% of patients who had partial LT tears had symptomatic improvement after undergoing arthroscopic debridement followed by 2 weeks of immobilization.[30] A review by Ritt et al supports similar conclusions; however, it is imperative that these patients do not have an associated VISI deformity.[15] However, not all studies are in concordance with these findings. Westkaemper et al found that four out of five patients treated with a similar protocol had poorer outcomes, and debridement was overall less effective for LT tears compared to scapholunate (SL) and triangular fibrocartilage complex (TFCC) tears.[31] The disparity in outcomes is most likely related to the definition of partial and complete injuries, the portion of the ligament that was addressed, and the degree of incompetence of the volar and dorsal ligaments.

20.4.2 Direct Ligament Repair

When feasible, direct LT ligament repair has been advocated with successful results. This is typically in the acute setting when surgery is performed within a few weeks of initial injury. It is performed through a dorsal incision with ligament-sparing capsulotomy.[32] Repair of the ligament may be done with either drill holes or suture anchors in the lunate or triquetrum, depending on where the ligament avulsed from. If utilizing drill holes, 3 to 4 parallel holes are created where the LT ligament avulsed from the bone, and then exit on the opposite dorsal cortex (▶ Fig. 20.1). Nonabsorbable sutures are passed through these holes, sutured into the remaining LT ligament, and passed back out through the drill holes.[17] A similar technique is employed if suture anchors are used, which are typically embedded into the dorsal aspect of the ligament avulsion site. Percutaneous K-wires hold the LT joint reduced for 8 to 12 weeks, at which point they are removed, and wrist range of motion is begun. The dorsal capsule can be imbricated into the repair to augment the repair.

Multiple prior studies have reported overall satisfactory results after direct LT repair. Reagan et al previously examined seven patients who underwent direct LT ligament repair; six of these patients had symptomatic improvement postoperatively.[10] Similarly, Favero et al reported a 90% satisfaction rate with only one failure in a cohort of 21 patients after undergoing direct LT ligament repair.[33] The largest series was reported on by Shin et al and found that patients reported similar DASH scores after both repair and reconstruction.[26] However, this study did report a 15% revision rate after direct LT repair, which has led many surgeons to consider ligament reconstruction after acute ligament injury.

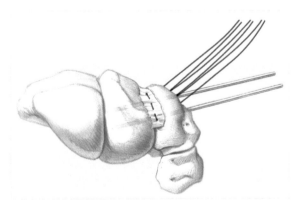

20.4.3 Ligament Reconstruction

As previously mentioned, direct ligament repair has a 15% revision rate despite symptomatic improvement.[26] Therefore, ligament reconstruction should be considered in virtually all patients. In addition, reconstruction should be the treatment of choice in manual laborers and athletes, given their increased risk of rerupture and attenuation after direct repair.[26] In this series by Shin et al, the only complication noted was neuritis in the distribution of the dorsal sensory branch of the ulnar nerve.[26] Ligament reconstruction is also the treatment of choice in chronic LT ligament injuries, as long as there is no evidence of static VISI deformity or carpal arthritis.

The most common variation of this technique of reconstruction uses a distally based strip of the ECU tendon. Reagan et al was the first to publish the outcomes of this technique in three patients, and found that all reported satisfactory outcomes.[10] In a large cohort study of chronic LT injuries by Shahane et al found that 40 out of 46 patients were satisfied with their outcome after reconstruction, with excellent or good Mayo Wrist Scores in 63% of patients.[34] An additional study by Pilný et al, reported that 90% of patients recorded good or excellent results after LT reconstruction with ECU tendon in their cohort of 19 patients.[35] However, it is important to note that most of these studies examined patients with chronic LT ligament injury rather than acute.

A recent study has suggested the utilization of an arthroscopic-assisted LT ligament reconstruction with the ECU tendon, allowing for smaller incisions and the potential for less scarring.[36] This technique has only been performed in two reported patients to date, with no available outcomes currently. Other graft options have also been proposed, including the palmar longus autograft; however, the number of patients is not yet robust enough to draw adequate conclusions on their outcomes.[37]

20.4.4 Arthrodesis

In patients with static VISI deformity or evidence of radiocarpal arthritis, arthrodesis remains the only viable surgical option. Unfortunately, surgical outcomes after arthrodesis for LT ligament injury are variable.[10,26,38,39] All four patients in Reagan's study who underwent arthrodesis continued to experience symptoms postoperatively.[10] In addition, Shin et al found that 78% of patients required reoperation after arthrodesis, with a less than 1% chance of remaining free from complications. Of those who underwent arthrodesis, nearly 41% went on to nonunion.[26] Despite this, arthrodesis continues to be recommended as a last resort for these patients and is typically not used in the acute setting unless preexisting carpal arthritis is identified.[15]

20

20.4.5 Augmentation

Dorsal Capsulodesis

Dorsal capsulodesis can be used to reinforce the LT ligament, typically after repair or reconstruction. This is done by using a portion radiotriquetral ligament to recreate the dorsal LT ligament, which is typically secured using additional suture anchors in the lunate and triquetrum. Antti-Poika et al previously examined 26 patients who underwent dorsal capsulodesis for LT instability and found that 64% reported no or mild pain postoperatively.[40] Most commonly, this is done in the chronic setting in patients with chronic dynamic LT instability with good results.[41]

Ulnar Shortening Osteotomy

Ulnar shortening osteotomy may be used alone or in combination with any of the above techniques. A prior biomechanical study found that an ulnar shortening osteotomy decreases motion between the lunate and triquetrum by increasing strain in the ulnolunate and ulnotriquetral ligaments.[42] Mirza et al examined this theory in 53 patients with acute LT ligament tears who were treated with isolated ulnar shortening osteotomy. They found that 83% reported good or excellent scores postoperatively.[27] However, additional data on this treatment is sparse and this should be put within the clinical context of each patient. Patients with ulnar positive wrists or those with evidence of ulnocarpal impaction are most likely to benefit from consideration of ulnar shortening osteotomy.

20.5 Authors' Preferred Technique/Tips and Tricks

20.5.1 Acute Lunotriquetral Ligament Repair vs Reconstruction with Distally Based Extensor Carpi Ulnaris Strip

Setup and Positioning

A preoperative long-acting regional block is typically performed prior to surgery to help with postoperative pain control. The patient is then positioned supine on the operating room table with the arm on a radiolucent hand table. A nonsterile tourniquet is applied prior to sterile prepping and draping. Standard intravenous antibiotics are administered prior to incision. It is important to perform an examination of both wrists under anesthesia to evaluate for range of motion, LT laxity, midcarpal and radioulnar clunks. Examination should always be performed on the contralateral, unaffected extremity, to determine what is normal for each patient. After prep and drape, the arm is exsanguinated and suspended in finger traps in preparation for the diagnostic arthroscopy.

Diagnostic Arthroscopy and Debridement

Arthroscopy should be done in less than 10 minutes if an open reconstruction is planned for at the same surgery. Standard dorsal 3–4 and 4–5 radiocarpal portals are first established. Diagnostic arthroscopy can then be performed to evaluate the status of the dorsal and volar LT ligaments, as well as the articular cartilage. Dorsal radial midcarpal and dorsal ulnar midcarpal portals are made. The integrity of the dorsal and volar LT ligament is inferred by the space between the lunate and triquetrum. If the scope is easily passed between the bones, the ligament is completely incompetent. An inventory of all other damaged structures is made and should be considered for reconstruction or repair as needed. Formal LT ligament debridement and removal of any loose bodies may then be performed using this combination of radiocarpal and midcarpal portals. The decision is then made to either proceed with reconstruction under the same anesthesia, or as a secondary procedure in a staged procedure.

Incision and Dissection

The skin incision is centered over the third dorsal compartment, in line with the third metacarpal, directly overlying the carpus (▶ Fig. 20.2). Subcutaneous dissection is

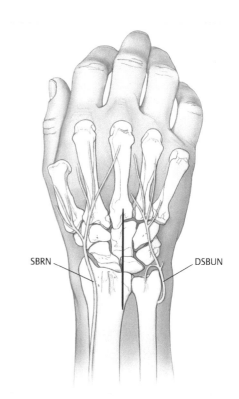

Fig. 20.2 Skin incision made in line with the third metacarpal. (By permission of Mayo Foundation for Medical Education and Research. All rights reserved.)

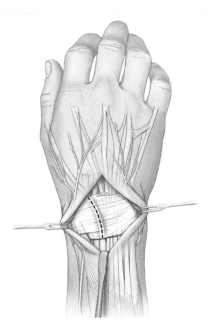

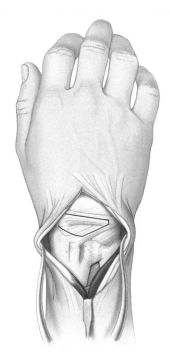

20

continued down to the level of the extensor retinaculum. Full-thickness flaps are developed. It is important to identify and protect the superficial branch of the radial nerve (SBRN) and the dorsal sensory branch of the ulnar nerve (DSBUN). The course of the extensor pollicis longus (EPL) and third dorsal compartment is identified, and the overlying extensor retinaculum is then divided from distal to proximal (▶ Fig. 20.3). An ulnarly based flap of retinaculum is reflected by dividing the septation between the 3–4 and 4–5 extensor compartments.

If it has not been previously performed, a posterior interosseous neurectomy is performed to prevent neuroma formation and to aid in pain control. A ligament-sparing capsulotomy, as previously described by Berger et al, is performed after proper identification of the dorsal radiocarpal and intercarpal ligaments (▶ Fig. 20.4, ▶ Fig. 20.5).[32] It is important to leave a cuff of tissue over the radius for later repair. The dorsal radiotriquetral ligament is intimately associated with the LT ligament and need to be meticulously separated. Careful dissection over the region of the dorsal LT ligament is crucial to avoid iatrogenic damage. The LT joint is identified, and any remaining LT ligament is debrided (▶ Fig. 20.6).

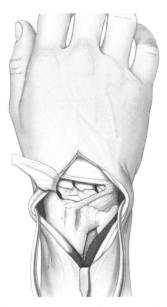

Direct Repair

If upon inspection of the LT joint, it is noted that the dorsal ligament is avulsed but the volar ligament remains intact, then a direct repair of the LT ligament may be performed. The authors' preference is to repair the ligament using suture anchors; however, bone tunnels may also be used. The site of avulsion of the dorsal LT ligament is examined, which is typically off of the triquetrum,

IV

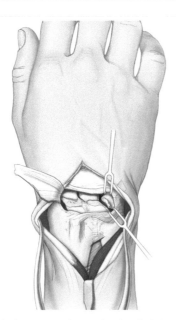

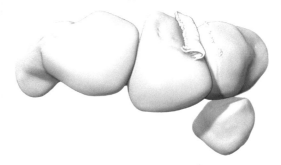

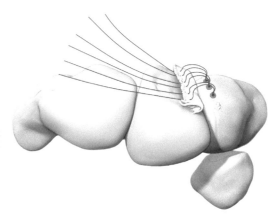

although it can also avulse off of the lunate (▶ Fig. 20.7). The site of attachment on the dorsal, nonarticular surface is debrided and prepared. Multiple horizontal suture anchors are then placed. The LT joint is reduced anatomically by direct visualization and palpation with a freer elevator, and two percutaneous 0.045 K-wires are then placed in a parallel fashion. The wires are cut and buried beneath the skin. With the reduction held by the K-wires, the ligament is then repaired. Sutures are typically placed in a horizontal mattress fashion, tensioned, and tied, and the needles are left on the sutures (▶ Fig. 20.8). The capsulotomy is closed, and the sutures can then be placed through the dorsal radiotriquetral ligament to augment the repair as needed.

Reconstruction with Distally Based Strip of ECU Tendon

If the LT ligament is completely incompetent, a reconstruction should be performed. A transverse 2 cm incision 6 to 8 cm proximal to the ulnar styloid is made over the ECU tendon.[43] The ECU tendon is identified, and the sheath is incised. A small retractor is then used to isolate the tendon circumferentially. The radial most 4 mm of the ECU tendon is transected in order to create the strip of graft. A 28-gauge wire is then tied to the distal end of the cut tendon. The ECU sheath is identified in the wrist incision in the distal ulnar wound, near the carpometacarpal joint. A tendon passer is placed into the ECU sheath distally, the 28-guage wire is grabbed proximally, and the wire is pulled distally creating a distally based tendon graft (▶ Fig. 20.9). Graft is then passed under the extensor retinaculum and the wire is left attached to the cut end of the tendon while the bone tunnels are prepared.

Bone Tunnel Creation and Graft Passage

Two 0.045-inch K-wires are used to obtain the starting points for the bone tunnels. This should be done while holding the joint properly reduced. One starting point should be on the dorsal ulnar aspect of the triquetrum and one on the dorsal radial edge of the lunate (▶ Fig. 20.10). The two K-wires should converge at the volar margin of the LT joint, without being intra-articular. Intraoperative fluoroscopic imaging should be used to confirm proper positioning. The tunnels are then drilled to a final size of 4 to 5 mm using a cannulated drill bit or a series of sharp awls (▶ Fig. 20.11, ▶ Fig. 20.12).

The wire attached to the ECU graft is passed through the tunnel in the triquetrum. An arthroscopic probe or a suture passer can then be used to guide the wire back through the lunate tunnel (▶ Fig. 20.13). The wire is used

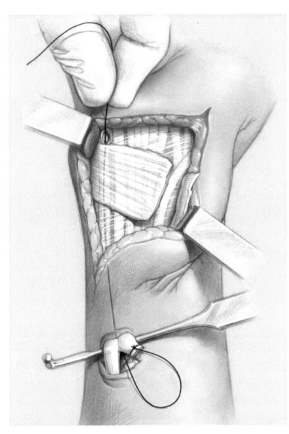

Fig. 20.9 Passage of the extensor carpi ulnaris (ECU) tendon from proximal to distal. (By permission of Mayo Foundation for Medical Education and Research. All rights reserved.)

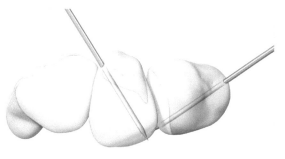

Fig. 20.10 Starting points on the dorsal ulnar border of the triquetrum and dorsal radial border of lunate converge on the volar aspect of the lunotriquetral (LT) articulation. (By permission of Mayo Foundation for Medical Education and Research. All rights reserved.)

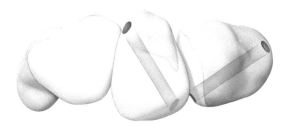

Fig. 20.12 Lunate and triquetrum bone tunnels. (By permission of Mayo Foundation for Medical Education and Research. All rights reserved.)

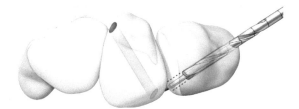

Fig. 20.11 Use of cannulated drill to create bone tunnels. (By permission of Mayo Foundation for Medical Education and Research. All rights reserved.)

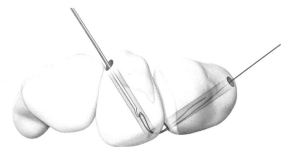

Fig. 20.13 Passage of wire through bone tunnels. (By permission of Mayo Foundation for Medical Education and Research. All rights reserved.)

to pull the graft through these tunnels. The LT joint is reduced under fluoroscopic imaging and two parallel 0.045-inch K-wires are placed percutaneously across the LT joint for stabilization while tension is placed on the ECU graft (▶ Fig. 20.14, ▶ Fig. 20.15). The ECU graft is tensioned appropriately and is woven back among itself over the dorsal aspect of the LT joint (▶ Fig. 20.16). This allows recreation of both the volar and dorsal aspects of the LT ligament (▶ Fig. 20.17). The construct is secured using nonabsorbable suture and any excess tendon is trimmed and K-wires are cut under the skin and buried.

Closure and Postoperative Care

The ligament-sparing capsulotomy is repaired over the ligament reconstruction using nonabsorbable suture. The EPL tendon is transposed, and the extensor retinaculum is closed. Skin can then be closed based on surgeon preference. A long-arm splint is applied postoperatively to prevent wrist flexion/extension as well as pronosupination.

IV

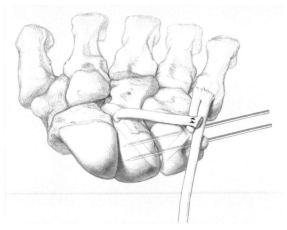

Fig. 20.14 Percutaneous K-wires are used for temporary stabilization. (By permission of Mayo Foundation for Medical Education and Research. All rights reserved.)

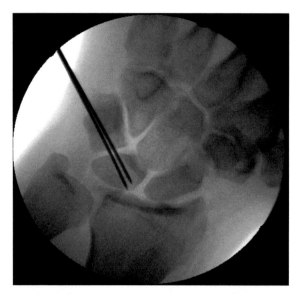

Fig. 20.15 Fluoroscopic imaging is used to ensure adequate reduction of the lunotriquetral (LT) interval. (By permission of Mayo Foundation for Medical Education and Research. All rights reserved.)

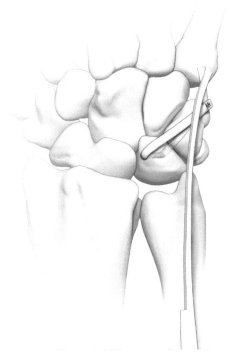

Fig. 20.16 The extensor carpi ulnaris (ECU) graft is weaved back through itself and secured with nonabsorbable sutures. (By permission of Mayo Foundation for Medical Education and Research. All rights reserved.)

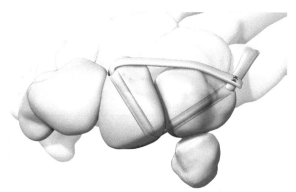

Fig. 20.17 Ligament reconstruction recreates both the dorsal and volar lunotriquetral (LT) ligaments. (By permission of Mayo Foundation for Medical Education and Research. All rights reserved.)

The patient is then transitioned to a long-arm neutral rotation cast approximately 10 to 14 days after surgery for an additional 6 weeks. They can then be transitioned to a short-arm Muenster cast for an additional 4 to 6 weeks, based on patient-specific considerations. Total immobilization is between 10 and 12 weeks, at which point the buried K-wires are removed and patients are permitted to begin range of motion exercises.

20.5.2 Tips and Tricks

- Place a moist sponge around the graft while preparing the bone tunnels to prevent desiccation.

- If repairing with suture anchors, be sure to place the anchors first, then reduce, then place K-wires. If the K-wires are placed first, they may obstruct placement of the suture anchors.

- When reducing the LT joint, ensure that the entire joint is visualized and reduced, to prevent dorsal-only or volar-only reduction. A freer elevator can be used to palpate if there are any step-offs or if the joint is adequately reduced.
- If you are able to easily visualize the entire LT joint, it is not reduced. The curvature of the joint should make it difficult to see when reduced.
- Additional K-wires can be placed into the lunate and triquetrum to act as joysticks to help achieve and maintain the reduction.
- A 14-gauge angiocatheter needle can be used as a trochar for 0.045-inch or 1-mm K-wires. This allows better control during wire placement and protects soft tissues.
- Bone tunnels need to be carefully placed. Reduce the LT interval and estimate the placement of tunnels and make sure they are in correct position to prevent distal/proximal translation when the ECU tendon is pulled taught.
- Create a loop on the 28-guage wire prior to passing through the triquetral tunnel. A hook can then be created on the end of a 0.035 K-wire to then hook the 28-guage wire and allow easier passing through the tunnels.
- It is crucial to maintain adequate reduction of the LT joint while tensioning and securing the graft. A Kocher or Allis can be used to grasp the free edge of the tendon to allow better control while weaving and securing the tendon to itself.

20.6 Essential Rehabilitation Points

Patients are typically immobilized for 10 to 12 weeks postoperatively. Finger range of motion and edema control begin immediately post-op. After the period of immobilization, the K-wires are removed, and wrist range of motion is begun under the direction of an experienced hand therapist. Ample immobilization is key to allowing proper healing of the ligament reconstruction and thereby achieving a successful outcome. Patients progress from wrist range of motion to wrist strengthening and stabilization over a course of several weeks postoperatively.

20.7 Conclusion

Once the diagnosis of an acute LT injury is made, it is imperative that treatment begin in the acute phase. Those patients with instability and lack of VISI deformity or arthritis should be considered for acute surgical intervention. Open treatment consisting of direct repair versus ligament reconstruction is typically utilized, with reconstruction having improved results compared to repair. The authors' preference is to perform reconstruction using a distally based ECU graft as it is a robust reliable repair. Second choice is ligament repair if a good remnant ligament is present. Arthrodesis should be avoided, given unreliable clinical improvement and high rate of nonunion. While reconstruction has shown satisfactory results, there still remains a lack of high-quality level I or level II clinical evidence to support one technique over the others.[44]

References

[1] Hessert W. XII. Dislocation of individual carpal bones, with report of a case of luxation of the scaphoid and semilunar. Ann Surg. 1903; 37 (3):402–414
[2] Mayersbach L v. Ein seltener Fall von Luxatio intercarpea. Deutsche Zeitschrift für Chirurgie. 1913; 123:79–189
[3] Chaput V, Vaillant C. Etude radiographique sur les traumatismes du carpe. Rev Orthop. 1913; 4:227–239
[4] Navarro A. Luxaciones del carpo. 1921:113–141
[5] Dunn AW. Fractures and dislocations of the carpus. Surg Clin North Am. 1972; 52(6):1513–1538
[6] Campbell RD, Jr, Lance EM, Yeoh CB. Lunate and perilunar dislocations. J Bone Joint Surg Br. 1964; 46(1):55–72
[7] Scaramuzza R. El movimiento de rotacion en el carpo y su relacion con la fisiopatologia de sus lesiones traumaticas. Bol Trab Soc Argent Ortop Traumatol. 1969; 34:337
[8] Linscheid RL, Dobyns JH, Beabout JW, Bryan RS. Traumatic instability of the wrist. Diagnosis, classification, and pathomechanics. J Bone Joint Surg Am. 1972; 54(8):1612–1632
[9] Taleisnik J, Malerich M, Prietto M. Palmar carpal instability secondary to dislocation of scaphoid and lunate: report of case and review of the literature. J Hand Surg Am. 1982; 7(6):606–612
[10] Reagan DS, Linscheid RL, Dobyns JH. Lunotriquetral sprains. J Hand Surg Am. 1984; 9(4):502–514
[11] Yu J. MRI of the wrist. Orthopedics. 1994; 17:1041–1048
[12] Weiss LE, Taras JS, Sweet S, Osterman AL. Lunotriquetral injuries in the athlete. Hand Clin. 2000; 16(3):433–438
[13] Osterman AL, Seidman GD. The role of arthroscopy in the treatment of lunatotriquetral ligament injuries. Hand Clin. 1995; 11(1):41–50
[14] Geissler WB, Freeland AE, Savoie FH, McIntyre LW, Whipple TL. Intracarpal soft-tissue lesions associated with an intra-articular fracture of the distal end of the radius. J Bone Joint Surg Am. 1996; 78(3):357–365
[15] Ritt MJ, Linscheid RL, Cooney WP, III, Berger RA, An KN. The lunotriquetral joint: kinematic effects of sequential ligament sectioning, ligament repair, and arthrodesis. J Hand Surg Am. 1998; 23(3):432–445
[16] Moran SL, Berger RA. Biomechanics and hand trauma: what you need. Hand Clin. 2003; 19(1):17–31
[17] Nicoson MC, Moran SL. Diagnosis and treatment of acute lunotriquetral ligament injuries. Hand Clin. 2015; 31(3):467–476
[18] Beckenbaugh RD. Accurate evaluation and management of the painful wrist following injury. An approach to carpal instability. Orthop Clin North Am. 1984; 15(2):289–306
[19] Culver JE. Instabilities of the wrist. Clin Sports Med. 1986; 5(4):725–740
[20] Sebald JR, Dobyns JH, Linscheid RL. The natural history of collapse deformities of the wrist. Clin Orthop Relat Res. 1974(104):140–148
[21] León-Lopez MM, Salvà-Coll G, Garcia-Elias M, Lluch-Bergadà A, Llusá-Pérez M. Role of the extensor carpi ulnaris in the stabilization of the lunotriquetral joint. An experimental study. J Hand Ther. 2013; 26(4): 312–317, quiz 317
[22] Hagert E, Lluch A, Rein S. The role of proprioception and neuromuscular stability in carpal instabilities. J Hand Surg Eur Vol. 2016; 41(1):94–101
[23] Esplugas M, Garcia-Elias M, Lluch A, Llusá Pérez M. Role of muscles in the stabilization of ligament-deficient wrists. J Hand Ther. 2016; 29 (2):166–174
[24] Weber E. Wrist mechanics and its association with ligamentous instability. The wrist and its disorders. Philadelphia, PA: WB Saunders; 1988:41–52

20

[25] Taleisnik J. Pain on the ulnar side of the wrist. Hand Clin. 1987; 3(1): 51–68

[26] Shin AY, Weinstein LP, Berger RA, Bishop AT. Treatment of isolated injuries of the lunotriquetral ligament. A comparison of arthrodesis, ligament reconstruction and ligament repair. J Bone Joint Surg Br. 2001; 83(7):1023–1028

[27] Mirza A, Mirza JB, Shin AY, Lorenzana DJ, Lee BK, Izzo B. Isolated lunotriquetral ligament tears treated with ulnar shortening osteotomy. J Hand Surg Am. 2013; 38(8):1492–1497

[28] Tomaino MM. The importance of the pronated grip x-ray view in evaluating ulnar variance. J Hand Surg Am. 2000; 25(2):352–357

[29] Imaeda T, Nakamura R, Shionoya K, Makino N. Ulnar impaction syndrome: MR imaging findings. Radiology. 1996; 201(2):495–500

[30] Weiss AP, Sachar K, Glowacki KA. Arthroscopic debridement alone for intercarpal ligament tears. J Hand Surg Am. 1997; 22(2):344–349

[31] Westkaemper JG, Mitsionis G, Giannakopoulos PN, Sotereanos DG. Wrist arthroscopy for the treatment of ligament and triangular fibrocartilage complex injuries. Arthroscopy. 1998; 14(5):479–483

[32] Berger RA, Bishop AT, Bettinger PC. New dorsal capsulotomy for the surgical exposure of the wrist. Ann Plast Surg. 1995; 35(1):54–59

[33] Favero K, Bishop A, Linscheid R. Lunotriquetral ligament disruption: a comparative study of treatment methods. In: 46th Annual Meeting of the American Society for Surgery of the Hand, Orlando, FL, October 2–5, 1991

[34] Shahane SA, Trail IA, Takwale VJ, Stilwell JH, Stanley JK. Tenodesis of the extensor carpi ulnaris for chronic, post-traumatic lunotriquetral instability. J Bone Joint Surg Br. 2005; 87(11):1512–1515

[35] Pilný J, Svarc A, Perina M, Siller J, Visna P. [Chronic lunotriquetral instability of the wrist. Presentation of our method of treatment]. Acta Chir Orthop Traumatol Cech. 2009; 76(3):208–211

[36] Haugstvedt JR, Rigó IZ. Arthroscopic assisted reconstruction of LT-ligament: a description of a new technique. J Wrist Surg. 2021; 10(1): 2–8

[37] Harper CM, Iorio ML. Lunotriquetral ligament reconstruction utilizing a palmaris longus autograft. J Hand Surg Asian Pac Vol. 2017; 22(4):544–547

[38] Sennwald GR, Fischer M, Mondi P. Lunotriquetral arthrodesis. A controversial procedure. J Hand Surg [Br]. 1995; 20(6):755–760

[39] Nelson DL, Manske PR, Pruitt DL, Gilula LA, Martin RA. Lunotriquetral arthrodesis. J Hand Surg Am. 1993; 18(6):1113–1120

[40] Antti-Poika I, Hyrkäs J, Virkki LM, Ogino D, Konttinen YT. Correction of chronic lunotriquetral instability using extensor retinacular split: a retrospective study of 26 patients. Acta Orthop Belg. 2007; 73(4): 451–457

[41] Omokawa S, Fujitani R, Inada Y. Dorsal radiocarpal ligament capsulodesis for chronic dynamic lunotriquetral instability. J Hand Surg Am. 2009; 34(2):237–243

[42] Gupta R, Bingenheimer E, Fornalski S, McGarry MH, Osterman AL, Lee TQ. The effect of ulnar shortening on lunate and triquetrum motion: a cadaveric study. Clin Biomech (Bristol, Avon). 2005; 20(8):839–845

[43] Shin AY, Bishop AT. Treatment options for lunotriquetral dissociation. Tech Hand Up Extrem Surg. 1998; 2(1):2–17

[44] Andersson JK, Rööser B, Karlsson J. Level of evidence in wrist ligament repair and reconstruction research: a systematic review. J Exp Orthop. 2018; 5(1):15

IV

21 Chronic Injury Management of the LT Joint: Open Treatment

Thomas Pillukat, Martin Langer, and Jörg van Schoonhoven

Abstract

A chronic lunotriquetral (LT) dissociation is considered when the ends of the ruptured ligament show degenerative changes. In this case they have no potential to heal and a repair would be without success. As the pattern of the injury depends not only on the disruption of the LT ligament but also on the involvement of the extrinsic ligaments, a broad spectrum of injuries appear. As far as no carpal collapse and volar-intercalated segment instability (VISI) exists or it is easily reducible, capsulodesis, LT-ligament reconstruction, and LT arthrodesis are recommendable. In fixed VISI with carpal collapse only salvage procedures are successful.

Keywords: lunotriquetral, tear, chronic instability, carpal collapse, ligament reconstruction

21.1 Introduction

A chronic lunotriquetral (LT) dissociation (Stage II and III according to the classification of Viegas and colleagues[1]) is recognized when the ends of the ruptured ligament show degenerative changes. In this case they have no potential to heal and a repair would be without success. It is assumed that healing is possible up to 6 months after a tear.[2]

In contrast to acute injuries, the symptoms are less specific and misleading. In addition, chronic LT dissociation is not an entity but a broad spectrum of sequential injuries. This was demonstrated by Horii and colleagues.[3] They showed that by sequential sectioning of the stabilizing ligaments, the typical symptoms like volar-intercalated segment instability (VISI), altered LT-motion and catch-up clunks first at all appear, when the dorsal radiocarpal (DRC) and dorsal intercarpal (DIC) ligaments are transsected as well. If these ligaments are preserved, disturbances of the LT kinematics are difficult to detect radiographically and clinically, but they can generate synovitis and kinematic alterations. These patients typically have no radiographic findings. They merely complain about weakness with ulnar-sided wrist pain distal to the triangular fibrocartilage complex (TFCC), clunking sensations, and other unspecific ulnar-sided symptoms. Therefore, in these cases the whole spectrum of causes for ulnar-sided wrist pain has to be considered. Vice versa in all conditions with ulnar-sided wrist pain without other reasons, there should be a reasonable degree of suspicion for a chronic undetected LT instability.

21.2 Clinical Examination

On clinical examination typically pain is located over the dorsal triquetrum. The classical tests (e.g., ballottement test, shear test) for LT instability may be positive. They are sensitive but less specific.[4] To discriminate LT pathologies from other causes of ulnar-sided wrist pain, corticosteroid injections into the LT articulation have been recommended.[5]

21.3 X-Rays

On plain X-rays the carpal and midcarpal alignment of the carpal bones (Gilula arcs) may be interrupted with a step-off between the lunate and triquetrum. On the lateral view the palmar flexion of the lunate is an indicator for LT lesions in cases of not only intrinsic LT ligament but additional extrinsic ligament (DRC and DIC ligament) disruption. This situation is defined as volar-intercalated segment instability (VISI), a carpal instability dissociative (CID). However, in less severe cases the plain X-ray will be normal.

In cases of suspected midcarpal instability, kinematography can be a useful additional diagnostic tool.

Computed tomography (CT) scans are helpful to detect other wrist pathologies like occult fractures or signs of osteoarthritis. CT scans after intra-articular arthrography (arthro-CT) are less specific since there is a high rate of age-related alterations of the LT ligament. This results in a high number of false-positive results. The same applies for magnetic resonance imaging (MRI) and arthro-MRI, which are less sensitive in LT lesions than in scapholunate tears.[6]

21.4 Arthroscopy

The diagnostic gold standard remains wrist arthroscopy. Direct ulnocarpal visualization of the LT ligament is limited and best performed using the 4–5 portal. Wrist arthroscopy helps to identify instability and rule out other intra-articular pathologies. A reducible step-off in the midcarpal view or an avulsion of the dorsal capsule from the triquetrum are easily detected.

21.5 Classification

The classification system of Viegas et al[1] (▶ Table 21.1) guides the treatment of chronic instability by defining two stages.

In Stage II, the chronic tear exists without carpal collapse. The carpal alignment remains relatively normal due to intact parts of the supporting intrinsic and extrinsic ligaments. A VISI position of the proximal row is easily reducible. There are no degenerative changes of adjacent joint surfaces.

Table 21.1 Stages of LT disruption according to Viegas et al[1]

Stage I	Partial or complete disruption of the LT interosseous ligament without clinical/radiological evidence of dynamic or static VISI
Stage II	Complete disruption of the LT interosseous and palmar ligaments with clinical and/or radiographical evidence of reducible VISI deformity
Stage III	Complete disruption of the LT interosseous and palmar ligaments, attenuation or disruption of the DRC with clinical and radiographical evidence of static VISI deformity

Abbreviations: DRC, dorsal radiocarpal; LT, lunotriquetral; VISI, volar-intercalated segment instability.

IV

Table 21.2 Open procedures in LT instability

LT dissociation No carpal collapse No ulnocarpal abutment	LT-ligament reconstruction and/or capsulodesis	Normal surfaces of adjacent joint Normal or near-normal carpal alignment No or easily reducible VISI position
	LT fusion	Osteoarthritic changes of the lunotriquetral junction Unreducible carpal alignment of the proximal row No or easily reducible VISI position
LT dissociation + carpal collapse No ulnocarpal abutment	Radiolunate (RL) fusion	Abnormal carpal alignment Unreducible VISI position Intact midcarpal joint surfaces. Intact radioscaphoidal joint
	Radioscapholunate (RSL) fusion	Abnormal carpal alignment Unreducible VISI position Intact midcarpal joint surfaces. Osteoarthritis of the radioscaphoidal joint
	Midcarpal fusion	Abnormal carpal alignment Unreducible VISI position Osteoarthritis of the midcarpal and radioscaphoidal joint surfaces Intact radiolunate joint surfaces
	Wrist fusion	Abnormal carpal alignment Unreducible VISI position Osteoarthritis of the midcarpal and radiocarpal joint surfaces
	Denervation	Painful wrist Good wrist mobility Patient not prepared for loss of mobility

Abbreviations: LT, lunotriquetral; VISI, volar-intercalated segment instability.

In Stage III, the chronic tear is accompanied by a carpal collapse. Predominantly, the DRC and the ulnar arcuate ligaments are additionally disrupted. This leads to rotational subluxation of the proximal row into a VISI position that becomes fixed over time. In addition, the midcarpal joint is subluxed and degenerative changes occur.

In this situation LT-ligament reconstructions fail, as they are not strong enough to correct this malalignment. LT fusion not only might correct the rotational-subluxation between triquetrum and lunate/scaphoid within the proximal row, but also does not alter or prevent the rotational subluxation of the complete proximal row, since the external stabilizers are left untreated.

21.6 Surgical Treatment

The goal of treatment is to stop further progression, reduce symptoms, restore stability, and avoid development of a carpal collapse. Before a surgical reconstruction is considered, nonoperative treatment for at least 3 months should be performed. If it fails a number of open operative procedures have been recommended (▶ Table 21.2).

Surgical procedures for LT injury can be divided into four groups: capsulodesis, ligament reconstruction, LT arthrodesis, and salvage procedures.

21.6.1 Soft Tissue Procedures

Indications for soft tissue procedures like LT-ligament reconstruction or capsulodesis are chronic-dynamic instability of the LT junction, when the adjacent joint surfaces are unaffected, the carpal alignment is normal or nearly normal, and the palmar flexion of the proximal row (VISI-position) is easily reducible.

Contraindications are a fixed VISI position, osteoarthritis of adjacent joint surfaces, ulnar impaction, rheumatoid arthritis, and crystal arthropathies.

21.6.2 Lunotriquetral Fusion

Indications for LT fusion are the same as for ligament reconstruction with additional presence of osteoarthritis of the LT junction. A step-off at the LT joint or a rotational subluxation between the lunate and scaphoid can be reduced. A VISI position is only reduced if the extrinsic stabilizers of the triquetrum are intact. A fixed VISI position cannot be reduced. The contraindications are similar to ligament reconstruction.

21.6.3 Radiolunate (RL) and Radioscapholunate (RSL) Fusion

The indication for radiolunate (RL) fusion is carpal collapse with an irreducible VISI position in the absence of osteoarthritis. An irreducible VISI position is combined with a subluxation of the midcarpal joint that results in osteoarthritis and decreased wrist extension. Fixing the lunate in a normal position corrects the rotational subluxation of the proximal row and—perhaps more important—of the midcarpal joint. Prerequisites are normal midcarpal and radioscaphoidal joint surfaces.

In a coexisting radioscaphoidal osteoarthritis the scaphoid should be included into the fusion (RSL fusion).

The indication for midcarpal fusion is a carpal collapse with osteoarthritic changes in the midcarpal joint as long as the radiolunate/radioscaphoidal joints are intact. The capitolunate and hamatotriquetral fusion corrects the VISI position and eliminates the arthritic part of the joint. In additional osteoarthritic changes of the radioscaphoidal joint, the scaphoid should be excised.

21.6.4 Total Wrist Fusion

Total wrist fusion is indicated in carpal collapse with osteoarthritic changes of the radiocarpal and the midcarpal joint.

21.6.5 Wrist Denervation

Wrist denervation is a therapeutical option for painful wrists, when other procedures would result in a significant loss of wrist mobility that the patient does not want to accept.

21.7 Literature Review

21.7.1 Soft Tissue Procedures

In contrast to scapholunate instability, there has been no enthusiasm for capsulodesis in chronic LT dissociation.

Only Omokawa and colleagues[7] treated 11 patients with K-wire stabilization of the LT joint, primary repair of the ligament using suture anchors, and DRC ligament capsulodesis. After a mean follow-up of 31 month outcomes were promising with an improvement of grip strength, pain, and Mayo wrist score. Though it was not a treatment of chronic instability, this procedure might be indicated in chronic instabilities without carpal collapse as well.

Antti-Poika and colleagues[8] continued after arthroscopic diagnosis with an open repair. They used an 8 to 10 mm wide and radial-based extensor retinacular split for dorsal capsular reinforcement. After a follow-up of 39 months (range: 14–84), 64% had no or only occasional mild pain and 36% had pain with overuse or lifting. Overall scoring including pain, patient satisfaction, range of motion, and grip strength was excellent in 24% and good in 64%. Only three patients had fair results: one after a further injury leading to distal radioulnar joint (DRUJ) instability and two with concurrent DRUJ stabilization.

In a study comparing repair, arthrodesis, and tendon graft reconstruction of reducible chronic instability due to complete disruption of the LT ligaments, Shin and colleagues[9] demonstrated that ligament reconstruction with a tendon graft was the most reliable technique. The technique consists of reconstructing the LT ligament with a strip of the extensor carpi ulnaris (ECU) tendon, left attached distally and passed through osseous channels in the lunate and triquetrum. Tightly looping the tendon graft around the LT joint immediately achieved stability. The reconstruction was further secured by transfixing the joint with one or two K-wires for 8 weeks, followed by 4 more weeks in a protective splint. A group of eight patients treated with this technique showed encouraging results.

Shahane and colleagues[10] published a different approach using an ECU strip in 46 patients. A distally based strip was passed through two drill holes in the triquetrum and sutured to itself. After an average follow-up of over 3 years, good and excellent results were noted in 29 patients, satisfactory in 11, and poor in 6. Five of the six complications were related to the pisotriquetral joint.

Wehbe and Whitaker[11] described a reconstructive procedure for the LT ligament using four strands of a 2.0 polyester suture guided through bony channels in the lunate and triquetrum. They reported encouraging results in 103 wrists with a follow-up period of up to 15 years.

21

In an own study,[12] the authors treated eight patients with a ligament reconstruction using an ECU-tendon strip. Two patients reported a severe sprain of the wrist; in the other patients no reason for the instability was detectable. The diagnosis was arthroscopically confirmed. Reducible VISI position was found in five patients. The ulnar variance measured −1 to −3 mm in four patients, neutral in three patients, and + 1 mm in one patient. Healing was uneventful. At the final follow-up after 43 ± 21 (19–83) months, all patients had returned to their prior occupation. A minor reduction in grip strength, pain at exercise, and a reduced range of motion persisted.

The procedure reliably restored the stability of the LT junction with no complications.

A bone–ligament–bone ligamentoplasty has been described by Berger.[13] After reposition and K-wire transfixation between triquetrum and lunate a transverse 4-mm broad groove is drilled into the dorsal cortex of the lunate and triquetrum. A bone–ligament–bone autograft is harvested from the dorsal capitohamate ligament. The autograft is press-fit, inserted into the groove, and secured by small screws. Clinical results of this method were not presented. The procedure resembles to the ligamentoplasty that has been described by Cuénod[14] for chronic scapholunate injury. The technique has obviously not been applied by other authors.

21.7.2 Lunotriquetral Fusion

Lunotriquetral arthrodesis is another alternative. The procedure has shown variable success and a high nonunion rate. According to Guidera and colleagues[15] most complications result from technical problems. The authors used cancellous bone grafts to fill a biconcave space created in the adjoining bones and stabilized the joint with multiple K-wires. They report a 100% fusion rate with this technique. In their series of 26 operations, postoperative flexion-extension averaged 78% of the contralateral side, with good or excellent pain relief in 83% of the cases and with 88% returning to their occupation. These excellent results with a 100% fusion rate have not been confirmed in the literature.[16] A meta-analysis of 143 LT fusions summarized that LT fusion is technically demanding and associated with a nonunion rate of 26% and an overall complication rate of 43% mostly in the form of persistent pain.[16]

Nelson and colleagues[17] noted in 22 patients, union rates were higher in those who were treated with a combination of compression screw and K-wire fixation (91%) than with K-wire alone (60%) and advocated immobilization for more than 6 weeks. The procedure should not be performed in the presence of a VISI deformity, as fusion would only convert a dissociative VISI into a nondissociative VISI.

Besides these classical studies the results of LT arthrodesis are discouraging. Larsen and colleagues[18] reported on low fusion rates in 1997. Van de Grift and Ritt[19] recently analyzed another 10 studies on LT arthrodesis and found an average nonunion rate of up to 57%. Therefore, they recommended this procedure only for selected cases.

The only study comparing ligament reconstruction with LT fusion[9] as noted above has been performed by Shin and colleagues. They retrospectively reviewed 57 patients with an average follow-up of 9.5 years. Patients who underwent tendon reconstruction had a more favorable subjective and objective outcome and a lower complication rate than patients with LT fusion.

21.7.3 Salvage Procedures

As carpal collapse due to LT instability is a rare condition, there seem to be no reports on this subject in contrast to an enormous literature on scapholunate advanced collapse. Halikis and colleagues[20] recommended RL fusion for static dissociative VISI.

21.8 Authors' Preferred Technique

21.8.1 Ligament Reconstruction

For their therapeutic strategy, the authors adapted the classification of Osterman and Seidman[21] as modified by Garcia-Elias[4] (▶ Table 21.3).

Table 21.3 Types of lunotriquetral injury and treatment options modified from Garcia-Elias[4]

Type 1	Acute injury without carpal collapse	Arthroscopically assisted lunotriquetral transfixation
Type 2	Chronic injury without carpal collapse	Ligament reconstruction capsulodesis Lunotriquetral arthrodesis
Type 3	Chronic injury with carpal collapse	Reducible: Ligament reconstruction lunotriquetral arthrodesis Unreducible: Partial/total wrist fusion
Type 4	Acute perilunate injury	Repair of ligaments and fractured bones
Type 5	Chronic perilunate injury	Partial/Total wrist fusion

For a chronic dynamic instability and a chronic static instability, the authors prefer ligament reconstruction instead of LT fusion, if the proximal row can be easily reduced. The authors are less enthusiastic about LT fusion due to the relatively high rate of nonunion. It is reserved for the rare cases, where the LT junction shows osteoarthritic changes.

The procedure was recommended and reported by Shin[9] and has been described by the authors as follows.[12]

The fourth extensor compartment is opened via a dorsal approach and the tendons are retracted radially. The capsule is raised by means of a radially based flap and the lunate and triquetrum are exposed. In the presence of a VISI position the reducibility of the proximal row is tested and the LT joint is assessed for osteoarthritic changes.

The ECU tendon is identified distally to the sixth extensor compartment and dissected up to its attachment at the base of the fifth metacarpal. The tendon is then identified proximal to the sixth compartment.

A distally based, about 5-mm-broad and 10-cm-long strip of the tendon is radially raised by blunt dissection of the tendon parallel to the fibers. Its proximal end is armed with a suture that is guided through the sixth compartment and the tendon strip can be pulled through the compartment without being opened (▶ Fig. 21.1).

Into the triquetrum and the lunate two K-wires are inserted. The tips of the K-wires should meet in the LT junction, following the reduction of the carpal bones (▶ Fig. 21.2).

These K-wires are used as drilling guides for a cannulated 3.2-mm drill.

Before the channels are created, two 1.4-mm K-wires are inserted parallel into the triquetrum for later LT transfixation (▶ Fig. 21.3).

The ECU-tendon slip is then guided through the bony channels in the triquetrum and lunate, the proximal row is reduced and the LT junction transfixed using the 1.4-mm K-wires (▶ Fig. 21.4).

Fluoroscopy is performed to confirm the position of the K-wires and the correct position of the proximal row. Finally, the ECU-tendon slip is pulled dorsally over the lunate and triquetrum and sutured to itself (▶ Fig. 21.5).

By this means the DIC ligament is reconstructed. The transfixing wires are shortened and the wound is closed.

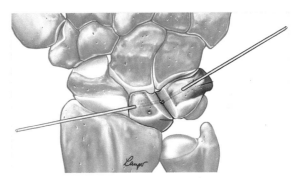

Fig. 21.2 K-wire insertion as drilling guides. The tips should meet in the lunotriquetral space. (Reproduced with permission from Pillukat T, Fuhrmann RA, Windolf J, van Schoonhoven J. [Ligament reconstruction for lunotriquetral instability using a distally based strip of the extensor carpi ulnaris tendon]. Oper Orthop Traumatol. 2015;27(5):404–413.)

21

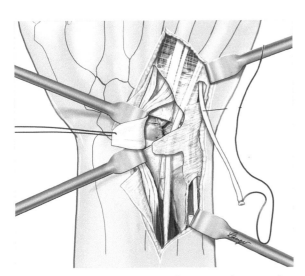

Fig. 21.1 Harvested extensor carpi-ulnaris strip. The proximal end is armed with a suture. (Reproduced with permission from Pillukat T, Fuhrmann RA, Windolf J, van Schoonhoven J. [Ligament reconstruction for lunotriquetral instability using a distally based strip of the extensor carpi ulnaris tendon]. Oper Orthop Traumatol. 2015;27(5):404–413.)

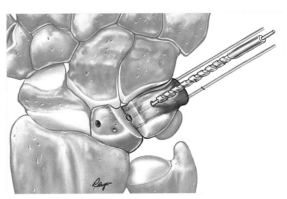

Fig. 21.3 Creating the channels using a cannulated drill. Note the two K-wires introduced into the triquetrum but not the lunate at this stage. (Reproduced with permission from Pillukat T, Fuhrmann RA, Windolf J, van Schoonhoven J. [Ligament reconstruction for lunotriquetral instability using a distally based strip of the extensor carpi ulnaris tendon]. Oper Orthop Traumatol. 2015;27(5):404–413.)

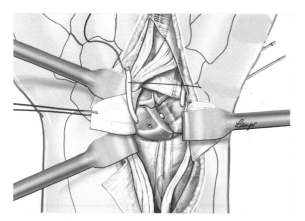

Fig. 21.4 The ECU strip has been introduced into the bony channels. (Reproduced with permission from Pillukat T, Fuhrmann RA, Windolf J, van Schoonhoven J. [Ligament reconstruction for lunotriquetral instability using a distally based strip of the extensor carpi ulnaris tendon]. Oper Orthop Traumatol. 2015;27(5):404–413.)

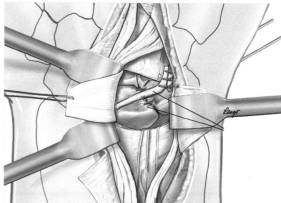

Fig. 21.5 The ECU strip is looped around the dorsal bones and sutured to itself to reconstruct the dorsal intercarpal ligament. (Reproduced with permission from Pillukat T, Fuhrmann RA, Windolf J, van Schoonhoven J. [Ligament reconstruction for lunotriquetral instability using a distally based strip of the extensor carpi ulnaris tendon]. Oper Orthop Traumatol. 2015;27(5):404–413.)

21.8.2 Postoperative Treatment

The wrist is immobilized for 8 weeks in a forearm cast including the metacarpophalangeal joint of the thumb. After 8 weeks, the transfixing K-wires are removed and the patient is encouraged to perform activities of daily life. ▸ Fig. 21.6, ▸ Fig. 21.7, ▸ Fig. 21.8, ▸ Fig. 21.9, ▸ Fig. 21.10, ▸ Fig. 21.11 demonstrate a typical case without loss of correction after 44 months.

21.8.3 Tips and Tricks

The ligament reconstruction can be enforced with a capsulodesis using a strip of the DIC ligament.

The sixth dorsal compartment should be closed, if it has been opened to avoid painful dislocation of the tendon.

Fractures of the lunate or triquetrum can occur during drilling or at the insertion of the tendon strip. Small partial fractures can be neglected. Simple complete fractures are reduced and fixed using the transfixing K-wires.

Extended fragmentations have less chance to heal, and salvage procedures should be considered. This possible complication has to be discussed with the patient prior to the procedure.

21.8.4 Lunotriquetral Fusion

Lunotriquetral fusion is performed using a similar dorsal approach. After removing the LT joint surfaces and exposing cancellous bone a preferable cortical iliac crest bone graft is interposed. Following a preliminary reduction and K-wire transfixation of the triquetrum and lunate and fluoroscopy, a headless compression screw is inserted. The authors agree with Guidera and colleagues[15] that exact restoration of the distance between the lunate

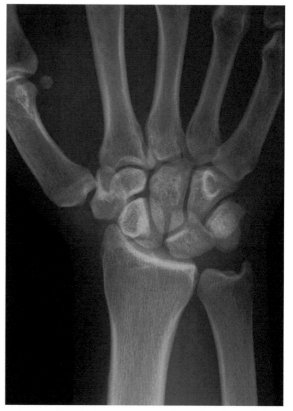

Fig. 21.6 Chronic lunotriquetral (LT) instability Type 2 (p.a. view).

and triquetrum is essential for bony healing. A compression screw, as recommended by Nelson and colleagues,[17] does not only offer compression of the fusion site (that

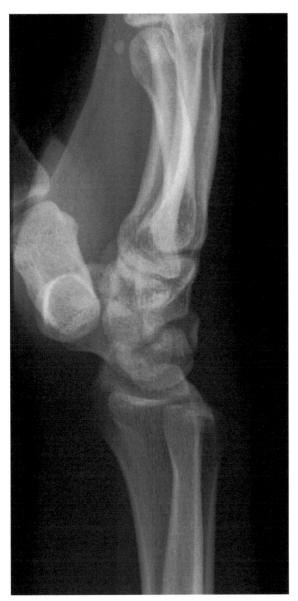

Fig. 21.7 Chronic lunotriquetral (LT) instability Type 2 (lateral view).

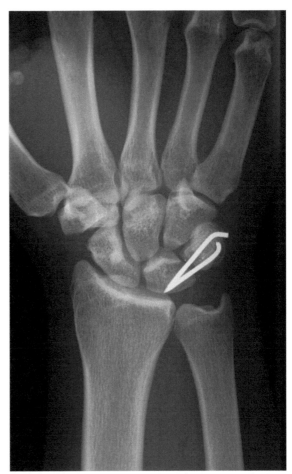

Fig. 21.8 Postop. after ligament reconstruction (p.a. view).

21

and in cases of ulnar neutral or minus variance. In contrast to four-corner fusion it preserves the valuable dart throw motion. In authors' experience, interposition of cancellous bone graft from the radius or an iliac crest bone graft is necessary to preserve the distance of the proximal row and the radius as well as to avoid ulnar impaction. The authors use two 1.6 K-wires for transfixation.

will decrease soon) but more rigidity than a second K-wire. It should be kept in mind that a VISI position is not addressed by the procedure.

Postoperatively the wrist is immobilized for 8 weeks in a forearm cast including the metacarpophalangeal joint of the thumb. After 8 weeks healing is confirmed by plain radiographs and the patient is encouraged to perform activities of daily life.

21.8.5 RL/RSL Fusion

For fixed VISI positions the authors prefer RL fusion, if the adjacent joint surfaces are without osteoarthritic changes

Essential rehabilitation points for RL/RSL fusion:
Postoperatively the wrist is immobilized in a forearm cast including the metacarpophalangeal joint of the thumb for 6 weeks. When healing is confirmed after 6 weeks the cast is omitted and exercise started. The implants are not removed routinely.

21.8.6 Midcarpal and Total Wrist Fusion

Other salvage procedures like four-corner fusion or arthrodesis are indicated according to the extent of osteoarthritis

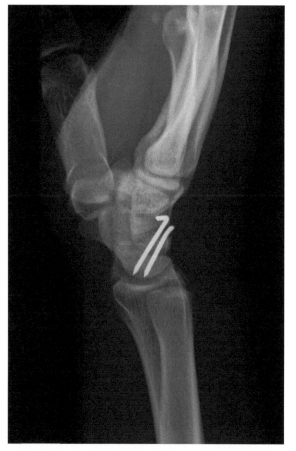

Fig. 21.9 Postop. after ligament reconstruction (lateral view).

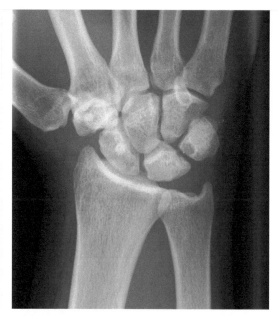

Fig. 21.10 Follow-up after 44 months (p.a. view).

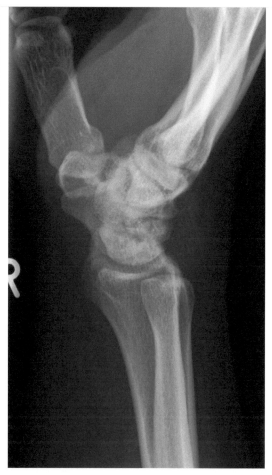

Fig. 21.11 Follow-up after 44 months (lateral view).

and are performed in the standard way. In midcarpal fusion the authors prefer an augmentation of the fusion site using a cancellous bone graft from the radius that can be easily harvested using the dorsal approach to the wrist. For stabilization of the reduced carpal bones the authors use 1.6 K-wires, which are routinely removed after 12 weeks following radiographic confirmation of bony healing of the fusion. For a midcarpal fusion in LT instability the authors apply four K-wires to promote fusion of the hamatotriquetral junction (▸ Fig. 21.12, ▸ Fig. 21.13, ▸ Fig. 21.14, ▸ Fig. 21.15).

Essential rehabilitations points for four-corner fusion:
Postoperatively the wrist is immobilized in a forearm cast including the metacarpophalangeal joint of the thumb for 6 weeks. When healing is confirmed after 6 weeks the cast is omitted and limited exercise started. Unlimited exercise is possible after implant removal after 12 weeks.

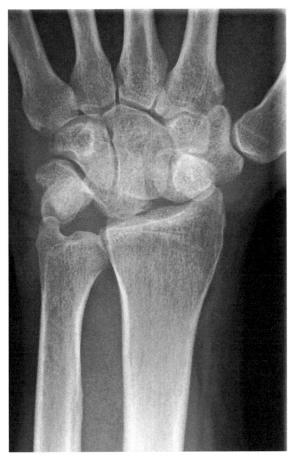

Fig. 21.12 Chronic lunotriquetral (LT) instability with carpal collapse (p.a. view).

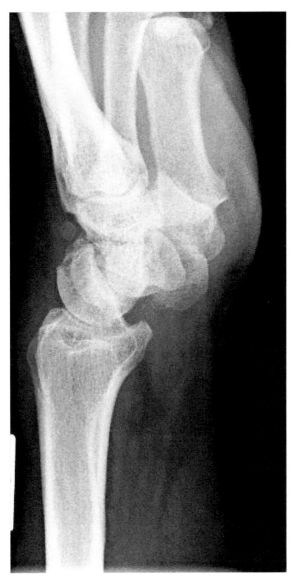

Fig. 21.13 Chronic lunotriquetral (LT) instability with carpal collapse (lateral view).

21.8.7 Wrist Denervation

In authors' experience denervation of the wrist is not a long-lasting solution but can give a valuable pain relief for a period of time until partial or complete fusion becomes necessary. Besides complete wrist denervation sectioning[22] of only the anterior and posterior nerve has been recommended.

21.9 Conclusion

Chronic LT instability consists of a broad spectrum of pathologies. Though not all procedures are completely satisfying, for all types of chronic instability an appropriate open procedure is available.

IV

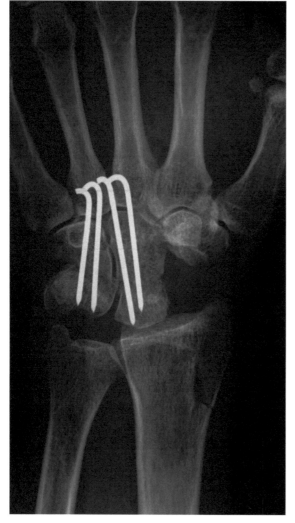

Fig. 21.14 Midcarpal fusion for carpal collapse (p.a. view).

References

[1] Viegas SF, Patterson RM, Peterson PD, et al. Ulnar-sided perilunate instability: an anatomic and biomechanic study. J Hand Surg Am. 1990; 15(2):268–278

[2] Ambrose L, Posner MA. Lunate-triquetral and midcarpal joint instability. Hand Clin. 1992; 8(4):653–668

[3] Horii E, Garcia-Elias M, An KN, et al. A kinematic study of luno-triquetral dissociations. J Hand Surg Am. 1991; 16(2):355–362

[4] Garcia-Elias M. Carpal instability. In: Green D, Hotchkiss R, Pederson W, Wolfe S, eds. Green's operative hand surgery. Philadelphia, PA: Churchill Livingston; 2011:465–522

[5] Wagner ER, Elhassan BT, Rizzo M. Diagnosis and treatment of chronic lunotriquetral ligament injuries. Hand Clin. 2015; 31(3):477–486

[6] Schmitt R, Christopoulos G, Meier R, et al. [Direct MR arthrography of the wrist in comparison with arthroscopy: a prospective study on 125 patients]. Röfo Fortschr Geb Röntgenstr Neuen Bildgeb Verfahr. 2003; 175(7):911–919

[7] Omokawa S, Fujitani R, Inada Y. Dorsal radiocarpal ligament capsulodesis for chronic dynamic lunotriquetral instability. J Hand Surg Am. 2009; 34(2):237–243

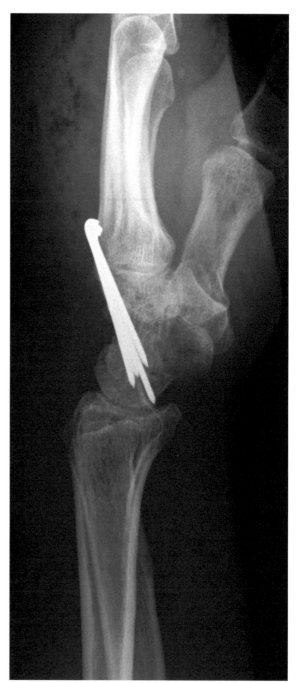

Fig. 21.15 Midcarpal fusion for carpal collapse (lateral view).

[8] Antti-Poika I, Hyrkäs J, Virkki LM, Ogino D, Konttinen YT. Correction of chronic lunotriquetral instability using extensor retinacular split: a retrospective study of 26 patients. Acta Orthop Belg. 2007; 73(4): 451–457

[9] Shin AY, Weinstein LP, Berger RA, Bishop AT. Treatment of isolated injuries of the lunotriquetral ligament. A comparison of arthrodesis, ligament reconstruction and ligament repair. J Bone Joint Surg Br. 2001; 83(7):1023–1028

[10] Shahane SA, Trail IA, Takwale VJ, Stilwell JH, Stanley JK. Tenodesis of the extensor carpi ulnaris for chronic, post-traumatic lunotriquetral instability. J Bone Joint Surg Br. 2005; 87(11):1512–1515

[11] Wehbé MA, Whitaker ML. A carpal ligament substitute part II: polyester suture for scapho-lunate and triqueto-lunate ligament reconstruction. Hand Clin. 2013; 29(1):149–154

[12] Pillukat T, Fuhrmann RA, Windolf J, van Schoonhoven J. [Ligament reconstruction for lunotriquetral instability using a distally based strip of the extensor carpi ulnaris tendon]. Oper Orthop Traumatol. 2015; 27(5):404–413

[13] Berger RA. Lunotriquetral joint. In: Berger RA, Weiss AP, eds. Hand surgery. Philadelphia, PA: Lippincott Williams & Wilkins; 2004:495–509

[14] Cuénod P. Osteoligamentoplasty and limited dorsal capsulodesis for chronic scapholunate dissociation. Ann Chir Main Memb Super. 1999; 18(1):38–53

[15] Guidera PM, Watson HK, Dwyer TA, Orlando G, Zeppieri J, Yasuda M. Lunotriquetral arthrodesis using cancellous bone graft. J Hand Surg Am. 2001; 26(3):422–427

[16] Wolfe S, Kakar P. Carpal instability. In: Wolfe S, Kozin S, Pederson W, Cohen M, eds. Greens operative hand surgery. Philadelphia, PA: Elsevier; 2022:531–537

[17] Nelson DL, Manske PR, Pruitt DL, Gilula LA, Martin RA. Lunotriquetral arthrodesis. J Hand Surg Am. 1993; 18(6):1113–1120

[18] Larsen CF, Jacoby RA, McCabe SJ. Nonunion rates of limited carpal arthrodesis: a meta-analysis of the literature. J Hand Surg Am. 1997; 22(1):66–73

[19] van de Grift TC, Ritt MJ. Management of lunotriquetral instability: a review of the literature. J Hand Surg Eur Vol. 2016; 41(1):72–85

[20] Halikis MN, Colello-Abraham K, Taleisnik J. Radiolunate fusion. The forgotten partial arthrodesis. Clin Orthop Relat Res. 1997(341):30–35

[21] Osterman AL, Seidman GD. The role of arthroscopy in the treatment of lunatotriquetral ligament injuries. Hand Clin. 1995; 11(1):41–50

[22] Berger RA, Bishop AT. A fiber-splitting capsulotomy technique for dorsal exposure of the wrist. Tech Hand Up Extrem Surg. 1997; 1(1):2–10

21

22 Acute and Chronic Management of LT Ligament Injury: Arthroscopic Treatment

Jan Ragnar Haugstvedt and István Zoltán Rigó

Abstract

An isolated lunotriquetral (LT) ligament lesion is relatively uncommon as the injury is usually part of a more extended carpal injury. Most of these injuries have been treated by open procedures with exposure through the skin, cutting carpal ligaments and opening the capsule with the risk of damaging vessels and nerves. For years we have used an arthroscopic-assisted technique, whenever possible, for treatment of these acute and chronic injuries. In this chapter we will share our experience and give tips and tricks for arthroscopic management of LT injuries and instabilities, techniques that provide lesser damage to other structures, less wounds, and could possibly give a faster and better rehabilitation.

Keywords: LT ligament injuries, arthroscopy, treatment, ligament repair, ligament reconstruction, arthrodesis

22.1 Introduction

In his classification, Viegas[1] divided the lunotriquetral (LT) ligament injuries into three stages: Stage I describing rupture of the interosseous ligament only without any signs of VISI (volar-intercalated segment instability), Stage II including rupture of the palmar ligament as well, with or without signs of VISI, while Stage III showing a complete disruption of the ligament including attenuation or disruption of the dorsal radiocarpal (DRC) ligament with evidence of VISI. Most of the LT ligament injuries are found to be dynamic; they are not visible on radiological examinations. When an LT ligament lesion is suspected, we find an arthroscopic evaluation of the wrist mandatory to access the carpal bones and ligaments. There are several options for treatment depending on the extent of and the time from the injury itself. Most of these treatment options could be managed by an arthroscopically assisted procedure.

22.2 Acute Injury

In an acute injury the patient will suffer from pain. Clinical examination, as described earlier in this book (Chapter 6) and in previous publications,[2] could reveal the diagnosis. If a patient suffers from a wrist injury, i.e., the patient tells about an injury with axial loading of the wrist in a radial-deviated and radial-pronated position[3] and suffers from ulnar-sided pain often with a "clunk" upon examination, an LT ligament injury should be considered. Clinical and radiological examinations should always be performed; however, these examinations could often raise suspicion of the injury only, while wrist arthroscopy will confirm the diagnosis. As stated by Cooney many decades ago,[4] wrist arthroscopy should be considered the gold standard for examining and diagnosing injuries of the wrist ligaments.

22.3 Acute Management

The goal of the treatment is to reduce pain, increase strength, and to reestablish normal alignment and stability. The literature has recommended a well-molded cast for 6 to 12 weeks. The cast should give support underneath the pisiform and over the dorsum of the distal radius. Forearm rotation should be prevented for at least the first 4 weeks.[5,7] It has been reported[5] that in more than 80% of patients who are treated in a cast the ligaments are healed; however, some symptoms may remain for as long as several months.

The authors always schedule a patient with this history and findings for wrist arthroscopy. They have the arm in a vertical tower that allows them easy access for using a drill or a fluoroscope. They establish portals for the radiocarpal and the midcarpal joints knowing that an LT ligament injury may often be part of a more extended injury that will need to be diagnosed and addressed. (See Chapters 24 and 25.) The authors often find a combination of injuries such as a scapholunate (SL) and an LT lesion (Video 22.1). If the LT lesion is the only injured ligament, the K-wires are predrilled into the triquetrum under fluoroscopic control.

With the arthroscope in the radial portal in the midcarpal joint, the LT interval is reduced and a transfixation of the joint is performed by entering the predrilled K-wires into the lunate (Video 22.2; ▶ Fig. 22.1a, b).

If the injury is acute and there is no bony avulsion of any ligament attachments, the authors do not perform any suture of the ligaments. If there is avulsion of a bony fragment, the authors consider using a bone anchor, a K-wire, or a small screw to fix this.

For an isolated LT ligament lesion, a cast is put to immobilize the wrist and include the condyles of humerus to prevent rotation of the forearm. The cast is changed after 2 weeks and a new similar cast is put on for another 6 weeks. Eight weeks after surgery the cast and the K-wires are removed, and the patient consults a hand therapist for rehabilitation.

(For more complex injuries with involvement of more ligaments and bones, see Chapters 24 and 25.)

22.4 Subacute Management

The authors have sometimes used plication of the ulnocarpal (UC) ligaments to shorten the length of the ligaments to try to prevent LT motion.[8] For this technique, the authors use the 3–4 portal for the arthroscope and establish a 6-U

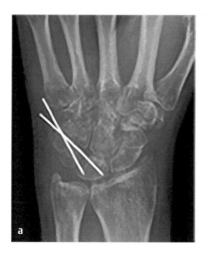
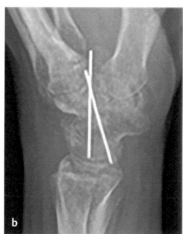

Fig. 22.1 Two K-wires and a cast will immobilize the wrist and prevent forearm rotation for 8 weeks followed by removal of the cast and the K-wires before the start of rehabilitation: **(a)** front view, **(b)** lateral view.

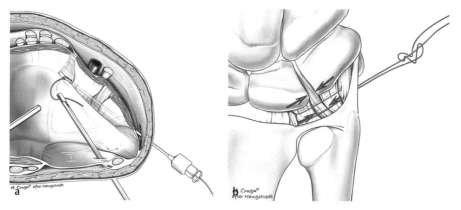

Fig. 22.2 (a) A needle with a suture inside is inserted through the 6-U portal volar of the capsule but dorsal to the artery, the nerves, and the tendons. It is passed in a radial direction and is viewed from the 3–4 portal as it passes the ulnocarpal (UC) ligaments. The tip of the needle is entered into the joint and the suture is forwarded to come into the joint where it is grasped by a mosquito. The suture is then passed back to the 6-U portal. **(b)** A suture is made, but before tightening it another suture is prepared in a similar manner. With two sutures in place, the sutures are tightened and viewed from the 3–4 that the interval between the UC ligaments is tightened in order to stabilize the LT joint.

portal. The skin is opened to make sure not to damage any nerve before inserting a needle with a suture inside through the 6-U portal. The needle with the suture is passed in a radial direction just palmar of the capsule but dorsal to other structures on the palmar side. It is then entered into the radiocarpal joint immediately radial to the UC ligaments, where a grasper is used to bring the suture back to the 6-U portal. When tightening the suture, it will make a loop around the UC ligaments and stabilization is achieved (▶ Fig. 22.2a, b).

22.5 Chronic Management

22.5.1 Ligament Reconstruction

To authors' knowledge, there are no prospective randomized studies comparing different treatment options for repair or reconstruction of the LT ligament. In 2001, a paper was published out of the Mayo Clinic comparing arthrodesis, ligament reconstruction, and ligament repair for isolated injuries of the LT ligament.[9] Five years following surgery, they found less complications, reoperations, in the group with ligament reconstruction as compared to the other groups. This led the authors to use the technique described by Shin et al using a slip of the extensor carpi ulnaris (ECU) tendon as their preferred method for the LT ligament reconstruction. The authors performed this technique as an open procedure for many years. To minimize the need for opening the joint spaces and the joint capsule, and to reduce exposing and cutting other ligaments to perform the open procedure, the authors developed a technique for arthroscopically assisted reconstruction of the LT ligament and the DRC ligament.[10,11]

22

Technique for Arthroscopic-Assisted Ligament Reconstruction

The patient is in general anesthesia, the arm in a tourniquet, and a vertical tower is used for traction. The authors use a dry technique. They verify the diagnosis by performing arthroscopy of the radiocarpal and midcarpal joints (Video 22.3). If it is decided to go on with the procedure, the arm is put down on the table and half of the ECU tendon is harvested, leaving the distal insertion attached (▶ Fig. 22.3).

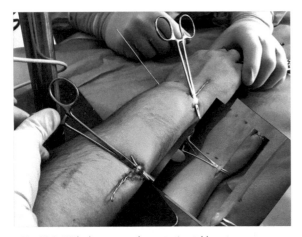

Fig. 22.3 With the arm on the operating table, a transverse incision is made on the dorsal side of the triquetrum and the extensor carpi ulnaris (ECU) tendon is identified. The tendon is freed distally to its insertion. A home-made device, a cerclage that has been twisted many times, is entered into the ECU tendon sheath and into the proximal part of the forearm where it can be palpated. Another incision is made at this level, the ECU tendon is identified, a graft is prepared with the width required, the part of the tendon that has to be used is cut and put into the device, and the graft is pulled down to the open wound over the triquetrum. The width of the graft is measured and it should be 2.8 to 3.0 mm. (Reproduced from Mathoulin C, ed. Wrist Arthroscopy Techniques. 2nd ed. Stuttgart: Thieme; 2019:94.)

They then bring the arm back up in the traction tower. They establish the 1–2 portal, and with the arthroscope in the 1–2 (or the 6-R) portal, insert a guidewire for a drill through the 3–4 portal. They can check the entrance point for the K-wire into the lunate (Video 22.4). As for the direction of the K-wire, the authors aim for the pisiform that can be palpated on the palmar, ulnar side of the wrist. They drill one K-wire through the lunate and then check the position using a fluoroscope in a horizontal position. If the position is not what they want, they use a drill guide (Parallel Drill Guide, 3.5 Compression FT Screw System; Arthrex Co., Naples, FL) to make another, parallel drill hole (▶ Fig. 22.4a, b). When the position is good, they drill a 2.8-mm hole (2.5–3.0) through the lunate using a cannulated drill bit.

They then enter a drill guide (Wrist Drill Guide; Arthrex Co., Naples, FL) with one end through the hole in the lunate and the other end placed on the dorsal side of the triquetrum (▶ Fig. 22.5a, b).

The authors once again check the position using the fluoroscope and then drill a K-wire through the triquetrum. The aim for these two holes is that the exit points on the palmar side of the carpus should almost touch each other. If the K-wire is in the right position, they drill another 2.8-mm hole using the same cannulated drill bit.

After having drilled the holes, the challenge is to pass the tendon graft from the dorsal side of the triquetrum, passing through the holes in the triquetrum and the lunate to exit on the dorsal, radial side of the lunate. They enter the free side of the tendon graft into a tendon shuttle (Quick Pass Tendon Shuttle, Arthrex Co., Naples, FL). They will not be able to push the tendon shuttle into the holes and make the turn on the palmar side. Thus, to facilitate the transfer, they enter from the lunate either a suture or a wire loop (Micro suture Lasso, Arthrex Co., Naples, FL) (▶ Fig. 22.6).

The suture can be fixed to the tendon shuttle by making a knot, or the tendon shuttle can be inserted into the

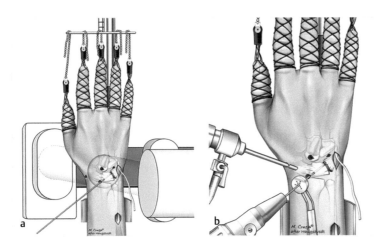

Fig. 22.4 (a) When viewing the entrance point for the K-wire into the lunate, a K-wire is drilled aiming for the pisiform. The position of the K-wire is checked using the fluoroscope. (b) If the direction or position of the K-wire has to be changed, a guide should be used to make a parallel hole to the first K-wire to have the exit point on the palmar side where it should be. When the position is good, a hole, 2.8 to 3.0 mm, is drilled using a cannulated bur. The size of the hole depends on the size of the wrist. (Reproduced from Mathoulin C, ed. Wrist Arthroscopy Techniques. 2nd ed. Stuttgart: Thieme; 2019:95.)

IV

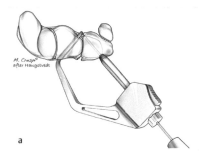
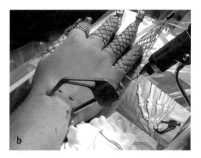

Fig. 22.5 **(a)** Using another guide, one arm of the guide is entered through the 3–4 portal and put into the drill hole in the lunate. Ensure that the tip of the guide arm is all the way through the lunate and goes just outside the lunate. **(b)** The other arm of the guide is placed on the dorsal side of the triquetrum close to the point where the graft from the extensor carpi ulnaris (ECU) tendon is attached. The position of this guide is important, and the fluoroscope should once again verify the position. If the two drill holes don't match, there will be difficulties in passing the graft through the bones. When this guide is in place, the second hole is drilled through the triquetrum. (Reproduced from Mathoulin C, ed. Wrist Arthroscopy Techniques. 2nd ed. Stuttgart: Thieme; 2019:96.)

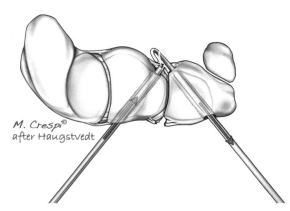

Fig. 22.6 Passing a suture or a wire loop through the lunate and the triquetrum will facilitate the transfer of the graft. The suture or the wire loop should be inserted into the lunate, then a hook or a micrograsper should be used through the second drill hole in the triquetrum to retrieve the suture or the wire loop. The suture or the wire loop should then be used to pull the tendon shuttle through the two bones from the dorsal side of the triquetrum to the dorsal side of the lunate. (Reproduced from Mathoulin C, ed. Wrist Arthroscopy Techniques. 2nd ed. Stuttgart: Thieme; 2019:96.)

suture lasso. The tendon shuttle can then be pulled through the carpal bones (▶ Fig. 22.7a, b; Video 22.5).

The authors have so far in their clinical practice never used an incision on the palmar side of the wrist to pass the tendon shuttle and the graft through the bones; however, if any problems occur by pulling the graft through the bones, a palmar incision could be performed.

At this time, the graft is passed through the triquetrum and the lunate to reconstruct the volar part of the LT ligament. The reconstruction can be checked by pulling the graft while viewing the LT interval from the midcarpal joint (Video 22.6). To fix the graft to the bones an interference screw is used (PEEK, Vented, 3 × 8 mm; Arthrex Co., Naples, FL, USA). While pulling the graft, a screw is first inserted into the triquetrum from the entrance point of the graft on the dorsal side of the triquetrum (▶ Fig. 22.8a, b). Then the second screw is inserted into the lunate through the 3–4 portal into the drill hole in the lunate.

To reconstruct the dorsal LT ligament, the graft is brought back to the triquetrum. From the dorsal side of the triquetrum, pass a mosquito, grasper, or a wire loop to the exit point of the graft through the lunate. The graft is then passed dorsal of the capsule, but volar of the extensor tendons, back to where the graft entered triquetrum to make the ligament reconstruction extracapsular (▶ Fig. 22.9).

To avoid too many holes in the carpal bones, another screw is not used; however, the graft is passed around the intact part of the ECU tendon and sutured back to itself. Nonresorbable sutures are used to finalize this reconstruction of the palmar and dorsal part of the LT ligament (▶ Fig. 22.10).

As mentioned in the introduction to this chapter, Viegas stated in his classification of LT ligament injuries that for Grade III, an injury of the DRC ligament is found. Thus, the authors always reconstruct this ligament as well. They plan for this and make the graft long enough for this last reconstruction. Using the fluoroscope, they identify the dorsal, ulnar corner of radius, make a small incision, and make a drill hole for a bone anchor. They pass the tendon graft from triquetrum to this latter drill hole; the graft is palmar of the extensor tendons. The tendon graft is then fixed to a bone anchor while the wrist is kept in a neutral position (▶ Fig. 22.11).

They close all wounds, put on a sterile dressing, and then put the arm in a cast that goes above the elbow (Video 22.7).

Postoperative Care

The patient will come back for a follow-up after 2 weeks. The stitches are removed and the patient is given a new cast that includes the wrist and the epicondyles

22

IV

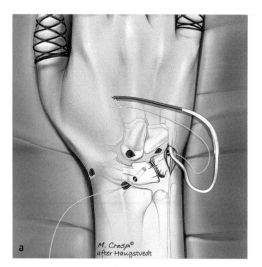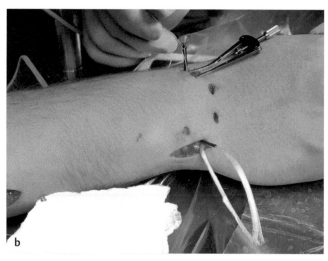

Fig. 22.7 (a) A suture is passed through the lunate and the triquetrum to help pull the tendon shuttle through the bones. **(b)** The tip of the tendon shuttle is coming out from the lunate and by pulling the tendon shuttle the graft will follow. (Reproduced from Mathoulin C, ed. Wrist Arthroscopy Techniques. 2nd ed. Stuttgart: Thieme; 2019:97.)

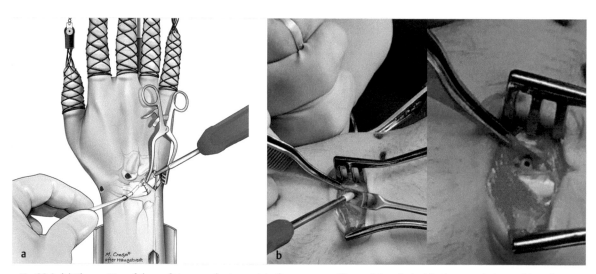

Fig. 22.8 (a) The position of the graft is secured using an interference screw. The graft is pulled while the screw is inserted into the triquetrum. **(b)** Close-up views of the interference screw in place. (Reproduced from Mathoulin C, ed. Wrist Arthroscopy Techniques. 2nd ed. Stuttgart: Thieme; 2019:98.)

(to prevent forearm rotation, however enabling elbow flexion-extension). The authors recommend immobilization for a total of 8 weeks before the cast is removed, and rehabilitation started.

Results

The authors have been able to use this reconstruction in several cases; however, they do not see many patients with the need of this reconstruction, and there are not many cases presented in the literature. They have only two patients with a follow-up for more than 5 years.

A young manual worker, born in 1993, had a preoperative Quick-DASH score of 31 and 100 (general and work-related scores, respectively), while 5 years postoperatively the scores are 15.9 and 0 (he changed his job and is no longer a heavy manual worker). The other patient, born in 1961, is an office worker with similar Quick-DASH scores of 61 and 75 (general and work-related scores, respectively), while 5 years postoperatively his scores are 25 and 19. (The latter patient had a stroke some years after the LT ligament reconstruction and this has probably affected his outcome.)

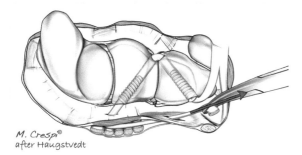

M. Crespi®
after Haugstvedt

Fig. 22.9 The tendon graft used for the reconstruction of the lunotriquetral (LT) ligament is secured in the carpal bones using a polyether ether ketone (PEEK) screw. The reconstruction is extracapsular, and the graft is passed between the extensor tendons and the capsule from the lunate to the triquetrum to reconstruct the dorsal part of the ligament. The graft is sutured back to the remaining part of the extensor carpi ulnaris (ECU) tendon on the dorsal side of the triquetrum. (Reproduced from Mathoulin C, ed. Wrist Arthroscopy Techniques. 2nd ed. Stuttgart: Thieme; 2019:99.)

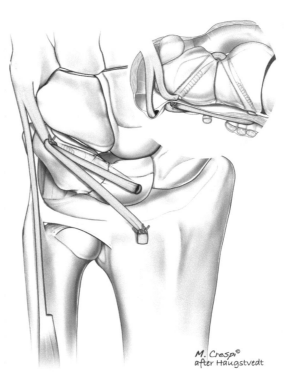

M. Crespi®
after Haugstvedt

22

Fig. 22.11 The reconstruction of the entire lunotriquetral (LT) ligament and the dorsal radiocarpal (DRC) ligament. It shows the tunnels through the triquetrum and the lunate, how the graft is passed on the palmar and the dorsal side of the carpal bones, all extracapsular. It should be noted that the DRC ligament is an important part of the reconstruction.

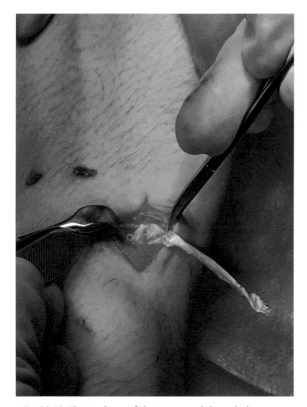

Fig. 22.10 The tendon graft having passed through the triquetrum and the lunate is brought back to the dorsal side of the triquetrum. The inserted polyether ether ketone (PEEK) screw is visible. The graft is passed around the extensor carpi ulnaris (ECU) tendon itself and secured with nonresorbable sutures.

The other patients do not have a long follow-up; however, the authors have not had any complications and have not needed to reoperate any patients.

22.5.2 Arthrodesis

As previously mentioned, Shin et al found more complications with arthrodesis for LT instability compared to ligament reconstruction. The authors have not performed LT arthrodesis as a standard procedure, but only in selected cases. Minnaar[12] published a classification of coalition of the LT joint and described four types: from type I as an incomplete fusion, like a pseudarthrosis, to type IV with a complete osseous fusion. The authors have seen patients with an incomplete fusion who had no pain until they sustained an injury of the wrist. Radiological examination revealed the coalition; most patients did not know about this before the injury. However, when experiencing pain after the injury, an instability is created and the patients suffer from this.[13] For these cases the authors performed an arthrodesis (▶ Fig. 22.12a, b).[14]

IV

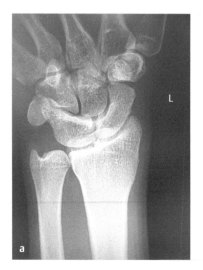
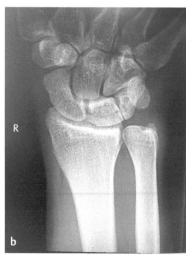

Fig. 22.12 These X-rays show to the left **(a)** a coalition of the lunotriquetral (LT) interval that shows a complete osseous fusion, while on the picture to the right **(b)** an incomplete coalition is shown. The patient complained suffering from pain following an injury of this wrist; an unstable situation had developed following the trauma, which was verified during arthroscopy.

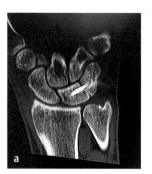
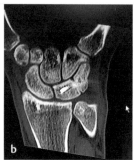
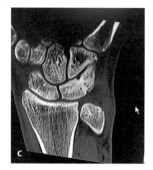
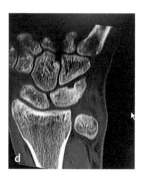

Fig. 22.13 In this patient one headless compression screw and one K-wire are used. The aim was to fuse the dorsal part of the lunotriquetral (LT) joint. The computed tomography (CT) scans 6 weeks postsurgery do not show a complete fusion of the joint; however, there are bone bridges crossing the gap and the fusion is considered healed **(a–d)**.

Technique for Arthroscopic-Assisted Arthrodesis

The authors use the same setup as previously mentioned with the hand in a vertical tower and the patient in general anesthesia. They use a tourniquet and a dry technique for arthroscopy. Portals are established to the radiocarpal and midcarpal joints. The joint is examined and the diagnosis is verified with an instability over the LT joint (Video 22.8).

To keep the configuration of the carpal bones, they enter the midcarpal joint and start shaving of the LT interval. They then enter a bur into the joint space; however, they resect only the dorsal part of the joint. Using fluoroscope, they are careful not to enter the radiocarpal joint. When they have the view of bleeding bone from both sides, they harvest cancellous bone preferably from the iliac crest; however, bone from the distal radius could also be used. The bone is transferred into the dorsal part of the joint space by passing the bone through small drill guides. Having done that, a small incision is made over the triquetrum, the soft tissue is spread to avoid the subcutaneous nerves, and two K-wires are drilled into the triquetrum crossing the LT-joint space. They aim for one wire going from the dorsal part of the triquetrum into the palmar part of the lunate, while the other is inserted from the palmar side of the triquetrum into the dorsal part of the lunate. When the position is good and checked in the fluoroscope, they enter headless compression screws over the K-wires. (If this is difficult, one compression screw and one K-wire could also be used.) They check the stability after the fixation (Video 22.9).

The patient is given a cast that is changed after 14 days when a new cast is applied for another 4 weeks. Six weeks following surgery, the authors ask for a computed tomography (CT) scan to verify healing of the bones. They typically check bone bridges at this time, and if 40 to 50% of the gap is filled with bone they consider it as healed and remove the cast and start rehabilitation (▶ Fig. 22.13a–d).

Results

The patients that authors have operated with arthrodesis for a coalition have all healed. If a K-wire is applied, it will be removed, but the headless compression screws are left in place. The authors have not had any complications with this technique.

References

[1] Viegas SF, Patterson RM, Peterson PD, et al. Ulnar-sided perilunate instability: an anatomic and biomechanic study. J Hand Surg Am. 1990; 15(2):268–278

[2] Haugstvedt JR. LT tears and arthroscopic repair. In: Piñal FD, Mathoulin C, Nakamura T, eds. Arthroscopic management of ulnar pain. Berlin; New York: Springer; 2012:213–236

[3] Murray PM, Palmer CG, Shin AY. The mechanism of ulnar-sided perilunate instability of the wrist: a cadaveric study and 6 clinical cases. J Hand Surg Am. 2012; 37(4):721–728

[4] Cooney WP. Evaluation of chronic wrist pain by arthrography, arthroscopy, and arthrotomy. J Hand Surg Am. 1993; 18(5):815–822

[5] Cohen MS. Ligamentous injuries of the wrist in the athlete. Clin Sports Med. 1998; 17(3):533–552

[6] Garcia-Elias M, Geissler WB. Carpal instability. In: Green DP, ed. Green's operative hand surgery. 5th ed. Philadelphia: Elsevier Inc.; 2005

[7] Shin AY, Battaglia MJ, Bishop AT. Lunotriquetral instability: diagnosis and treatment. J Am Acad Orthop Surg. 2000; 8(3):170–179

[8] Levine JW, Savoie FH III, Moskal MJ. Arthroscopic plication of lunotriquetral ligament tears. In: Slutsky DJ, Nagle DJ, eds. Techniques in wrist and hand arthroscopy. Philadelphia, PA: Elsevier Inc.; 2008

[9] Shin AY, Weinstein LP, Berger RA, Bishop AT. Treatment of isolated injuries of the lunotriquetral ligament. A comparison of arthrodesis, ligament reconstruction and ligament repair. J Bone Joint Surg Br. 2001; 83(7):1023–1028

[10] Haugstvedt JR, Rigo IZ. Arthroscopic-assisted reconstruction of LT-ligament. In: Mathoulin C, ed. Wrist arthroscopy techniques. 2nd ed. Stuttgart; New York: Thieme; 2019:93–101

[11] Haugstvedt JR, Rigó IZ. Arthroscopic assisted reconstruction of LT-ligament: a description of a new technique. J Wrist Surg. 2021; 10(1):2–8

[12] Devilliers Minnaar AB. Congenital fusion of the lunate and triquetral bones in the South African Bantu. J Bone Joint Surg Br. 1952; 34-B(1):45–48

[13] Spaans AJ, Beumer A. Carpal coalitions: failures of differentiation of the carpus: a description of cases. Open J Radiol. 2013; 3:1–6

[14] Weinzweig J, Watson HK, Herbert TJ, Shaer JA. Congenital synchondrosis of the scaphotrapezio-trapezoidal joint. J Hand Surg Am. 1997; 22(1):74–77

22

23 LT Ligament Injury (Disorders) and Instability Associated to Ulnocarpal Abutment Syndrome: Ulnar-Shortening Osteotomy

Toshiyasu Nakamura

Abstract

Lunotriquetral (LT) ligament can be damaged with shearing and compression force applied from the longer ulna relative to the radius in the ulnocarpal abutment syndrome, representing relatively chronic and degenerative damages on the LT ligament with degenerative disorders of the triangular fibrocartilage complex (TFCC) and articular cartilage of the lunate, triquetrum, and ulnar head. Radiographs, magnetic resonance imaging (MRI), arthrogram, or arthro-CT (computed tomography) are useful in diagnosing LT ligament disorders due to ulnocarpal abutment syndrome. Midcarpal arthroscopic exploration confirms LT disorders, while radiocarpal arthroscopy indicates degenerative changes on the TFCC and ulnar carpal bones. Ulnar-shortening procedure is the primary option for LT ligament disorders with ulnocarpal abutment syndrome. Additional temporary pinning with arthroscopic debridement associated with ulnar shortening is effective in severely unstable LT interval.

Keywords: LT ligament, ulnocarpal abutment syndrome, ulnar shortening osteotomy, TFCC injury, DRUJ instability

23.1 Ulnocarpal Abutment Syndrome

Ulnar variance is the relative length of the ulna with respect to the radius.[1] Longer ulnar length relative to the radius corresponds to the "positive ulnar variance," same length of the ulna to the radius indicates the "neutral or null ulnar variance," and lesser length of the ulna relative to the radius is the "minus ulnar variance."[1] Ulnocarpal abutment syndrome is the disorders of the ulnar-side wrist due to compression force produced by long ulna, associated with degenerative triangular fibrocartilage complex (TFCC) tears, chondromalacia of the lunate, triquetrum and ulnar head, lunotriquetral (LT) ligament tears, first reported by Trumble in 1988.[2] There are two types of ulnocarpal abutment syndrome: (1) caused by congenital positive ulnar variance with/without minor trauma; (2) caused by shortening deformity of the radial shaft fracture/malunion. Synonyms of the ulnocarpal abutment syndrome is ulnar (ulnocarpal) impaction syndrome.[3,4]

In the ulnocarpal abutment syndrome, most of the cases indicate more than 2-mm positive ulnar variance, while some of the neutral to minus ulnar variance cases demonstrate similar pathology on the lunate and/or triquetrum. During pronation-supination motion, the ulnar variance changes longer by 2 mm in pronation and shorter by 1 to 2 mm in supination[4] that produces shearing stress from severely unstable ulnar head to the ulnar carpus through the TFCC.[5]

Ulnar impingement syndrome is the different category which indicates the impingement of the ulnar stump to the radial shaft in the Darrach procedure or Sauvé-Kapandji procedure.[6] Avoiding confusion between ulnocarpal abutment syndrome or ulnocarpal impingement syndrome and ulnar impingement syndrome, the name radioulnar impingement syndrome or radioulnar convergence syndrome may be adequate. The other similar name to the ulnocarpal abutment syndrome is ulnar styloid impaction syndrome reported by Topper et al in 1997.[7] The longer ulnar styloid impacts on the triquetrum indicating ulnar-side pain in ulnar-deviated position with pronosupination.

23.2 Lunotriquetral Ligament (LT) Injury

The LT ligament consists of the dorsal portion, proximal membranous portion, and the volar portion that is the strongest portion among three portions.[8] When the LT ligament is ruptured, the scaphoid and lunate have a tendency to flex, while the triquetrum has a tendency to extend, where the lunate bone shows flexion deformity which is called volar intercalated segment instability (VISI) deformity.[9] The LT ligament injury can be caused by severe hyperextension or flexion trauma. Widening of the LT interval is seen in some patients. Mayfield et al biomechanically analyzed the perilunate injury pattern that was started from the scapholunate (SL) ligament injury, through the midcarpal joint to the LT ligament.[10] In its variation, reverse Mayfield mechanism can occur starting from the LT ligament.

The other scenario is the LT ligament can be damaged with the longer ulna in the ulnocarpal abutment syndrome.[11] There are wear or degenerative changes especially on the membranous portion of the LT ligament with the degenerative changes on the TFCC.[11] The latter normally does not indicate tear or avulsion of the ligamentous part of the LT ligament, such as the dorsal or volar portion, and widening of the LT gap or VISI deformity is seldom seen.

23.3 Symptom of the LT Ligament Injury with the Ulnocarpal Abutment Syndrome

Symptom of the LT ligament injury due to the ulnocarpal abutment syndrome indicates ulnar-side wrist pain during pronosupination with ulnar deviation or in push-up. Typical motion of pain is twisting doorknob or opening pet bottle.[12,13] These are quite similar symptoms of degenerative tear of the TFCC.

23.4 Diagnosis of the LT Injury with Ulnocarpal Abutment Syndrome

In physical examination, the ulnocarpal stress test,[14] forced ulnar deviation or forced ulnar deviation with pronosupination, is useful in diagnosing LT ligament injury with ulnocarpal abutment syndrome. However, the ulnocarpal stress test can be also positive in fresh TFCC injury or extensor carpi ulnaris (ECU) tendon disorder, so this test indicates lower specificity. Tenderness point on the ulnotriquetral gap is also positive in LT ligament disorders.

Radiographs demonstrates more than 1-mm positive ulnar variance and the cystic lesion in the lunate, triquetrum, or ulnar head in the posteroanterior view (▶ Fig. 23.1). The lateral radiographs indicate dorsal transposition of the ulnar head in excessive positive ulnar variance wrist.

Magnetic resonance imaging (MRI) demonstrates low signal intensity on the lunate, triquetrum, and ulnar head in T1-weighted images, mid to high signal intensity on the same lesion in T2-weighted images.[15] T2*-weighted images delineates degenerative TFCC injury with bone edema in the ulnar carpus or ulnar head (▶ Fig. 23.2).

Arthrogram indicates intrusion of the radiographic dye passing through the LT interval from radiocarpal injection.[16] Arthrogram in forced radial- or ulnar-deviated position is useful to demonstrate increase in the LT gap (▶ Fig. 23.3). Arthro-CT that is the CT image soon after the arthrogram is taken, can indicate the hidden LT ligament injury[17] (▶ Fig. 23.4).

Arthroscopy is the gold standard diagnostic tool for the LT disorders, cartilage damages on the lunate, triquetrum or ulnar head, degenerative tears on the TFCC. In radiocarpal arthroscopy, degenerative changes on the cartilage of the lunate and triquetrum and degenerative changes

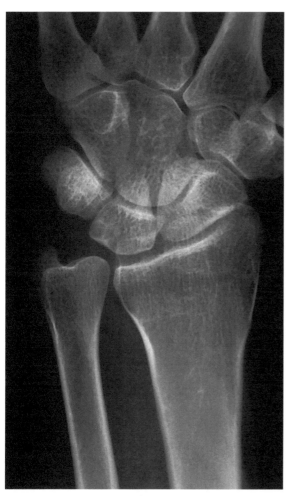

Fig. 23.1 Posteroanterior radiograph of ulnocarpal abutment syndrome. Cystic changes occur on the ulnar side of the lunate with positive 3-mm ulnar variance.

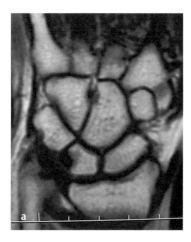
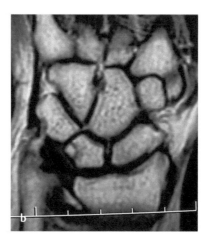

Fig. 23.2 Magnetic resonance imaging (MRI) of the same patient of Fig. 24.1. Note the low-signal-intensity area in the lunate at the site of cyst in T1-weighted image **(a)** and high-signal-intensity area in the lunate due to fluid inside the cyst in T2-weighted image **(b)**.

23

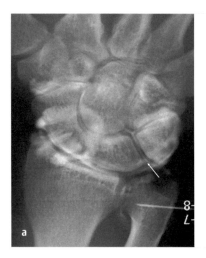
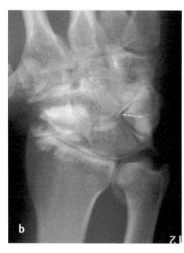

Fig. 23.3 Arthrogram indicates peripheral triangular fibrocartilage complex (TFCC) injury with radiologic dye passing through the lunotriquetral (LT) interval (*arrow*) in the neutral wrist position **(a)**. Step forms at the LT interval in the same patients (*dashed arrow*) that indicates LT ligament instability in the radial-deviated position **(b)**.

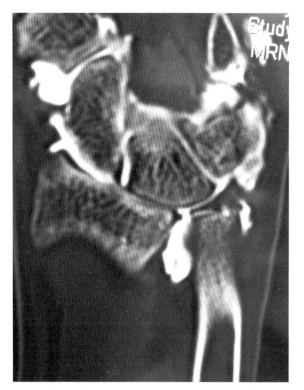

Fig. 23.4 Arthro-CT (computed tomography) images indicate radiologic dye passing both through the LT and SL interval with an avulsion of the radioulnar ligament at the fovea and slit tear in the triangular fibrocartilage.

Table 23.1 Modification of Geissler's SL ligament injury classification to LT ligament injury

Grade	Description
0	LT interval is stable
1	Floating of the triquetrum or lunate with the probe
2	The 2-mm diameter probe can be inserted into the LT gap
3	The 2-mm diameter probe can be rotated inside the LT interval
4	The 2.7-mm diameter arthroscope can be driven through the interval and radiocarpal joint can be seen from ulnar midcarpal portal

Abbreviations: LT, lunotriquetral; SL, scapholunate.

modified Geissler's classification for LT injury, Grade 1 indicates instability of the LT gap with probe; in Grade 2, the 2-mm diameter probe can be inserted into the LT gap; in Grade 3, the 2-mm diameter probe can be rotated in the LT interval; in Grade 4, 2.7-mm diameter arthroscope can be driven through the interval and radiocarpal joint can be seen from ulnar midcarpal portal (▸ Fig. 23.5). In this classification, Grades 3 and 4 may be an indication for surgical treatment.

23.5 Treatments

23.5.1 Conservative Treatment

Conservative treatment includes brace and supporter that immobilize the wrist for rest. Normally, it takes 3 months for the patients to achieve successful clinical result with conservative treatment. If conservative treatment results in failure after 3 months, surgical treatment should be considered.

on the TFCC, such as perforation or fibrillation, are popular findings of the ulnocarpal abutment syndrome.[11,12] Midcarpal arthroscopy reveals information of the distal cartilage surface of the scaphoid, lunate, and triquetrum and condition of the SL and LT interval. The Geissler's classification for the SL ligament injury[18,19] can be converted into the LT ligament injury (▸ Table 23.1). In

23.5.2 Surgical Treatment

Ulnar-Shortening Procedure

Ulnar-shortening procedure is the primary surgical treatment for both primary and secondary ulnocarpal abutment syndrome.[11,12,21,22] Ulnar shortening can decompress the ulnocarpal interval thereby leverizing the positive ulnar variance, restoring the articulation of the distal radioulnar

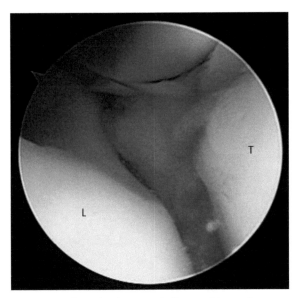

Fig. 23.5 Midcarpal arthroscopy indicates wide gap formation between lunotriquetral (LT) interval where the scope can be driven through (Geissler Grade 4). L, lunate; T, triquetrum.

joint (DRUJ) for smooth pronosupination inside the joint, and stabilizing the DRUJ with pulling effect to the TFCC[23] that normalizes the stress and its function. The ulnar-shortening procedure can reduce ulnar-side wrist pain.[11,12,20,21,22] In neutral variance wrist, ulnar shortening can reduce pressure upon the ulnocarpal joint and stabilize the DRUJ, while joint incongruity can occur.[24] The ulnar shortening can also stabilize the LT interval[25] with pulling effect of the 3D structure of the TFCC (▸ Fig. 23.6). There is a little problem that at least half of the joint congruity can remain after ulnar shortening. Excessive shortening is a risk for destruction of the DRUJ surface.[26]

Osteotomy methods reported are horizontal cut,[13] oblique cut,[27] or step-cut for diaphyseal osteotomy. Horizontal cut has a disadvantage for area of the contact after shortening, while oblique cut or step-cut has increased contact area.[27] Advantage of horizontal cut is intentional rotational realignment for supinating or pronating to adjust pronosupination range in the forearm rotation contracture patients. Metaphyseal ulnar shortening is also indicated in the ulnocarpal abutment syndrome,[28,30] while this technique has less effect on stabilizing the DRUJ or LT interval.[30]

Shortening length can be determined to neutralize the positive ulnar variance. In neutral variance case, shortening length should be within 2 mm.

Additional treatments for TFCC injury are arthroscopic partial resection of the degenerative triangular fibrocartilage disk, arthroscopic capsular repair for peripheral injury, and arthroscopic or open repair for foveal avulsion of the radioulnar ligament (RUL).[13] Those additional treatments can be determined by arthroscopic exploration before or after ulnar shortening.[13]

23

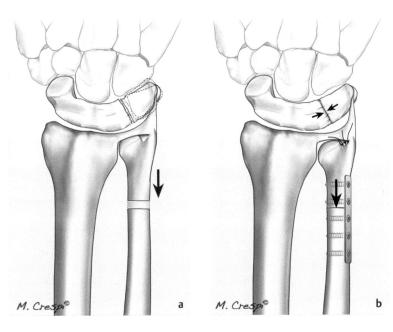

Fig. 23.6 Illustrations of how the ulnar-shortening procedure can tighten the lunotriquetral (LT) interval. Before ulnar shortening, the LT interval (or the triquetrum) can be unstable with the LT ligament rupture (**a**), the ulnar shortening pulls the TFCC to tighten the LT interval (**b**).

Author's Technique of Ulnar Shortening

After arthroscopic exploration on the radiocarpal joint, midcarpal joint, and DRUJ, longitudinal incision of 8 cm is made on the ulnar shaft. Subcutaneous tissue is separated with surgical knife, and ECU sheath is separated from the periosteum of the ulna (▶ Fig. 23.7a). A low contact-locking compression plate (LC-LCP; Depuy-Synthes, Raynham, PA, USA) with five holes is placed on the ulnar shaft to determine the osteotomy site. Normally osteotomy is done 6 cm proximal from the ulnar styloid, but proximal or distal arrangement of the plate setting may occur due to the natural angulation of the ulnar shaft. Minimum of 2 cm longitudinal splitting of the periosteum is done for osteotomy (▶ Fig. 23.7b). Care should be taken not to rotate the distal fragment to proximal fragment. Hence, marking on the osteotomy site is very useful in controlling rotation of the distal fragment and determining the shortening length (▶ Fig. 23.7c). Free-hand parallel osteotomy of 2 mm or simulated shortening length is performed on the ulna (▶ Fig. 23.7d), then ulnar shortening can be done with bone clump forceps (▶ Fig. 23.7e). Compression plate holes are used to fix the ulna, then rest of the screw is inserted with buttress plate holes (▶ Fig. 23.7f, g).

If the patients are male or female smokers more than 60 years of age, a plate with six holes is preferable to avoid nonunion.

Arthroscopic Debridement of the LT Lesion with Temporary Pinning

After ulnar shortening, arthroscopic exploration of the radiocarpal joint and DRUJ for confirmation of decompression of the TFCC and exploration of the midcarpal joint were performed. If the LT joint interval is unstable with probing, arthroscopic debridement may be performed with shaver and temporary pinning of the LT joint is done under fluoroscopy control. Be aware of the cutaneous nerve of the ulnar nerve, so longitudinal incision of 2 cm is made on the triquetrum to retract dorsal branch of the ulnar nerve avoiding any damage with the pins. Normally, ulnar-shortening procedure is required for degenerative changes on TFCC with LT pinning (▶ Fig. 23.8). Eight weeks after pinning, K-wire will be removed.

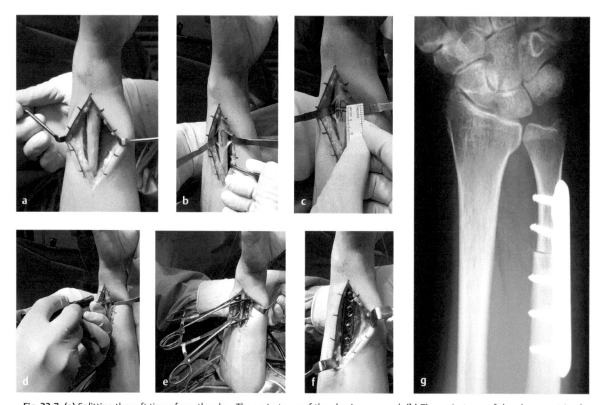

Fig. 23.7 **(a)** Splitting the soft tissue from the ulna. The periosteum of the ulna is preserved. **(b)** The periosteum of the ulna was striped longitudinally, approximately 2 cm. **(c)** To set the shortening length, the measure is used. Note the longitudinal three markings to control the rotation of the distal fragment. **(d)** Free-hand horizontal section of the ulna is made by oscillator. **(e)** The five-hole Synthes low contact-locking compression plate (LC-LCP) are clumped on the ulna and adequate shortening is applied manually. **(f)** Plate is fixed on the ulna by screws. In the second and third holes, dynamic compression hole was used. **(g)** Postoperative posteroanterior radiograph of ulnar shortening.

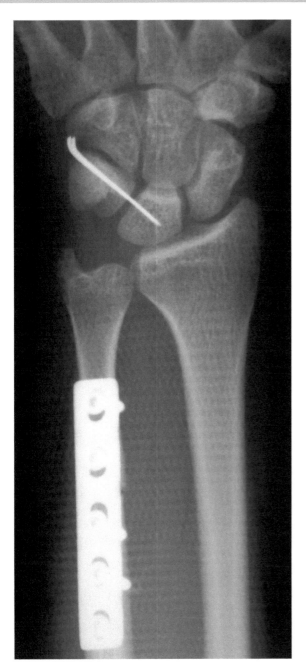

Fig. 23.8 Postoperative posteroanterior radiograph of arthroscopic debridement of the lunotriquetral (LT) lesion with temporary pinning and ulnar shortening.

Author's Case Series

Since 2014, 26 wrists of 26 patients of unstable LT joint underwent LT pinning with arthroscopic debridement on the dorsal surface of the LT ligament. Perilunate dislocation and lunate dislocation were excluded. There were 19 males, 6 females with average age of 34 (range 17–67). Cause of the LT ligament injury was strong axial force, such as fall on outstretched hand in 14 wrists, tennis in 6, and unknown in 6. Period from initial injury to the surgery was average 26 months (range 3 mo to 30 y). All patients claimed ulnar-side wrist pain, especially on the LT site. DRUJ instability was obvious in 22 wrists and clicking was noted in 8 wrists. Ulnar variance was neutral in 10 wrists and positive in 16 (range 2–5), with an average of 1.3 mm.

Arthrogram delineated connection between radiocarpal and midcarpal joints through LT interval and step of the LT joint was found in 11 wrists. Arthroscopic exploration revealed Geissler Grade 3 in 23 wrists and Grade 4 in 3, all indicated unstable triquetrum with the lunate, and among them, 9 wrists demonstrated avulsion of the dorsal portion of the LT ligament. Additional slit tear of the TFCC was found in 8 wrists and degenerative TFCC lesion was noted in 23 wrists. All patients underwent pinning of the LT interval with fluoroscopic control. Ulnar shortening was done in 18 wrists and open RUL repair to the fovea was performed in 3 wrists. Two wrists required additional SL pinning and 4 wrists underwent arthroscopic synovectomy. Final clinical results obtained were excellent in 22 wrists and good in 4.

Arthroscopic Wafer Procedure

Arthroscopic Wafer procedure[31] is a popular technique for ulnocarpal abutment syndrome to reduce compression force of the ulnar head to the TFCC or ulnar carpus. In LT ligament injury, as the arthroscopic Wafer procedure has no effect to stabilize the LT joint, the author does not prefer to perform this technique.

References

[1] Schuurman AH, Maas M, Dijkstra PF, Kauer JM. Assessment of ulnar variance: a radiological investigation in a Dutch population. Skeletal Radiol. 2001; 30(11):633–638

[2] Trumble TE, Easterling KJ, Smith RJ. Ulnocarpal abutment after wrist arthrodesis. J Hand Surg Am. 1988; 13(1):11–15

[3] Friedman SL, Palmer AK. The ulnar impaction syndrome. Hand Clin. 1991; 7(2):295–310

[4] Tomaino MM. Ulnar impaction syndrome in the ulnar negative and neutral wrist. Diagnosis and pathoanatomy. J Hand Surg [Br]. 1998; 23(6):754–757

[5] Nakamura T, Yabe Y, Horiuchi Y. Dynamic changes in the shape of the triangular fibrocartilage complex during rotation demonstrated with high resolution magnetic resonance imaging. J Hand Surg [Br]. 1999; 24(3):338–341

[6] Bell MJ, Hill RJ, McMurtry RY. Ulnar impingement syndrome. J Bone Joint Surg Br. 1985; 67(1):126–129

[7] Topper SM, Wood MB, Ruby LK. Ulnar styloid impaction syndrome. J Hand Surg Am. 1997; 22(4):699–704

[8] Ritt MJ, Linscheid RL, Cooney WP, III, Berger RA, An KN. The lunotriquetral joint: kinematic effects of sequential ligament sectioning, ligament repair, and arthrodesis. J Hand Surg Am. 1998; 23(3):432–445

[9] Linscheid RL, Dobyns JH, Beabout JW, Bryan RS. Traumatic instability of the wrist. Diagnosis, classification, and pathomechanics. J Bone Joint Surg Am. 1972; 54(8):1612–1632

23

[10] Mayfield JK, Johnson RP, Kilcoyne RK. Carpal dislocations: pathomechanics and progressive perilunar instability. J Hand Surg Am. 1980; 5(3):226–241

[11] Palmer AK. Triangular fibrocartilage complex lesions: a classification. J Hand Surg Am. 1989; 14(4):594–606

[12] Minami A, Kato H. Ulnar shortening for triangular fibrocartilage complex tears associated with ulnar positive variance. J Hand Surg Am. 1998; 23(5):904–908

[13] Nakamura T, Yabe Y, Horiuchi Y, Kikuchi Y, Makita A. Ulnar shortening procedure for the ulnocarpal and distal radioulnar joints disorders. J Jpn Soc Surg Hand. 1998; 15:119–126

[14] Nakamura R, Horii E, Imaeda T, Nakao E, Kato H, Watanabe K. The ulnocarpal stress test in the diagnosis of ulnar-sided wrist pain. J Hand Surg [Br]. 1997; 22(6):719–723

[15] Imaeda T, Nakamura R, Shionoya K, Makino N. Ulnar impaction syndrome: MR imaging findings. Radiology. 1996; 201(2):495–500

[16] Zinberg EM, Palmer AK, Coren AB, Levinsohn EM. The triple-injection wrist arthrogram. J Hand Surg Am. 1988; 13(6):803–809

[17] Moritomo H, Arimitsu S, Kubo N, Masatomi T, Yukioka M. Computed tomography arthrography using a radial plane view for the detection of triangular fibrocartilage complex foveal tears. J Hand Surg Am. 2015; 40(2):245–251

[18] Geissler WB. Arthroscopically assisted reduction of intra-articular fractures of the distal radius. Hand Clin. 1995; 11(1):19–29

[19] Löw S, Erne H, Strobl U, Unglaub F, Spies CK. Significance of scapholunate gap width as measured by probe from midcarpal. J Wrist Surg. 2017; 6(4):316–324

[20] Darrow JC, Jr, Linscheid RL, Dobyns JH, Mann JM, III, Wood MB, Beckenbaugh RD. Distal ulnar recession for disorders of the distal radioulnar joint. J Hand Surg Am. 1985; 10(4):482–491

[21] Boulas HJ, Milek MA. Ulnar shortening for tears of the triangular fibrocartilaginous complex. J Hand Surg Am. 1990; 15(3):415–420

[22] Bilos ZJ, Chamberland D. Distal ulnar head shortening for treatment of triangular fibrocartilage complex tears with ulna positive variance. J Hand Surg Am. 1991; 16(6):1115–1119

[23] Nishiwaki M, Nakamura T, Nakao Y, Nagura T, Toyama Y. Ulnar shortening effect on DRUJ stability: a biomechanical study. J Hand Surg Am. 2005; 30:719–726

[24] Deshmukh SC, Shanahan D, Coulthard D. Distal radioulnar joint incongruity after shortening of the ulna. J Hand Surg [Br]. 2000; 25(5):434–438

[25] Mirza A, Mirza JB, Shin AY, Lorenzana DJ, Lee BK, Izzo B. Isolated lunotriquetral ligament tears treated with ulnar shortening osteotomy. J Hand Surg Am. 2013; 38(8):1492–1497

[26] Nishiwaki M, Nakamura T, Nagura T, Toyama Y, Ikegami H. Ulnar-shortening effect on distal radioulnar joint pressure: a biomechanical study. J Hand Surg Am. 2008; 33(2):198–205

[27] Labosky DA, Waggy CA. Oblique ulnar shortening osteotomy by a single saw cut. J Hand Surg Am. 1996; 21(1):48–59

[28] Slade JF, III, Gillon TJ. Osteochondral shortening osteotomy for the treatment of ulnar impaction syndrome: a new technique. Tech Hand Up Extrem Surg. 2007; 11(1):74–82

[29] Hammert WC, Williams RB, Greenberg JA. Distal metaphyseal ulnar-shortening osteotomy: surgical technique. J Hand Surg Am. 2012; 37(5):1071–1077

[30] Kubo N, Moritomo H, Arimitsu S, Nishimoto S, Yoshida T. Distal ulnar metaphyseal wedge osteotomy for ulnar abutment syndrome. J Wrist Surg. 2019; 8(5):352–359

[31] Wnorowski DC, Palmer AK, Werner FW, Fortino MD. Anatomic and biomechanical analysis of the arthroscopic wafer procedure. Arthroscopy. 1992; 8(2):204–212

IV

Section V

Extrinsic Ligament Injuries

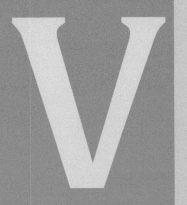

24 Perilunate Injuries

Bo Liu and Feiran Wu

Abstract

Perilunate injuries are highly unstable carpal dissociations characterized by a complete loss of contact between the lunate and capitate. Closed reduction and cast treatment of perilunate dislocations and fracture dislocations are associated with unacceptably poor results. For a successful outcome, early anatomical reduction must be achieved and preserved until healing. Open reduction and stabilization can be performed through a volar, dorsal, or a combined approach. To minimize morbidity, arthroscopic-assisted techniques can minimize adjacent soft tissue injury, while facilitating accurate anatomic reduction and percutaneous fixation of the carpus. This chapter describes refinements of the existing methods in order to present the most up-to-date techniques to treat this condition.

Keywords: perilunate dislocation, perilunate fracture dislocation, lunate, scaphoid fracture, scapholunate, lunotriquetral, percutaneous fixation, wrist arthroscopy, carpal fracture

24.1 Introduction

Perilunate injuries are severe, highly unstable carpal dissociations characterized by a complete loss of contact between the lunate and surrounding carpal bones. Such injuries represent a spectrum of conditions that include purely ligamentous injuries in the so-called perilunate dislocations (PLDs), through to bone and ligament injuries caused by transscaphoid perilunate fracture dislocations (PLFDs).[1,3] It is caused by excessive radiocarpal hyperextension and ulnar deviation coupled with intercarpal supination, which has been proven to be the principal pathologic forces that disrupt the key osseous and ligamentous components of the wrist.[1] The basic defining feature is the loss of contact between the head of the capitate and the distal surface of the lunate. Due to its high-energy mechanism, up to 10% of these injuries are open, 26% are associated with polytrauma, and 11% have concomitant injuries of the upper limb.[4]

Because the lunate is strongly bound to the radius and ulna by the volar capsular ligaments, PLDs and PLFDs are uncommon but devastating injuries, with the severity often underestimated. The capitolunate joint is the most congruent part of the midcarpal joint, and the pressure of the dorsal rim of the lunate on the capitate cartilage at the time of the dislocation explains the frequent cartilage erosions or cartilaginous fractures observed.[4] This phenomenon also explains the frequency of posttraumatic arthritis of the midcarpal joint occurring after PLD-PLFD.[5]

The key to success is to achieve early anatomical reduction and maintain the carpal alignment in both fractures and dislocations.[6] Nonoperative management with closed reduction and cast treatment has been shown to result in unacceptable outcomes; therefore, surgical intervention with open reduction, ligament repair or reconstruction, and internal fixation of any fractures is the current gold standard.[3,6,14]

In this chapter, the authors discuss the surgical techniques of open and arthroscopic treatment of PLDs and PLFDs. They aim to describe refinements of the existing methods and key steps in their favored approach in order to present the most up-to-date techniques to treat this condition.

24.2 Classification

Mayfield et al[1] described progressive perilunate instability where the four stages of progressive ligamentous damage occurred with the wrist hyperextended, in variable degrees of ulnar deviation and the forearm supinated. In their seminal study, 32 cadaveric wrists were loaded onto two machines until ligamentous or bony failure. There was a predictable pattern of injury as the scapholunate (SL) ligament was torn followed by a sequence of ligaments around the lunate in an ulnar direction until dislocation of the carpus occurred with or without a fracture of one of the carpal bones (▶ Table 24.1). In Stage I, there is disruption of the SL and radiocapitate ligaments. In Stage II, the traumatic force disrupts the lunocapitate

Table 24.1 Mayfield stages of perilunar instability

	Joints disrupted	Ligaments torn/attenuated
Stage 1	Scapholunate	Radioscaphoid scapholunate Radiocapitate
Stage 2	Scapholunate Capitolunate	Radioscaphoid Scapholunate Radial collateral radiocapitate
Stage 3	Scapholunate Capitolunate Triquetrolunate	Radioscaphoid scapholunate Radial collateral radiocapitate Lunotriquetral Palmar radiotriquetral +/− Ulnotriquetral
Stage 4	Scapholunate Capitolunate Triquetrolunate Radiolunate	Radioscaphoid scapholunate Radial collateral radiocapitate Lunotriquetral Palmar radiotriquetral +/− Ulnotriquetral +/− Dorsal radiocarpal

24

215

association. In Stage III, there is failure of the lunotrique-tral (LT) and ulnotriquetral ligaments, where the entire carpus essentially separates from the lunate. Finally, Stage IV involves palmar lunate dislocation into the carpal tunnel. Mayfield demonstrated that slower application of load produced fractures (radial styloid, scaphoid, and/or capitate) prior to the lunate dislocation, termed "greater arc injuries." Conversely, a more rapidly applied force caused purely ligamentous disruptions, termed "lesser arc injuries."

24.3 Assessment and Investigations

The deformity in PLD-PLFDs can be variable, from subtle to obvious.[9] A retrospective study reported that diagnosis was initially missed in 25% of patients, even in isolated trauma.[5] Clinically, there is invariably pain and swelling, but an obvious visible abnormality may not be apparent. The carpus is usually displaced dorsally. Signs of median nerve injury, particularly sensory, should be examined for, and can be present in up to 16% of patients.[15] The most common demographic is young males, with a typical mechanism as a result of a fall from two to three stories of height or road traffic accidents.[15]

For investigation, plain posterior-anterior (PA) and lateral radiographs of the wrist are almost always sufficient, without the need for advanced imaging.[6] On PA radiographs the space between individual carpal bones should be uniform. Uneven gapping between the carpal bones indicates disruption of their ligamentous connections. The articular surfaces of proximal and distal carpal rows should form smooth arcs at the radiocarpal and midcarpal articulations, i.e., Gilula's arcs. With PLD these arcs are disrupted and an unusual overlap of adjacent bones is seen. On lateral radiographs, the distinctive moon shape of the lunate can be identified with careful inspection, and should be seated in the convexity of the proximal capitate. In PLDs, the lunate-capitate articulation is disrupted, and the concave distal lunate no longer articulates with the capitate.

24.4 Treatment

The definitive treatment of these complex injuries is operative. Nonoperative management of perilunate injuries has unacceptably high rates of loss of reduction with poor eventual outcomes.[15,16] The key principles of treatment are to reduce the carpus as soon as possible, followed by repair of the SL and LT ligaments. The authors recommend a single attempt of closed manual reduction of capitolunate joint dislocations, which is helped by suspending the hand in finger traps and applying 10 to 15 lb of countertraction. For acute PLDs, usually more than 50% of cases are successfully reduced with closed manipulation after one attempt. If reduction fails, further repeated attempts are generally unsuccessful and should be

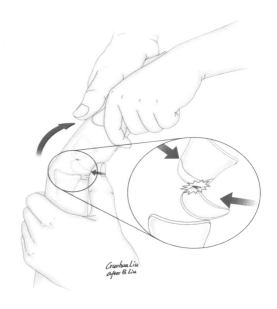

Fig. 24.1 Damage of the capitolunate articular cartilage from blind repeated forceful closed reduction attempts.

avoided. Repeated blind and forceful attempts can lead to further damage of the proximal capitate cartilage, an area that is already vulnerable from the index injury (▶ Fig. 24.1). The rate of successful closed manual reductions of capitolunate dislocations significantly reduces when there is a delay of 3 days or longer following initial injury. In this situation, open or arthroscopic surgery should be arranged without delay.

Treatment for PLDs and PLFDs can be managed through an arthroscopic-assisted or open technique. The majority of patients that present with acute or early subacute PLDs (within 4 wk of injury) are suitable for arthroscopic-assisted intervention. For patients presenting > 4 weeks after injury, the existing scarring would impede the likelihood of arthroscopic-assisted fracture reduction of the capitolunate joint, necessitating an open approach. Open injuries, or lunate dislocations that has migrated a significant distance away from the lunate fossa, will also require an open approach.

24.4.1 Perilunate Dislocations

Open Reduction and Fixation of PLDs

Open reduction and internal fixation of PLDs can be performed through three basic surgical approaches: volar, dorsal, or combined dorsal-volar approaches. The volar approach is used for lunate dislocations and carpal tunnel decompression. In addition, the space of Poirier and LT ligament can also be repaired directly.[17]

The dorsal approach can be utilized to restore carpal alignment and to repair the SL ligament, the key to ensuring long-term successful outcomes by mitigating against chronic instability.[18]

A combined method is described to incorporate the advantages of both approaches.[10,17] An extended carpal tunnel incision is used on the volar side, commencing 2 to 3 cm proximal to the wrist crease in line with the ulnar border of the palmaris longus tendon. The brachial fascia and transverse carpal ligament are released, and the flexor tendons and median nerve are retracted to expose the lunate. This can be reduced by retraction of interposed capsular tissue and gentle direct pressure on the bone itself. The volar capsuloligamentous tissue is repaired with a 3–0 or 4–0 suture to prevent redislocation. The dorsal approach is performed with a standard midline incision. The extensor retinaculum is opened through the third compartment, and the second and fourth compartments are raised off the periosteum. A ligament-sparing capsulotomy is performed along the fibers of the dorsal intercarpal ligament. After inspection of joint surfaces and clearing of debris, K-wires are placed into the scaphoid and lunate and used as joysticks to correct malrotation. Percutaneous intercarpal pinning using 1.1-mm K-wires is then placed in the lunate from the scaphoid and triquetrum to hold the reduction. A further wire can be placed from the scaphoid into the capitate for added stability. Suture anchors can then be placed under vision into the scaphoid, lunate, and/or triquetrum, depending upon the site of ligament avulsion, and used to repair the SL and LT ligaments.

Arthroscopic Reduction and Fixation of PLDs

Recently, arthroscopic-assisted minimally invasive management of these injuries has been gaining prominence.[6,19,23] Combined with fluoroscopy, wrist arthroscopy allows anatomic reduction and precise percutaneous internal fixation of the carpal bones with minimal tissue dissection. This technique may encourage healing with less stiffness, and recent publications have shown encouraging outcomes.[23,25]

Under regional or general anesthesia, the arm is positioned in a wrist traction tower with traction applied by sterile finger-traps. A dorsal 3–4 radiocarpal portal is used for initial inspection of the joint. There is usually sufficient space for scope placement as the lunate is commonly tilted volarly and impinged against the proximal volar aspect of the capitate. It can also be trapped by interposed and torn palmar capsular ligaments, which is a cause for the failure of closed reduction. The initial arthroscopic view is usually obscured by traumatic synovitis, intra-articular hematoma, bony/chondral debris, and torn capsuloligamentous tissue. As a result, wet arthroscopy is required for initial joint debridement to facilitate establishment of a working view. Joint insufflation also helps to compress small capillaries within the capsule and synovium, which helps to control intra-articular bleeding to achieve a clearer image.

Once a clear view is obtained, an additional 4–5 radiocarpal portal is made and the radiocarpal joint systematically examined. The triangular fibrocartilage complex (TFCC), volar and intercarpal ligaments are assessed by direct inspection and manual probing. TFCC tears are addressed according to their injury type. The volar ligament injuries are treated with debridement after the dislocations and/or fractures have been reduced and fixed. Radial and ulnar midcarpal portals are then made to examine the midcarpal joint. The SL and LT ligaments are assessed by manual probing, and concomitant chondral injuries are identified and debrided. Any soft tissue or bony fragments interposed between the SL and LT intervals are excised to facilitate reduction of the intercarpal joint.

Following assessment, an arthroscopic probe is introduced into the radiocarpal joint through the dorsal 4–5 portal. This portal is most convenient for this maneuver because it allows the probe to directly face the subluxated lunate. The force of wrist traction is gently increased at the point so the tip of the probe can be hooked onto the dorsal rim of the lunate (▶ Fig. 24.2). Two K-wires are advanced toward the lunate from the scaphoid and triquetrum, initially without crossing the SL and LT intercarpal intervals (▶ Fig. 24.3). Next, the "shoehorn maneuver" is employed to reduce the dislocated lunate, by using the probe to pull the lunate dorsally under the proximal capitate (▶ Fig. 24.4). This can be conducted entirely under direct arthroscopic visualization without requiring any forceful movements, which protects against further compromise of the articular cartilage. Once the capitolunate joint is reduced, traction is reduced and any abnormal lunate angulation is corrected by passively flexing or extending the wrist and transfixing the radiolunate joint with a temporary K-wire, advanced through the dorsal distal radius. Further correction of the rotation deformity of the scaphoid and lunate can be obtained by using a probe or depressor through the midcarpal portals. Once the SL and LT intervals are reduced, the K-wires in the scaphoid and triquetrum are advanced under direct vision into the lunate and the alignment verified by fluoroscopy (▶ Fig. 24.5).

Despite K-wire fixation, more than half of PLDs will have grossly unstable SL joints that are easily redislocated, due to incompetence of both the primary and secondary stabilizers from the trauma. In this situation, augmentation of the SL ligament through a dorsal mini-invasive approach is advocated, by reinforcing the dorsal SL complex. The dorsal SL complex, including dorsal capsuloscapholunate septum (DCSS) and the dorsal extrinsic ligament, is a key structure for the maintenance SL stability and subsequent long-term successful results.[26,27] To perform the augmentation, the 3–4 portal is extended transversely along the skin crease creating a 2 cm opening. After retracting the extensor tendons, a suture anchor is

24

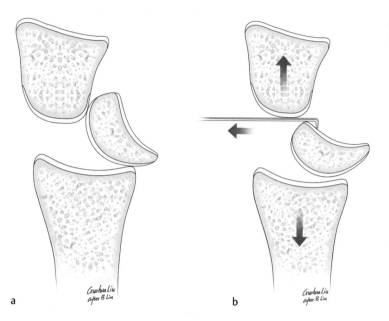

Fig. 24.2 (a,b) The shoehorn maneuver in reducing perilunate dislocations.

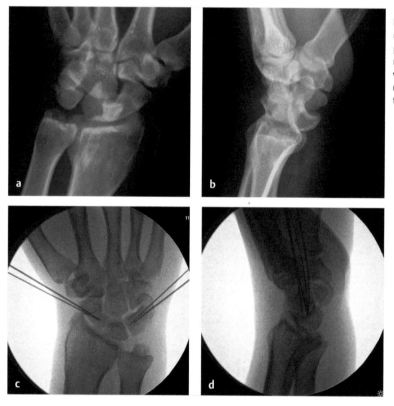

Fig. 24.3 (a) Posterior-anterior (PA) and **(b)** lateral radiographs demonstrating a perilunate dislocation. **(c)** PA and **(d)** lateral radiographs showing the position of the K-wires before fixation of the scapholunate (SL) and lunotriquetral (LT) intervals. Note the dorsal tilting of the lunate.

placed into the scaphoid and lunate at a distance of 1 cm from the SL interval under fluoroscopic guidance. Following joint fixation using two K-wires as described, both sutures are delivered through the dorsal capsule and tied together superficial to the dorsal capsule to create an extra-articular reinforcement of the dorsal SL complex.

Associated Injuries in PLDs

Traditionally, PLDs are often thought of as purely ligamentous injuries. However, it is not uncommon to find concomitant carpal fractures in these patients, as the mechanism is generally of high energy. Associated displaced fractures of the triquetrum or capitate may require open or arthroscopic-assisted reduction and percutaneous fixation. Other associated injuries that are typically seen include tears of the TFCC, which can be debrided or repaired as appropriate.

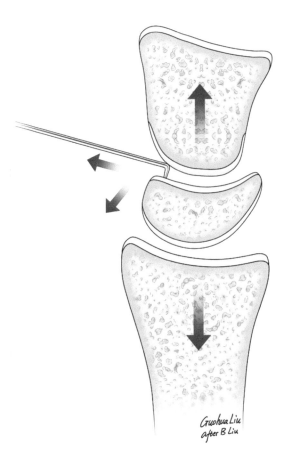

Fig. 24.4 The outcome of the shoehorn maneuver once the capitolunate joint is reduced.

24.4.2 Perilunate Fracture Dislocations

Open Reduction and Fixation of PLFDs

Similar to the treatment of PLDs, PLFDs can be approached through a volar, dorsal, or combined incision, although a dorsal approach alone is usually sufficient.[4] A dorsal midline incision is used and the retinaculum is opened at the third compartment. After capsulotomy, the carpus and radial styloid is exposed and the articular surfaces inspected.

The scaphoid fracture is the initial surgical target after capitolunate reduction. Temporary joystick K-wires can aid in the reduction of the scaphoid fracture, and fixation is performed using a retrograde headless compression screw along the central axis of the scaphoid. In cases with marked comminution of the proximal fragment, 1.1-mm K-wires can be used for definitive fixation instead. After scaphoid fixation, the lunate is stabilized using a radiolunate K-wire, before placing SL, scaphocapitate, and LT K-wires for fixation of the carpus.

Arthroscopic Reduction and Fixation of PLFDs

With the arm suspended in a wrist traction tower, a thorough arthroscopic examination and debridement of the radiocarpal and midcarpal joints are initially performed in transscaphoid PLFDs. In patients who failed closed reduction or presented 3 days or later after the initial injury, the shoehorn maneuver is performed to reduce the capitolunate dislocation. In PLFDs, the probe can also be hooked onto the SL ligament to reduce the dislocation. Similar to the open approach, the scaphoid fracture is the initial surgical target after reduction. This fracture frequently remains significantly displaced with varying degrees of comminution even after the capitolunate dislocation is reduced. Arthroscopic-assisted scaphoid fracture reduction and fixation is typically the most challenging step and critical in the success of the overall surgical outcome. In displaced scaphoid fractures, a

24

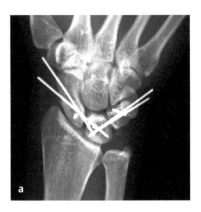
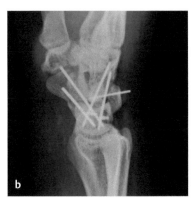

Fig. 24.5 (a) Posterior-anterior and (b) lateral radiographs confirming the position of the K-wire fixation of the scapholunate and lunotriquetral joints.

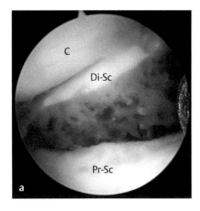
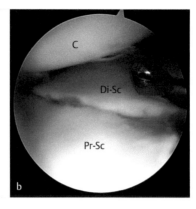

Fig. 24.6 (a) Pre- and (b) post-reduction midcarpal joint view of a scaphoid fracture. C, capitate; Di-Sc, distal scaphoid fragment; Pr-Sc, proximal scaphoid fragment.

guidewire is advanced along the central axis of the distal fragment from the scaphoid tubercle in a retrograde direction, not crossing the fracture line. Further temporary K-wires can be inserted into the distal and proximal fracture fragments, and by using the ulnar midcarpal portal for visualization, the scaphoid fracture can be reduced by manipulating these K-wire joysticks (▶ Fig. 24.6). Attention should be paid to both the sagittal and coronal planes when checking the adequacy of reduction to ensure both the rotational and translational displacements are corrected. Once the scaphoid is reduced anatomically, the surgical assistant drives the central axis guidewire into the proximal scaphoid (▶ Fig. 24.7). An antirotation K-wire is also placed across the fracture site for added stability.

If a residual gap persists between the proximal and distal fracture fragments after K-wire reduction, a cannulated headless compression screw may be used for fracture compression. In these situations, the traction is released and the wrist placed horizontally on a hand table to allow ease of fluoroscopic guidance. The scaphoid is reamed over a central guidewire and the headless screw is inserted retrograde. For proximal third or proximal pole fractures, the central guidewire is advanced proximally through the dorsal skin. A percutaneous incision is made over the dorsal skin, and reaming and screw insertion are then performed in an antegrade direction through this incision. In cases where a screw is used, a supplemental antirotation K-wire is added in the scaphoid for added stability. All K-wires are cut short and buried under the skin for both PLDs and PLFDs.

Associated Injuries in PLFDs

In contrast to the commonly held belief that the SL ligament remains intact in PLFD injuries, the authors found that hemorrhage and attenuation of this ligament can be observed arthroscopically in almost all patients. Most of these injuries are Geissler Grade 1 or 2, which can be managed with immobilization only. A few patients will have more severe SL ligament avulsions from the lunate or gross ruptures of the SL ligament (▶ Fig. 24.8). In these

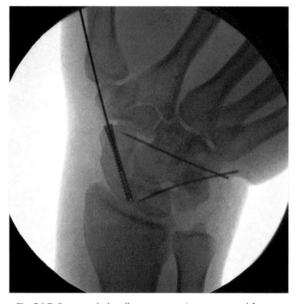

Fig. 24.7 Retrograde headless compression screw used for fixation of the scaphoid in a perilunate fracture dislocation (PLFD).

cases, a Geissler Grade 3 or 4 disruption will be revealed during arthroscopic midcarpal inspection, and SL pinning is required following an accurate reduction of the SL interval.

24.4.3 Postoperative Care

Postoperatively, the wrists are immobilized in a short-arm thermoplastic splint. The proximal phalanx of the thumb is included in the splint for PLFDs, but left free in PLDs. In those with TFCC injuries, a long-arm thermoplastic splint is used with the forearm in semisupination for 6 weeks, followed by a short-arm splint for a further 2 weeks.

K-wires are removed at 8 weeks postoperatively. Active wrist motion is initiated at this point under the guidance of hand therapy. In PLFDs, weight loading and sporting

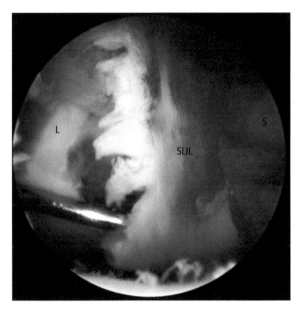

Fig. 24.8 Scapholunate ligament avulsion from the lunate in a patient with transscaphoid perilunate fracture dislocation (PLFD). L, lunate; S, scaphoid.

activities are started only after confirmation of scaphoid union.

24.5 Clinical Results

In their unit, authors routinely employ an arthroscopic approach for the management of suitable PLDs and PLFDs. In 31 patients with 26 transscaphoid PLFDs and 5 dorsal PLDs, arthroscopic-assisted reduction and percutaneous fixation was successful in reducing the dislocation and maintaining carpal alignment. Despite nine patients having median nerve symptoms preoperatively, none required carpal tunnel decompression, as median nerve symptoms due to nerve stretching will usually resolve with reduction of the capitolunate joint.

At a mean final follow-up of 14.8 months (range 12–32), normal carpal alignment was restored and maintained for all patients. The mean flexion-extension arc of the wrist was 115 degrees (range 80–150), which was 86% of the contralateral side. The mean grip strength was 33 kg (range 8–48 kg), which was 83% of the contralateral wrist. Patient-reported outcome measures showed the mean Mayo wrist score to be 87 (range 40–100)— excellent in 17 patients, good in 9, fair in 4, and poor in 1. The mean Disabilities of the Arm, Shoulder, and Hand (DASH) score was 7 (range 0–65). The mean Patient-Rated Wrist Evaluation (PRWE) score was 10 (range 0–63). All patients returned to their preinjury occupations at a mean of 4 months after surgery (range 1–12 mo). There were 15 manual laborers, of which only 3 required reduced workloads.

24.6 Conclusion

The optimal management of perilunate injuries is challenging, and the decision for the "best" approach can frequently be controversial. The authors' philosophy is to employ the method that is associated with the least surgical morbidity in order to achieve a successful outcome, which has led them to utilize an arthroscopic approach for the majority of these injuries in recent years. Open surgery involves extensive soft tissue dissection which could lead to capsular scarring, joint stiffness, and further impair the already tenuous vascular supply to the scaphoid and intrinsic ligaments. Arthroscopic treatment of such injuries, when combined with intraoperative fluoroscopy, offers a more precise alternative to assist with anatomic reduction and enable percutaneous fixation. Although technically challenging, once mastered, an arthroscopic approach can offer a favorable alternative to the traditional open treatment of this condition.

References

[1] Mayfield JK, Johnson RP, Kilcoyne RK. Carpal dislocations: pathomechanics and progressive perilunar instability. J Hand Surg Am. 1980; 5(3):226–241

[2] Johnson RP. The acutely injured wrist and its residuals. Clin Orthop Relat Res. 1980(149):33–44

[3] Herzberg G. Perilunate and axial carpal dislocations and fracture-dislocations. J Hand Surg Am. 2008; 33(9):1659–1668

[4] Herzberg G. Acute dorsal trans-scaphoid perilunate dislocations: open reduction and internal fixation. Tech Hand Up Extrem Surg. 2000; 4(1):2–13

[5] Herzberg G, Comtet JJ, Linscheid RL, Amadio PC, Cooney WP, Stalder J. Perilunate dislocations and fracture-dislocations: a multicenter study. J Hand Surg Am. 1993; 18(5):768–779

[6] Weil WM, Slade JF, III, Trumble TE. Open and arthroscopic treatment of perilunate injuries. Clin Orthop Relat Res. 2006; 445(445):120–132

[7] Cooney WP, Bussey R, Dobyns JH, Linscheid RL. Difficult wrist fractures. Perilunate fracture-dislocations of the wrist. Clin Orthop Relat Res. 1987(214):136–147

[8] Herzberg G, Forissier D. Acute dorsal trans-scaphoid perilunate fracture-dislocations: medium-term results. J Hand Surg [Br]. 2002; 27(6):498–502

[9] Budoff JE. Treatment of acute lunate and perilunate dislocations. J Hand Surg Am. 2008; 33(8):1424–1432

[10] Trumble T, Verheyden J. Treatment of isolated perilunate and lunate dislocations with combined dorsal and volar approach and intraosseous cerclage wire. J Hand Surg Am. 2004; 29(3):412–417

[11] Knoll VD, Allan C, Trumble TE. Trans-scaphoid perilunate fracture dislocations: results of screw fixation of the scaphoid and lunotriquetral repair with a dorsal approach. J Hand Surg Am. 2005; 30(6):1145–1152

[12] Forli A, Courvoisier A, Wimsey S, Corcella D, Moutet F. Perilunate dislocations and transscaphoid perilunate fracture-dislocations: a retrospective study with minimum ten-year follow-up. J Hand Surg Am. 2010; 35(1):62–68

[13] Kremer T, Wendt M, Riedel K, Sauerbier M, Germann G, Bickert B. Open reduction for perilunate injuries: clinical outcome and patient satisfaction. J Hand Surg Am. 2010; 35(10):1599–1606

[14] Souer JS, Rutgers M, Andermahr J, Jupiter JB, Ring D. Perilunate fracture-dislocations of the wrist: comparison of temporary screw versus K-wire fixation. J Hand Surg Am. 2007; 32(3):318–325

[15] Adkison JW, Chapman MW. Treatment of acute lunate and perilunate dislocations. Clin Orthop Relat Res. 1982(164):199–207

24

[16] Apergis E, Maris J, Theodoratos G, Pavlakis D, Antoniou N. Perilunate dislocations and fracture-dislocations. Closed and early open reduction compared in 28 cases. Acta Orthop Scand Suppl. 1997; 275:55–59

[17] Najarian R, Nourbakhsh A, Capo J, Tan V. Perilunate injuries. Hand (N Y). 2011; 6(1):1–7

[18] Moran SL, Ford KS, Wulf CA, Cooney WP. Outcomes of dorsal capsulodesis and tenodesis for treatment of scapholunate instability. J Hand Surg Am. 2006; 31(9):1438–1446

[19] Liu B, Chen SL, Zhu J, Tian GL. Arthroscopic management of perilunate injuries. Hand Clin. 2017; 33(4):709–715

[20] Park MJ, Ahn JH. Arthroscopically assisted reduction and percutaneous fixation of dorsal perilunate dislocations and fracture-dislocations. Arthroscopy. 2005; 21(9):1153

[21] Wong TC, Ip FK. Minimally invasive management of trans-scaphoid perilunate fracture-dislocations. Hand Surg. 2008; 13(3):159–165

[22] Kim JP, Lee JS, Park MJ. Arthroscopic reduction and percutaneous fixation of perilunate dislocations and fracture-dislocations. Arthroscopy. 2012; 28(2):196–203.e2

[23] Liu B, Chen SL, Zhu J, Wang ZX, Shen J. Arthroscopically assisted mini-invasive management of perilunate dislocations. J Wrist Surg. 2015; 4(2):93–100

[24] Herzberg G, Burnier M, Marc A, Merlini L, Izem Y. The role of arthroscopy for treatment of perilunate injuries. J Wrist Surg. 2015; 4(2):101–109

[25] Kim JP, Lee JS, Park MJ. Arthroscopic treatment of perilunate dislocations and fracture dislocations. J Wrist Surg. 2015; 4(2):81–87

[26] Wahegaonkar AL, Mathoulin CL. Arthroscopic dorsal capsulo-ligamentous repair in the treatment of chronic scapho-lunate ligament tears. J Wrist Surg. 2013; 2(2):141–148

[27] Mathoulin C. Treatment of dynamic scapholunate instability dissociation: contribution of arthroscopy. Hand Surg Rehabil. 2016; 35(6):377–392

V

25 Perilunate Injuries Non-Dislocated

Guillaume Herzberg, Marion Burnier, and Lyliane Ly

Abstract

Perilunate injury non-dislocated (PLIND) is a recently recognized pattern of spontaneously reduced perilunate dislocations and fracture-dislocations (PLDs-PLFDs). The injury pattern is characteristic of PLD-PLFD but there is no dislocation of the capitate from the lunate on the initial lateral radiographs because it was spontaneously reduced. PLIND is easily missed which implies that one may be faced with an acute or chronic form of this tricky injury. The purpose of this chapter is to provide practical examples of acute and chronic types of PLIND along with the key diagnostic role of arthroscopy in each case. Through clinical examples, the diagnostic issues of this rare but severe injury are emphasized.

Keywords: wrist trauma, perilunate dislocations, PLIND

25.1 Introduction

Perilunate dislocations and fracture-dislocations (PLDs-PLFDs) are high-energy traumatic injuries to the wrist localized at the midcarpal joint and proximal carpal row.

They consist of a combination of wrist ligaments (intrinsic and extrinsic) tears with or without associated carpal bones fractures producing a midcarpal dislocation allowed by a double rent into the proximal row on each side of the lunate. Indeed, it is impossible for a trauma to produce a dorsal or volar midcarpal dislocation without a double dissociation of the proximal row.

PLD and PLFD create an acute major dissociative destabilization of the carpal construct.

Their main defining feature is a dorsal dislocation of the head of the capitate from the distal facet of the lunate. The dislocation occurs dorsally in more than 90% of the cases but may occur palmarly.[1,3]

A typical dorsal PLD is a pure extrinsic and intrinsic wrist ligamentous midcarpal and proximal row injury which creates not only a dorsal dislocation of the capitolunate joint but also a combination of scapholunate and lunotriquetral dissociation.

A typical dorsal PLFD is a combined osseous and ligamentous midcarpal and proximal row injury which creates not only a dorsal dislocation of the capitolunate joint but also a markedly displaced scaphoid fracture and a lunotriquetral dissociation.

PLD and PLFD present as a myriad of variants and pathology associations. Despite the major extent of the injury, PLD-PLFD may be missed at the acute stage, especially in polytrauma patients, producing chronic unreduced cases. In the past up to 25% of PLDs-PLFDs were reported to be missed at the acute stage. Nowadays, one can estimate that less than 2% are missed at the acute stage in developed countries because the main clue to PLD-PLFD using lateral standard initial radiograph (which shows the capitate dislocated from the lunate and sometimes the lunate itself dislocated volarly) is rarely missed.

The degrees of displacements (i.e., amount of dislocation) of PLD-PLFD may also vary to a great extent. The possibility of spontaneously reduced PLD-PLFD was first quoted by Green and O'Brien.[4] Moreover several papers reported chronic[5,7] then acute[8] combinations of scapholunate and lunotriquetral dissociations (double rent into the proximal row on each side of the lunate) not associated with capitolunate joint disruptions.

In 2013, the authors described the perilunate injury non-dislocated (PLIND), a new entity gathering all equivalent, spontaneously reduced PLD-PLFD, whether these variants are pure ligamentous or osseous and ligamentous.[8,9] The floating lunate described by Badia[5] was classified as a pure ligamentous PLIND.

If PLD-PLFD can be missed at the acute stage, it is not surprising that PLIND may be easily missed, leading to major posttraumatic carpal disorders. This is why the authors emphasized PLIND clinical clues (high-energy wrist trauma in young individuals similar to accidents producing PLD-PLFD), radiological clues (midcarpal chip fractures on the initial posteroanterior [PA] radiographs), and the usefulness of wrist arthroscopy for the diagnosis of PLIND.[5,10]

The purpose of this chapter is to show four didactic examples of acute and chronic ligamentous/osteoligamentous PLIND in which wrist arthroscopy was key as a final diagnosis tool.

25.2 Acute PLIND Cases

Acute pure ligamentous PLIND case (▶ Fig. 25.1): This 26-year-old man sustained a high-energy car accident and was seen in our emergency department with a combination of fracture of the radial diaphysis of the right dominant forearm and a high suspicion of PLIND injury. After standard open reduction internal fixation (ORIF) of the radial diaphysis, an arthroscopy was performed. Wrist arthroscopy confirmed a pure ligamentous PLIND (▶ Fig. 25.1) which was surgically fixed like a dorsal perilunate dislocation.

Acute transscaphoid PLIND case (▶ Fig. 25.2): This 20-year-old male sustained a high-energy fall while playing soccer and was seen in our emergency department with a high suspicion of transscaphoid PLIND injury in his right dominant wrist. An arthroscopy was performed. Wrist arthroscopy confirmed a transscaphoid PLIND (▶ Fig. 25.2)

V

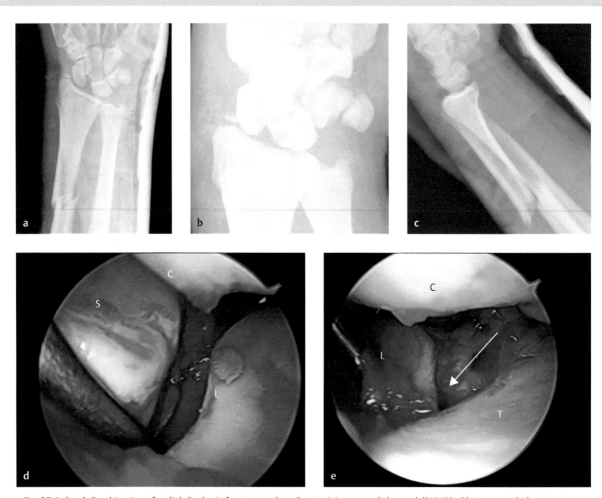

Fig. 25.1 (a–c) Combination of radial diaphysis fracture and perilunate injury non-dislocated (PLIND). Obvious scapholunate dissociation and radial styloid chip fracture and suspicion of lunotriquetral dissociation. Yet there is no capitolunate dislocation. **(d,e)** A complete scapholunate dissociation was confirmed at arthroscopy as well as a complete lunotriquetral dissociation (*white arrow*) confirming an acute pure ligamentous PLIND that could be treated at the acute stage like a perilunate dislocation. C, capitate; L, lunate; S, scaphoid.

which was surgically fixed like a dorsal transscaphoid perilunate dislocation.

25.3 Chronic PLIND Cases

Chronic missed pure ligamentous PLIND case (▶ Fig. 25.3): This 45-year-old right-handed male sustained a high-energy car accident (steering wheel) with significant left wrist pain that was left untreated. The patient was referred 4 months later with incapacitating radial dorsal wrist pain (VAS 7/10), wrist flexion/extension 50/50 degrees, and 45% grip strength compared with normal contralateral side. An arthroscopy was performed. Wrist arthroscopy confirmed a pure ligamentous chronic missed PLIND (▶ Fig. 25.3).

Chronic transscaphoid PLIND case (▶ Fig. 25.4): This 43-year-old male sustained a high-energy fall while falling off a bike with significant left wrist pain that was left untreated. The patient was referred 7 months later with

incapacitating radial dorsal wrist pain (VAS 6/10), wrist flexion/extension 70/70 degrees, and 60% grip strength compared with normal contralateral side. An arthroscopy was performed. Wrist arthroscopy confirmed a chronic missed transscaphoid PLIND (▶ Fig. 25.4).

25.4 Discussion

Clinical examples of acute and chronic missed perilunate injuries where the capitate had spontaneously reduced after dislocation. All cases exhibited features of a "perilunate-like" coronal path of injury.

These PLD-PLFD variants can be classified as a PLIND and included in a perilunate injuries classification[8] which covers both dislocated and spontaneously reduced PLD-PLFD. The concept of PLIND lesions is consistent with lesser arc, greater arc, and translunate types of perilunate injuries.

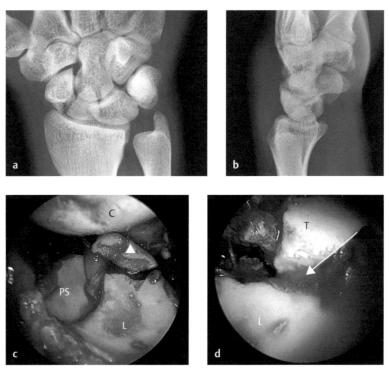

Fig. 25.2 (a, b) Obvious widely displaced waist scaphoid fracture with a high suspicion of trans-scaphoid perilunate injury non-dislocated (PLIND) injury. There is no capitolunate dislocation. **(c,d)** A displaced fracture of the volar lip of the lunate along with a complete lunotriquetral dissociation (*white arrow*) confirming an acute transscaphoid PLIND that could be treated at the acute stage like a dorsal transscaphoid perilunate dislocation. C, capitate; L, lunate; PS, proximal scaphoid; T, triquetrum; *white triangle*, volar rim fracture of the lunate.

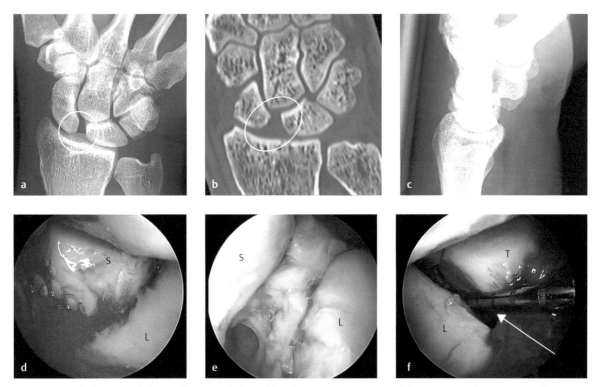

Fig. 25.3 (a–c) Obvious scapholunate dissociation (*white circle*) and suspicion of lunotriquetral dissociation. Yet there is no capitolunate dislocation. **(d–f)** Complete scapholunate dissociation was confirmed at arthroscopy as well as a complete lunotriquetral dissociation (*white arrow*) confirming a chronic pure ligamentous perilunate injury non-dislocated (PLIND). C, capitate; L, lunate; S, scaphoid; T, triquetrum.

25

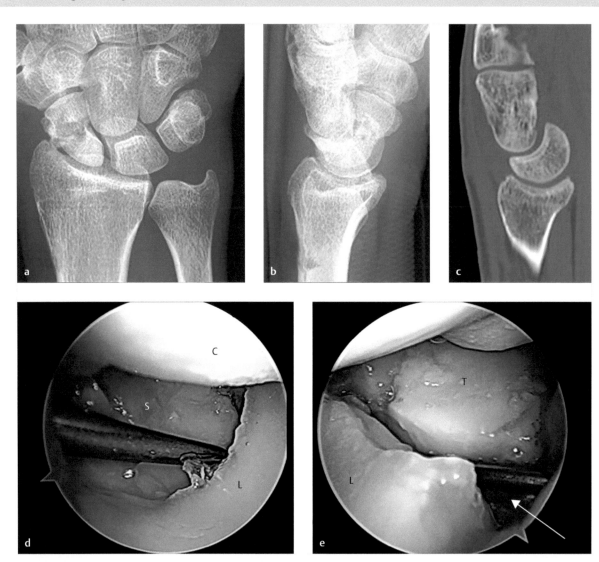

Fig. 25.4 (a–c) Obvious widely displaced waist scaphoid nonunion with a marked dorsal intercalated segment instability (DISI) of the lunate. **(d,e)** A complete lunotriquetral dissociation (*white arrow*) confirming a chronic missed transscaphoid perilunate injury nondislocated (PLIND). C, capitate; L, lunate; S, scaphoid; T, triquetrum.

Spontaneously reduced PLD or PLFD have been previously described as isolated entities in the literature.

Pin et al[7] were the first to describe eight cases showing chronic coincident ruptures of scapholunate and lunotriquetral ligaments without perilunate dislocation.

Badia described 13 cases of "floating lunate" (12 chronic, 1 acute) where complete scapholunate and lunotriquetral dissociations were demonstrated.[5,11] These are examples of pure ligamentous PLIND lesions.

Bain et al[12] described the translunate type of wrist injury. They described a subcategory of translunate injuries (subluxation group) where there was no true dislocation of the capitate from the fractured lunate. The authors believe that translunate injuries of the subluxation group should be considered as PLIND injuries.

Chee et al[6] described a chronic perilunate injury treated by trispiral tenodesis that is consistent with a chronic PLIND lesion that was missed at the acute stage.

The authors described 11 cases of acute PLIND injuries, 10 osseous and ligamentous, and 1 purely ligamentous.[8]

It is very important to recognize PLIND injuries at the acute stage in order to be able to provide a perilunate dislocation treatment and obtain a good clinical and radiological results as in most modern PLD-PLFD series.

The diagnostic and therapeutic issues raised by these cases are similar to those of classic acute PLDs-PLFDs but the diagnosis at the acute stage is even more difficult.

The common features of an acute PLIND lesion include a history of high-energy trauma combined with the physical findings of marked wrist swelling and diffuse wrist

V

tenderness that is suggestive of a more global injury. This clinical presentation requires a high index of suspicion of PLIND injury and demands further investigation.

The primarily common radiographic feature would be a coronal perilunate-type path of injury on the PA view. There would be no dislocation of the capitate from the lunate in the sagittal plane. This would be a secondary feature that would differentiate a "dislocated" perilunate injury from an equivalent PLIND lesion. A good clue is the presence of midcarpal osteochondral loose bodies. The use of arthroscopy is the preferred method to confirm the diagnosis of a PLIND lesion.

References

[1] Apergis E, Maris J, Theodoratos G, Pavlakis D, Antoniou N. Perilunate dislocations and fracture-dislocations. Closed and early open reduction compared in 28 cases. Acta Orthop Scand Suppl. 1997; 275 suppl 275:55–59

[2] Jones DB, Jr, Kakar S. Perilunate dislocations and fracture dislocations. J Hand Surg Am. 2012; 37(10):2168–2173, quiz 2174

[3] van der Oest MJW, Duraku LS, Artan M, et al. Perilunate injury timing and treatment options: a systematic review. J Wrist Surg. 2021; 11 (2):164–176

[4] Green DP, O'Brien ET. Open reduction of carpal dislocations: indications and operative techniques. J Hand Surg Am. 1978; 3(3): 250–265

[5] Badia A, Khanchandani P. The floating lunate: arthroscopic treatment of simultaneous complete tears of the scapholunate and lunotriquetral ligaments. Hand (N Y). 2009; 4(3):250–255

[6] Chee KG, Chin AYH, Chew EM, Garcia-Elias M. Antipronation spiral tenodesis: a surgical technique for the treatment of perilunate instability. JHSA. 2012; 37:2611–2618

[7] Pin PG, Nowak M, Logan SE, Young VL, Gilula LA, Weeks PM. Coincident rupture of the scapholunate and lunotriquetral ligaments without perilunate dislocation: pathomechanics and management. J Hand Surg Am. 1990; 15(1):110–119

[8] Herzberg G. Perilunate injuries, non dislocated (PLIND). J Wrist Surg. 2013; 2(4):337–345

[9] Herzberg G, Cievet-Bonfils M, Burnier M. Arthroscopic treatment of translunate perilunate injury non dislocated (PLIND). J Wrist Surg. 2019; 8(2):143–146

[10] Corella F, Del Cerro M, Ocampos M, Larrainzar-Garijo R. The rocking chair sign for floating lunate. J Hand Surg Am. 2015; 40(11):2318–2319

[11] Yassa R, Syed MA, Smith A. Atraumatic dislocation of the lunate: floating lunate syndrome. J Hand Surg Eur Vol. 2013; 38(5):559–560

[12] Bain GI, Pallapati S, Eng K. Translunate perilunate injuries-a spectrum of this uncommon injury. J Wrist Surg. 2013; 2(1):63–68

25

26 Axial Carpal Dislocations and Fracture Dislocations

Alex Lluch, Ana Scott-Tennent, Mireia Esplugas, and Marc Garcia-Elias

Abstract

Axial carpal injuries are rare but severe lesions that occur after high-energy trauma, in which an axially oriented disruption in the carpometacarpal joint and distal carpal row occurs. Although the dislocations are most of the time in a radial or ulnar pattern, other injury combinations are possible. These are frequently open injuries with a great variety of associated soft tissue lesions and always require surgical treatment. Debridement, anatomical reduction, stable fixation, and early management of associated lesions are key points for surgery. Long-term outcomes are seldom excellent, mainly due to the functional impairment of the hand caused by the soft tissue lesions. Decreased range of motion is to be expected in the wrist.

Keywords: carpal bones, axial carpal dislocation, fracture dislocation, axial carpal injuries.

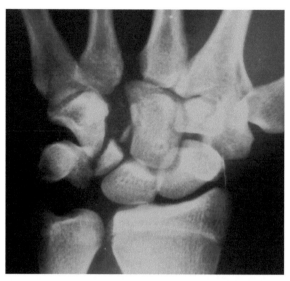

Fig. 26.1 Example of axial ulnar fracture-dislocation. The radial column is aligned and stable with the radius, whereas the ulnar column is ulnarly and proximally displaced. The injury pathway crosses the joint between the base of the third and fourth metacarpals, capitate and hamate with an avulsion fragment, and extends proximally through the triquetrum in a "trans" way.

26.1 Introduction

Axial carpal dislocations (ACDs) and fracture-dislocations are complex instabilities in which the carpometacarpal joint, the distal carpal row, and, sometimes, the proximal row longitudinally disrupt. As the primary injury pattern is parallel to the longitudinal axis of the wrist and forearm, both "axial dislocation" and "longitudinal disruption" are appropriate terms to describe these lesions. ACD is a rare type of carpal dislocation, with an incidence of 1.1 to 2%.[1,2] In the majority of cases, the wrist splits into two columns, one remaining normally aligned with the radius and the other shifting in a radial or ulnar direction, with the metacarpal bones following their corresponding carpal bones (▶ Fig. 26.1).

26.1.1 Mechanism of Injury

When axially seen the carpus resembles an arch, with the flexor retinaculum and some extrinsic ligaments at its base, and the capitate acting as a keystone in the center of the arch. Only an intense load can affect the weakest points of the structure, as it happens to any bridge.[3] Thus, due to the amount of force required to axially disrupt the carpus, an ACD occurs mostly after high-energy injuries and is frequently associated with extensive soft tissue trauma.[1,2]

The classically described mechanism of injury is not only a high-energy dorsopalmar compression (crush), twist, or blast to the wrist,[3,4] but also a true axial force that can produce an axial injury pattern.[2] Combined axial ulnar-radial injuries may need two or more consecutive injury mechanisms to occur.[5] Most of the time ACD is the result of industrial accidents, related to unsafe use of the press, wringer, or roller machinery.[4] The resulting axial force transmits through the intermetacarpal space, distal and proximal carpal rows. If the traumatic energy is parallel to the intercarpal joints, it will go around the carpal bones in a "peri" manner, often leading to dislocation. Obliquely directed forces may lead to dislocation with associated sagittal plane fractures in a "trans" way.

In a compression mechanism, the flexor retinaculum is always disrupted or avulsed from its lateral insertions, creating a traumatic decompression of the carpal tunnel. Also a flattering of the carpal and metacarpal arches appears, secondary to the ligamentous injury and associated bony lesions[3,4] (▶ Fig. 26.2, ▶ Fig. 26.3, ▶ Fig. 26.4, ▶ Fig. 26.5).

26.1.2 Historical Perspective and Classification

Axial ulnar dislocations were first described by Oberst in 1901, but it was not until 1985 that Garcia-Elias et al identified two weak areas in the ulnar side of the wrist and defined the axial ulnar injury pattern.[6] A new revision by Garcia-Elias et al in 1989 expanded the classification and, based on plain radiographs, defined three major groups of ACD that described the displaced, unstable

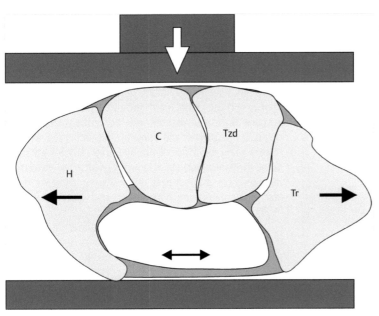

Fig. 26.2 A crush mechanism means that the palmar concavity of the carpus is involved in a high-energy dorsopalmar compression.

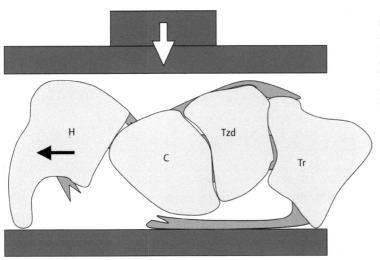

Fig. 26.3 If the compressive or axial force affects mainly the ulnar side of the wrist, the ligaments stabilizing the ulnar column will disrupt or the hamate or triquetrum will break. The flexor retinaculum will also be disrupted or avulsed from its insertions, and the carpal arches will flatten.

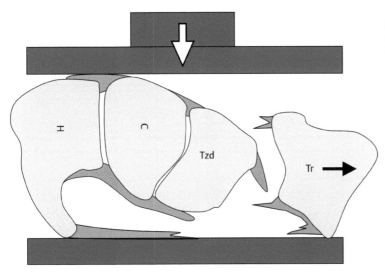

Fig. 26.4 As in ▶ Fig. 26.3, the forces can affect the radial side of the distal carpus and destabilize the radial column.

26

column of the carpus: (1) axial ulnar, (2) axial radial, and (3) combined or mixed axial ulnar-radial.[1] Axial ulnar

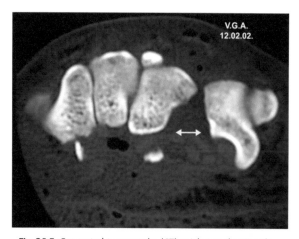

Fig. 26.5 Computed tomography (CT) axial view showing the injury pathway between capitate and hamate, and the avulsion fracture in the insertion of the flexor retinaculum in the triquetrum in a case of an ulnar axial lesion.

and axial radial injuries have a similar incidence in the largest published patient cohort (46% vs 54%[2]).

In *axial ulnar injuries*, the carpus splits into two columns, with the radial column aligned and stable with respect to the radius and the ulnar column unstable and displaced, usually proximally and ulnarly. In *axial radial injuries*, on the other hand, the ulnar part of the carpus remains normally aligned and the radial aspect of the carpus is displaced and unstable. In this type of ACD, attrition and exposure of the first web muscles are common. In *axial ulnar-radial injuries*, which are extremely rare, only the central part of the carpus remains stable and components of both ulnar and radial coexist[5,7] (▶ Fig. 26.6, ▶ Fig. 26.7).

The most common types of axial ulnar injuries are transhamate peripisiform, perihamate peripisiform, and perihamate transtriquetrum, whereas the most common axial ulnar-radial injuries are peritrapezoid peritrapezium, peritrapezium, and transtrapezium (▶ Fig. 26.8). Among all of them, transhamate peripisiform and transtrapezium are the most frequent patterns in each group.[2] The association of axial dislocations and perilunate injuries has been described.[8,10]

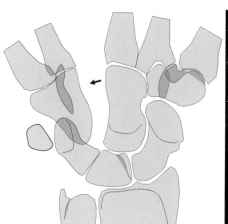
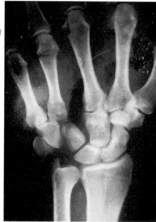

Fig. 26.6 Schematic representation of a perihamate peripisiform ulnar axial lesion, and the corresponding posteroanterior (PA) view in a plain X-ray.

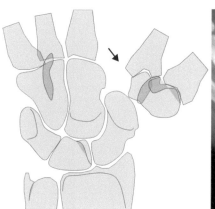
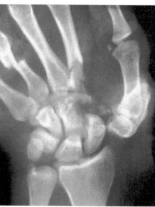

Fig. 26.7 Schematic representation of a peritrapezoid peritrapezium radial axial lesion, and the corresponding posteroanterior (PA) view in a plain X-ray.

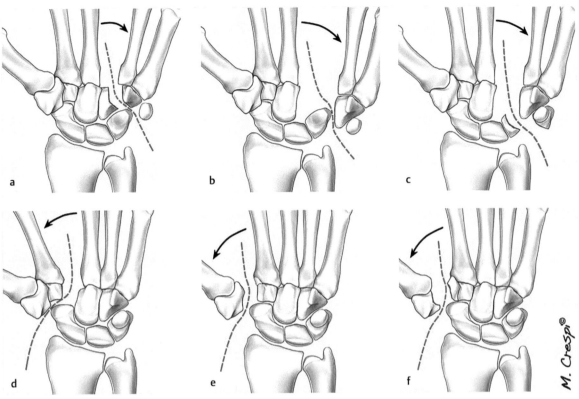

Fig. 26.8 The most common types of axial dislocations and fracture-dislocations. (1) Axial ulnar dislocations: **(a)** transhamate peripisiform, **(b)** perihamate peripisiform, and **(c)** perihamate transtriquetrum. (2) Axial radial dislocations: **(d)** peritrapezoid peritrapezium, **(e)** peritrapezium, and **(f)** transtrapezium. (Adapted with permission from Garcia-Elias M, Dobyns JH, Cooney WP, Linscheid RL. Traumatic axial dislocations of the carpus. J Hand Surg Am. 1989;14(3):446–457[1].)

26.2 Indications and Contraindications for Surgery

Axial carpal injuries need surgical treatment, without any room for conservative options. In general terms, ACDs have to be considered an emergency, especially if they present as an open injury. Only cases without displacement, reduced, partially treated and without vascular injury, severe swelling, and no risk of compartment syndrome may be treated with some delay.[5,10]

26.3 Literature Review and Different Surgical Treatment

Surgical repair should address all the components of the injury path within the carpus and the associated soft tissue injuries. Initial radiographic evaluation should include standard radiographs (posteroanterior [PA], lateral, and oblique). In order to fully understand the lesion pathway, dynamic views or fluoroscopic exam (frequently under anesthesia) are helpful. Computed tomography (CT) is extremely useful and recommended, especially in cases of axial ulnar-radial injuries.[3,5]

From the literature review and the authors' experience, treatment of ACD can be standardized.[3,4,8] After clearly defining the carpal injury, the neurovascular, muscular, and tendinous injuries and the potential risk for compartment syndrome should be assessed. Extending the existing traumatic wounds, and through a palmar (and dorsal if needed) approach, debridement of nonviable tissue is the first step. Fasciotomies of the forearm and hand are then performed if required. At that point, the authors prefer to continue with an open reduction and fixation of the carpal injuries using a dorsal approach, in order to have a stable and well-aligned wrist when performing the repair of nerves, vessels, tendons, or soft tissue coverage that may be needed. Closed reduction and percutaneous pinning, although possible, may not end with an anatomical reduction due to soft tissue interposition.[11]

Once anatomically reduced, the intermetacarpal joints and the distal carpal row are fixed with Kirschner wires, unless there are fractures that can be fixed with screws. Repair of the damaged intermetacarpal ligaments and intercarpal ligamentous structures of the distal carpal row is not necessary[4,8,11] (▶ Fig. 26.9, ▶ Fig. 26.10, ▶ Fig. 26.11, ▶ Fig. 26.12, ▶ Fig. 26.13, ▶ Fig. 26.14). However, if the injury extends to the proximal carpal row, repair of the

26

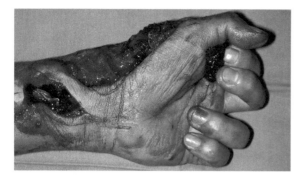

Fig. 26.9 Clinical aspect of a patient's hand and wrist who suffered an industrial accident with an injector machine. Thenar muscles are protruding through the first web and there's an evident divergence in the long fingers.

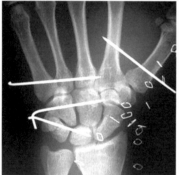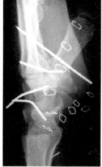

Fig. 26.11 The carpal lesion was treated with an open reduction and fixation with Kirschner wires. A K-wire was used to maintain the first web open. Nowadays, if the surgeon has enough arthroscopic skills, an axial lesion like this case can be treated with arthroscopic support as in the case shown in Video 26.1.

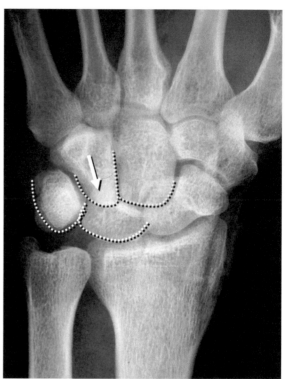

Fig. 26.10 Posteroanterior (PA) view of the patient from ▶ Fig. 26.9. Longitudinal disruption in the ulnar aspect, at the level of the carpometacarpal (CMC) joint, distal and proximal row in a perihamate peritriquetrum manner, which is not a common path for an axial ulnar injury. *Dotted lines* show the proximal contour of hamate, capitate, triquetrum, and lunate. Computed tomography (CT) scan from this patient is shown in ▶ Fig. 26.5.

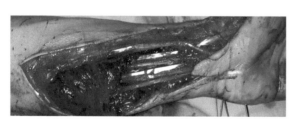

Fig. 26.12 After wrist stabilization, debridement of nonviable soft tissues is mandatory. Primary treatment of associated lesions is highly recommended.

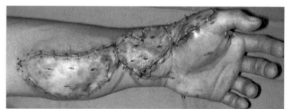

Fig. 26.13 In this case, skin loss didn't affect any critical zone for motion or there was no tendinous or neurovascular exposure, so a skin graft was used for coverage.

intercarpal ligaments is needed.[8] Proximal row carpectomy has also been described in the acute setting in complex injuries in which repair of proximal row injuries has not been possible.[9]

In closed injuries without important soft tissue involvement whose treatment can be delayed, and especially if the ACD is associated with a proximal row injury,

arthroscopically assisted reduction and fixation is a less invasive option that can prevent some scar formation (Video 26.1).

All damaged soft tissue structures should then be repaired or grafted primarily. Skin loss resulting from initial trauma or debridement needs to be grafted or covered with local or distant flaps. Although the flexor retinaculum is often injured already, in case of doubt, inspection of the carpal tunnel is recommended.[4] Interestingly, in

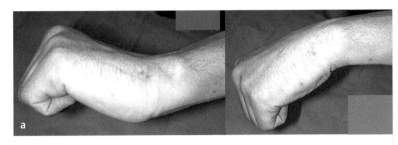

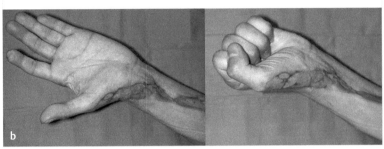

Fig. 26.14 (a,b) Clinical long-term result. Limited wrist flexion and extension, as expected in this type of lesion. Good finger motion and no sensory impairment is crucial for a good functional result. (With gratitude to Dr. Alberto Pérez; Valdivia, Chile.)

the largest clinical cohort from the 1980s,[1] the incidence of nerve injuries was higher (10/16 patients) than in the largest cohort from the 1990s and first decade of this century (3/37 patients), with only one case requiring nerve repair. Free flaps and fasciotomies were also more frequently performed.[2]

In general, patients suffering from an ACD shouldn't be expected to have an excellent outcome. Of the 37 patients in the Mayo Clinic series, 20 experienced a poor outcome, 14 had a satisfactory outcome, and only 3 had a good outcome, with no patient with an excellent outcome. Factors associated with poorer outcomes seem to be axial radial patterns of injury, probably because of involvement of the thumb column, the extent of soft tissue injury, and the ability to achieve normal carpal anatomy.[1,2,8]

26.4 Essential Rehabilitation Points

The heterogeneity of injury patterns and associated lesions in ACD doesn't allow to standardize a postoperative rehabilitation treatment. Due to the extensive damage, these injuries usually require long periods of wrist immobilization. As an example, the 37 patients from the Mayo Clinic cohort were immobilized for 63 days on average.[2]

Rehabilitation should be focused on early recovery of finger motion, decreasing swelling, and allowing gentle wrist motion as soon as possible. In these lesions, due to carpal damage, a restricted range of motion is more likely to happen than residual wrist instability. The functional result is many times conditioned by the associated lesions, and reoperations are not infrequent.

26.5 Conclusion

Axial carpal injuries are uncommon lesions produced by high-energy mechanisms and are frequently associated with a variety of soft tissue injuries. Understanding the affected carpal structures, restoring the normal anatomy, and proper and early treatment of associated injuries are the key points for treatment.

References

[1] Garcia-Elias M, Dobyns JH, Cooney WP, III, Linscheid RL. Traumatic axial dislocations of the carpus. J Hand Surg Am. 1989; 14(3):446–457

[2] Shannon SF, Boe CC, Shin AY. Comparison of outcomes between axial radial and axial ulnar carpal injuries. J Hand Surg Eur Vol. 2018; 43 (7):712–717

[3] Reinsmith LE, Garcia-Elias M, Gilula LA. Traumatic axial dislocation injuries of the wrist. Radiology. 2013; 267(3):680–689

[4] Garcia-Elias M, Lluch AL. Wrist instabilities, misalignments and dislocations. In: Wolfe SW, Hotchkiss RN, Pederson WC, et al, eds. Green's operative hand surgery, 7th ed. Vol. 1. Philadelphia, PA: Elsevier; 2017:418–478

[5] López-Cervantes RE, García-Elias M, Soto IB. Divergent axial carpal dislocation and its pathomechanics. J Wrist Surg. 2018; 7(3):253–257

[6] Garcia-Elias M, Abancó J, Salvador E, Sanchez R. Crush injury of the carpus. J Bone Joint Surg Br. 1985; 67(2):286–289

[7] Freeland AE, Rojas SL. Traumatic combined radial and ulnar axial wrist dislocation. Orthopedics. 2001; 24(12):1161–1163

[8] Herzberg G. Perilunate and axial carpal dislocations and fracture-dislocations. J Hand Surg Am. 2008; 33(9):1659–1668

[9] Gvozdenovic R, Nielsen NS, Garcia-Elias M. Combined perilunate and axial ulnar dislocation of the wrist. J Wrist Surg. 2012; 1(2):173–176

[10] Khurana S, Chen Z, Dowdle J. Perihamate-peripisiform-transtriquetrum axial ulnar fracture dislocation of the hand with an associated perilunate injury. J Hand Surg Am. 2018; 43(3):292.e1–292.e6

[11] Grabow RJ, Catalano L, III. Carpal dislocations. Hand Clin. 2006; 22(4): 485–500, abstract vi–vii

26

27 Classification and Treatment of Nondissociative Proximal Row Instability

Andrea Atzei, Riccardo Luchetti, Pedro J. Delgado, and Carlos Heras-Palou

Abstract

The clunking wrist has puzzled both patients and surgeons for a long time. Midcarpal instability is not instability of the midcarpal joint, but instability of the proximal row of the carpus as one block, without dissociation between scaphoid, lunate, and triquetrum.

A better name is nondissociative proximal row instability. This is constituted by a group of different conditions where the proximal row suddenly jumps into extension, or into flexion or both, as it loses its normal alignment or as it reduces its normal alignment.

Nondissociative carpal instabilities are a broad spectrum of poorly understood disorders. Proper understanding is complicated by confusing nomenclature and poor evidence due to paucity of cases. The authors describe the mechanics, staging, clinical presentation, investigation, and treatment of this group of conditions.

The management of these conditions includes conservative measures like muscle and proprioception retraining, soft tissue procedures where tendons or ligaments are used to provide stability, and bony operations, mainly partial arthrodesis.

Keywords: nondissociative proximal row instability, carpal instability, midcarpal instability, clunking wrist, proximal carpal row, treatment, classification, assessment

27.1 Introduction and Historical Perspective

The nondissociative instability of the wrist includes a group of carpal dysfunctions whose key feature is represented by the integrity of the bones and interosseous ligaments of the proximal carpal row (PCR).[1]

It is also referred to as carpal instability nondissociative (CIND).[2] In the CIND wrist, the scaphoid, lunate, and triquetrum move like one unit (the "intercalated segment" of the carpus), but not in a predictable, smooth manner, and may become malaligned, or even subluxate, relative to the radius and/or to the distal row.[1] According to the different tilting of the "intercalated segment" as seen on lateral views of the wrist, the instability pattern was divided into dorsal CIND (CIND-DISI), volar CIND (CIND-VISI), or a combination of both (combined-CIND).[2] In a further attempt to clarify the different subtypes of CIND according to the location of the kinematic abnormalities, three main patterns were identified: radiocarpal, midcarpal, and combined radiocarpal-midcarpal.

Radiocarpal instability (RCI) is defined when the entire carpus subluxates in relation to the radius. Commonly, RCI is referred to as carpal translocation (CTx). It may occur in any direction: palmar, dorsal, and most frequently in the ulnar direction.[3] Before the improvements in the medical treatment of the rheumatoid arthritis, CTx was a common condition for the rheumatoid wrist. However, currently it is a less common condition in the clinical practice.

In 1981, the publication by Lichtman and colleagues[4] helped raise awareness of midcarpal instability (MCI). Since then, the term "MCI" has been echoed in numerous publications as the most common form of CIND, although this name is rather misleading. Indeed, the term "MCI" appears to focus specifically on the kinematic dysfunction of the midcarpal joint only, assuming that radiocarpal kinematics remain unaffected. However, essentially the PCR tilts relative to both the radius and the distal carpal row and this implies that the dysfunction occurs at both the radiocarpal and midcarpal joint.[5] This observation was confirmed by biomechanical and clinical studies which found that the actual pattern of MCI results from the ligamentous disruption at both radiocarpal and midcarpal level.[6,15] Thus, these findings contradict the definition proposed by Lichtman et al[4] of MCI as an isolated midcarpal dysfunction. In fact, this definition refers to kinematic models of combined radiocarpal-midcarpal instability (CRMI) or instability of the proximal row as one block.

The lack of understanding of pathomechanics has added confusion to the misunderstanding of the definition proposed by Lichtman et al.[4] Therefore, early authors labelled several conditions as separate clinical entities, although in reality they were only describing some different aspects of MCI, such as snapping wrist,[16] capitate-lunate instability pattern (CLIP),[17] medial anterior midcarpal instability (MAMI),[18] chronic capitolunate instability (CCI),[19] localized medial triquetral-hamate instability (LMTHI),[20] and clunking wrist.[6] In order to minimize confusion around the definition of CIND and MCI, which are currently often used interchangeably, recent publications[11,15] propose the use of the definition of proximal row instability (PRI) to define the different subtypes of CIND, as suggested in the early publication by Wright et al.[2]

Consequently, the definition of MCI proper, i.e., isolated dysfunction of the midcarpal joint, should be reserved for the wrist with incompetent midcarpal ligaments after radiocarpal fusion or hemi-implant arthroplasty[10,15] or for those even more uncommon conditions (of mild CLIP or CCI) in which stress maneuvers can dislocate only the capitate dorsally from the lunate (while the proximal row still maintains normal alignment). Although the discussion on semantics and pathomechanics of CIND is still open,[21] it seems that the term "PRI" has the advantage of limiting the redundancy of the numerous kinematic and clinical scenarios and allows to assemble all CIND patterns, except CTx, into a single definition.

This chapter aims to provide an update on the different types of nondissociative instability of the PCR, which will be unified under the definition of PRI, and summarize the authors' recommendations on the treatment of the different subtypes.

27.2 Kinematic Dysfunction of the Unstable Proximal Row

During most activities of daily living, the wrist moves along an oblique plane, rotating from an extended-radial deviated position to a flexed-ulnar deviated position. This motion is referred to as the "dart-throwing" motion (DTM).[22] A number of laboratory and in vivo studies demonstrated that, during the DTM, the lunate shows no or minimal movement, as carpal rotation develops almost exclusively at the midcarpal joint.[23,24] Conversely, the PCR is subject to gross rotational forces during radioulnar deviations in the frontal plane and, more remarkably, when the wrist moves along the so-called "reversed dart-throwing" plane of motion, i.e., from an extended-ulnar deviated position to a flexed-radial deviated position. Therefore, PRI develops when the wrist moves either in the frontal plane of motion or along the "reverse-DTM." In order to facilitate the understanding of the carpal

dysfunction occurring in PRI, it is easier to consider PCR kinematics in the frontal plane of motion only, thus avoiding the more complicated analysis of the composite motions that produce along the oblique planes of movement (▶ Fig. 27.1). When a normal wrist moves from radial to ulnar deviation, the PRC moves smoothly from flexion to extension. In maximal radial deviation, the PCR is flexed due to compressive forces acting on the scaphoid-trapezium-trapezoid joint.[25] Inversely, in maximal ulnar deviation, compression forces on the helicoidally shaped triquetrohamate (TH) joint generate the extension moment to the PCR.[26] In PRI the smooth transition of the carpus during radioulnar deviation is lost. The PCR remains in a flexed position until extreme ulnar deviation. Then, the entire PCR suddenly reduces into the extended final position, taking the distal row with it. Classically, this abrupt reduction of carpal alignment is associated with a painful thud, known as the catch-up clunk[25] that can be seen and heard. The locked position assumed by the PCR in radial deviation and the pattern of the reduction of the distal row may vary according to three major patterns of carpal clunking,[5,9] which are described as follows[6]:

- *Anterior midcarpal clunking:* The PRC remains tilted into flexion (VISI) until near the end of ulnar deviation, when it suddenly rotates into extension, producing the typical "catch-up clunk."[27,28] This pattern is considered distinctive of the condition described by Lichtman as palmar midcarpal instability.[4,29]
- *Posterior midcarpal clunking:* The PCR is normally aligned, or slightly extended (DISI), in most wrist positions. PCR hyperextension is generated by the dorsal dislocation of the capitate over the edge of the

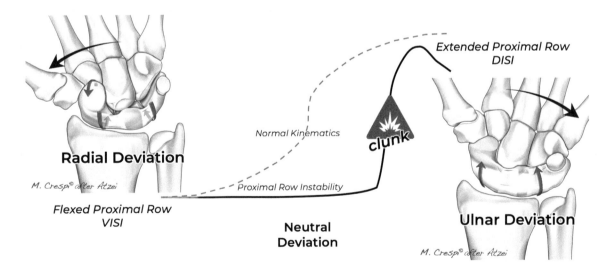

Fig. 27.1 Diagram demonstrating wrist motion on the frontal plane (radial and ulnar deviations) in normal conditions and in proximal row instability (PRI). When a normal wrist (*interrupted line*) moves from radial to ulnar deviation, the proximal carpal row moves smoothly from flexion (volar intercalated segment instability [VISI] posture) to extension (dorsal intercalated segment instability [DISI] posture). In PRI (*continuous line*), the smooth transition of the carpus during radioulnar deviation is lost, producing the catchup clunk.

scapholunate socket. The more the wrist deviates ulnarwards, the more the capitate displaces dorsally, the more the PCR extends. As an end result, PCR hyperextension triggers a protective contraction of extensor carpi ulnaris (ECU) and extensor carpi radialis longus and brevis (ECRL and ECRB) muscles, so that the distal row abruptly returns to its normal alignment, often with an audible clunk. This pattern was described as the typical finding of the CLIP wrists described by Louis et al[17] and of the CCI described by Johnson and Carrera.[19]

- *Combined radiocarpal-midcarpal clunking:* This pattern of clunking is similar to the anterior midcarpal clunking, but an increased mobility at the radiocarpal joint is associated. Thus, in full radial deviation the PCR shows an abnormal flexion (VISI) and ulnar translocation. Then, ulnar deviation produces abnormal extension of the PCR with capitate dorsal subluxation. This pattern is common among young patients with hyperlax radioulnocarpal ligaments, particularly those with an increased frontal slope of the distal articular surface of the radius and ulnar minus.[30,31] It is worth asking the patients about generalized joint laxity, examine the patient for laxity in other joints, since this can be a presentation of Ehlers-Danlos syndrome. According to the appearance of the locked position assumed by the PCR in the lateral X-ray views, the instability pattern is divided into dorsal (D-PRI) and volar (V-PRI).

Evidence is scarce on what structures may be injured in order to cause loss of the smooth and progressive transition of the PCR from flexion to extension during radioulnar deviations. Garcia-Elias[6] suggested that at least five ligamentous complexes are involved: (1) triquetrum-capitate-hamate ligament, also known as "ulnar arm of the palmar arcuate ligament (UAL)"[32]; (2) scaphotrapezio-trapezoid (STT) ligaments and radioscaphocapitate (RSC) ligaments; (3) dorsal radiocarpal (DRC) ligament, also known as the dorsal radiotriquetral ligament; (4) dorsal intercarpal (DIC) ligament and especially its deepest and most proximal portion connecting the scaphoid to the triquetrum, i.e., the dorsal scaphotriquetral (STq) ligament; (5) palmar radiolunate (RL) and ulnolunate ligaments, including specifically, the long radiolunate (LRL) ligament and the ulnocarpal ligament complex (UCLC). (▶ Fig. 27.2). Early studies attempting to illustrate the genesis of PRI considered only the kinematic dysfunction of the midcarpal joint. Only recently, the importance of the ligaments spanning the radiocarpal joint was given due attention. Deficiency of the UAL was considered the key in the "oval ring" pathoanatomical model proposed by Lichtman et al.[4] PRI, especially in the form of palmar MCI (or V-PRI), was considered as the result of the disruption of the "ulnar mobile link" of the wrist at the midcarpal level, i.e., the UAL. On the other hand, the oval ring

concept considers the disruption of the radial side of the ring (viz. following scaphoid fracture, scapholunate dissociation, etc.) as the cause of scapho-lunate-capitate complex instabilities.[4] This pathoanatomical model was investigated by other studies that confirmed the role of UAL in the development of (V-)PRI, although these were not able to fully replicate the carpal dysfunction.[33,34] Conversely, the division of the DRC ligament was essential to lock the PCR in VISI during ulnar deviation[33] and to produce a static VISI deformity.[34] More recently, animated computer-generated three-dimensional models of the wrist showed that the ligamentous connections between triquetrum and hamate are not isometric constraints, but rather loose bindings.[35,36] The lack of a fixed link between triquetrum and hamate confirms the works of Moritomo et al,[37,38] suggesting the ovoid pattern of motion at the midcarpal joint. Shiga et al[10] showed in a biomechanical study that, along with the UAL and the DRC ligament, the STT ligament complex need to be divided in order to replicate the V-PRI pattern.

The role of the STT ligament complex in PRI is not well understood. As a major stabilizer of the scaphoid, the STT ligament complex stabilizes the whole PCR to the distal row, provided the intercarpal ligaments are preserved.[39] Thus, it acts as a ligamentous restraint to both V-PRI and D-PRI.[40] The distal part of the RSC ligament, i.e., the scaphocapitate (SC) ligament, acts as an accessory STT collateral ligament. When tensioned, it extends and supinates the scaphoid. If these ligaments are insufficient, or torn, the scaphoid remains flexed.[6,11] The DIC ligament plays a twofold role, as a stabilizer of both the PCR and the distal row. The DIC ligament insertions on the scaphoid and mostly on the lunate prevent hyperextension of the PCR. Biomechanical studies in scapholunate-deficient wrists show that lunate extension occurs only after division of the insertions of the DIC ligament on the lunate.[40] Similarly, on a series of posttraumatic PRI, avulsion of the scapholunate attachments of the DIC caused hyperextension of the PCR and the development of D-PRI.[15] Yet, the most proximal portion of the DIC ligament, i.e., the STq ligament, prevents dorsal dislocation of the distal row. Spanning from the scaphoid to the triquetrum, the STq ligament acts as a labrum that increases the depth of the scapholunate socket, thus preventing dorsal dislocation of the capitate over the hyperextended PCR.[41] Albeit often underestimated, the LRL ligament plays an important role as a restraint to lunate extension.[42] The division of the LRL ligament produces significant lunate extension in the cadaveric scapholunate-deficient wrist[40]; however, its contribution in the generation of V-PRI, and particularly of the combined radiocarpal–midcarpal clunking, is not yet fully understood. To the best of our knowledge, the role of the UCLC in the development of PRI has never been studied thoroughly. The UCLC originates from the volar band of the TFCC and is formed by the ulnocapitate, ulnotriquetral, and ulnolunate ligaments. Since its ulnar

Volar Proximal Row Instability

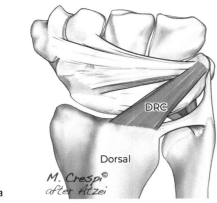
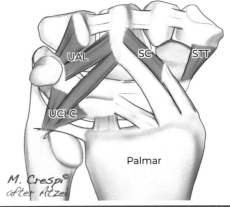

Dorsal Proximal Row Instability

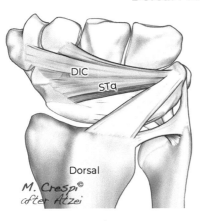
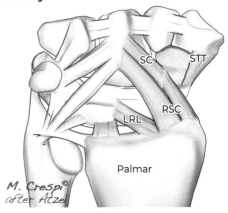

Fig. 27.2 Diagram demonstrating wrist ligaments involved in the volar **(a)** and dorsal **(b)** proximal row instability (PRI) from a palmar and dorsal perspective. DIC, dorsal intercarpal ligament; DRC, dorsal radiocarpal; LRL, long radiolunate ligament; RSC, radioscaphocapitate ligaments; STq, scaphotriquetral ligament; STT, scaphotrapeziotrapezoid ligaments; UAL, ulnar arm of the palmar arcuate ligament; UCLC, ulnocarpal ligament complex.

insertions are eccentric from the center of forearm rotation (fovea), the fascicles of the UCLC are tensioned with radial extension of the wrist and with forearm supination,[43] and are relaxed in ulnar flexion and pronation. The UCLC restrains palmar displacement of the PCR[44] and its rupture may be responsible for the development of ulnocarpal supination deformity, as classically seen with rheumatoid arthritis.[45] Furthermore, the possible contribution of the UCLC in PRI may be inferred by the observation that the clunking occurs and/or is exacerbated in forearm pronation (which decreases UCLC tautness), and limited in forearm supination (which increases UCLC tautness). Arthroscopic reports have confirmed the flabby appearance of the UCLC in those patients showing V-PRI with significant carpal supination.[46] The combination of laboratory studies, analysis of computationally derived models of carpal motion,[47] and clinical observations of PRI (developmental and posttraumatic) has permitted development of a comprehensive approach to the stabilizers of the intercalated segment, which was described by Wolfe as the "mooring lines" concept.[15,48] According to this concept, just as mooring lines secure a vessel in a stable position, while allowing adaptation to the forces of waves, wind, and currents, the ligaments inserting onto the PCR offer stability without sacrificing mobility (▶ Fig. 27.3). We propose that the ligamentous restraints to V-PRI (CIND-VISI) are dorsal at the radiocarpal joint (DRC) and volar at the midcarpal joint (UAL and STT ligaments). Conversely, the ligamentous restraints to D-PRI (CIND-DISI) are dorsal at the midcarpal joint (DIC) and volar at the radiocarpal joint (LRL ligament). In addition, the STT, RSC, and UCLC provide further support to the global stability of the wrist.

27

V

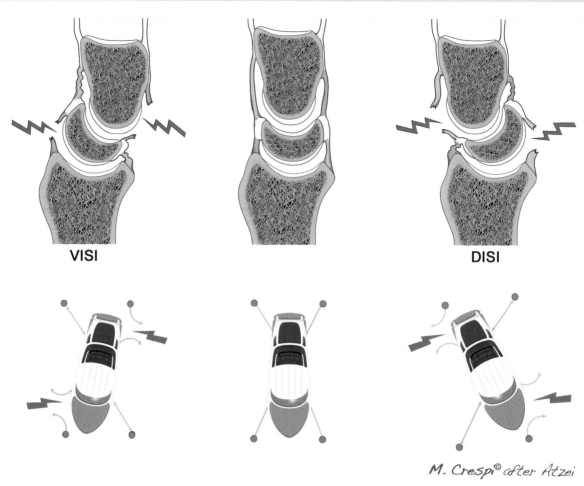

M. Crespi© after Atzei

Fig. 27.3 Diagram demonstrating the "mooring lines" concept according to Wolfe.[15,48] The ligamentous restraints to V-PRI (*green*) are dorsal at the radiocarpal joint and volar at the midcarpal joint. Conversely, the ligamentous restraints to D-PRI (*yellow*) are dorsal at the midcarpal joint and volar at the radiocarpal joint.

27.3 Classification of Proximal Row Instability

Based on recent laboratory and clinical findings, the use of the concept of PRI is a reasonable option to avoid confusion arising from the use of CIND and MCI. An updated PRI classification should highlight carpal dysfunction patterns and where possible provide a correlation with the pathoanatomy (▶ Table 27.1; ▶ Fig. 27.4). Previous classifications of MCI included the definition of "extrinsic midcarpal instability (EMCI)" to indicate some adaptative patterns, whose etiology was secondary to posttraumatic bone deformation (commonly a distal radius malunion). However, this definition may generate some equivocation with those PRI patterns secondary to the injury of "extrinsic ligaments of the PCR." Actually, since the carpal malalignment is secondary to bone abnormalities outside the carpus, the pattern of EMCI falls within the definitions of the general category of "carpal instabilities adaptive" (CIA), as classically described by the Mayo Clinic classification of carpal instabilities,[49] and it cannot be considered as a subtype of (primary) PRI. The increasing number of posttraumatic case reports has prompted a differentiation between nontraumatic (congenital or developmental) PRI and posttraumatic PRI.[15] According to the direction of dislocation of the PCR, also evidenced by the PCR posture in the lateral view of plain radiographs, the VISI and DISI subtypes are recognized. The VISI subtype of PRI (V-PRI) is the most common form. V-PRI is further divided according to the location of the ligamentous damage at the midcarpal joint. When the STT and the RSC ligaments are involved, the radial-sided V-PRI (V-R-PRI) subtype is defined. Instead, when the UAL is attenuated on the ulnar midcarpal joint, the ulnar-sided V-PRI (V-U-PRI) subtype is defined. Less frequently, a combined pattern of PRI may be present in hyperlax wrists or following high-energy traumatic injuries.

▶ Table 27.1 summarizes the subtypes of PRI correlating with the definitions from the previous classification.

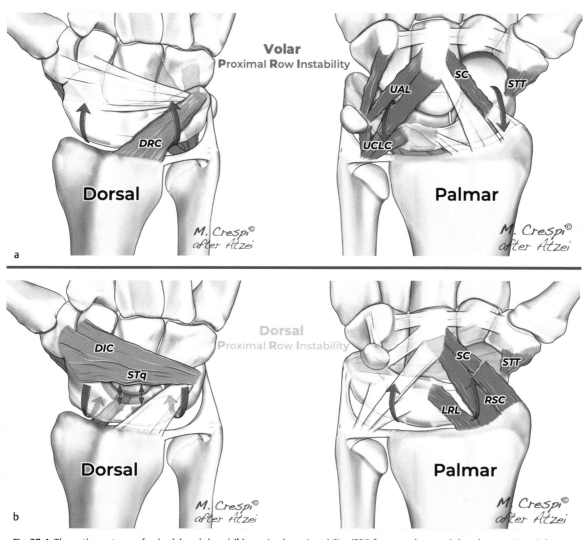

Fig. 27.4 The pathoanatomy of volar **(a)** and dorsal **(b)** proximal row instability (PRI) from a palmar and dorsal perspective. Palmar damaged ligaments are colored in green; dorsal damaged ligaments are colored in purple. DIC, dorsal intercarpal ligament; DRC, dorsal radiocarpal; LRL, long radiolunate ligament; STq, dorsal scaphotriquetral ligament; STT, scaphotrapeziotrapezoid ligament; UAL, ulnar arm of the palmar arcuate ligament; UCLC, ulnocarpal ligament complex.

Description of the ligaments involved and the clinical presentation of each subtype is also provided.

27.4 Clinical Presentation of Proximal Row Instability

Clinical presentation of patients with PRI varies from vague ulnar-sided exertional wrist pain, quickly relieved with rest, to a debilitating painful subluxation during activities requiring radioulnar deviation.[50,52] Ulnar-sided wrist pain is generally associated to a clunk, which sometimes patients can demonstrate voluntarily "to the amusement of friends, and consternation of doctors."[53] Patients report an insidious onset, often after immobilization for a trivial injury or no trauma. In the latter case, they report being normal until they perform repetitive loading activities of the wrist, thus starting to experience pain and instability which increases with muscle fatigue. This presentation is typical for developmental PRI patients, who are not aware that they suffer from some form of congenital laxity or ligamentous attenuation. PRI becomes obvious following the loss of muscular control either after prolonged immobilization or with muscular fatigue. More recently, a growing number of cases of posttraumatic PRI have been described—following fall from standing height or sports/road accident that apply a rotational axial force onto the outstretched hand.[14,15,54,55] PRI may also appear after intra-articular distal radius[14,55] and scaphoid fracture,[15] in which bone morphology is still preserved (therefore they cannot be considered as an adaptative PRI).

27

Table 27.1 The definition of proximal row instability (PRI) is used to define the different subtypes of carpal instability nondissociative (CIND), according to Mayo Clinic Classification of carpal instability

	Subtypes			Ligaments involved	Previous definitions	
RCI, radiocarpal instability	*Palmar* *Dorsal* *Ulnar (carpal translocation [CTx])*			*Palmar and/or dorsal radiocarpal ligaments*		
MCI, midcarpal instability	*Palmar* *Dorsal* *Ulnar*			*Palmar and/or dorsal midcarpal ligaments*	*CLIP or CCI (mild clinical forms)*	
CRMI, combined radiocarpal-midcarpal instability **PRI, proximal row instability**	Developmental/ Posttraumatic	**VISI** alignment	Ulnar sided	**Dorsal Lig.** *DRC	Palmar MCI[4]	Snapping wrist[16] Anterior medial midcarpal instability (MAMI)[18]
			V-U-PRI	**Palmar Lig.** [^UAL] *UCLC		
		V-PRI	Radial sided	**Dorsal Lig.** *DRC	Anterior midcarpal clunking[6]	Anterolateral midcarpal instability (ALMI)[6]
			V-R-PRI	**Palmar Lig.** ^STT ^SC *UCLC		
		DISI Alignment		**Dorsal Lig.** ^DIC	Dorsal MCI[4] Posterior midcarpal clunking[6] Capitate-lunate instability pattern (CLIP)[17] Chronic capitolunate instability (CCI)[19]	
		D-PRI		**Palmar Lig.** *LRL. *RSC [*UCLC]		
		Combined PRI		*Combination of Palmar and/or Dorsal Radiocarpal and/or Midcarpal Lig*	Combined MCI[4] Combined radiocarpal-midcarpal clunking[6]	

*Indicates a ligament of the radioulnocarpal joint.
^Indicates a ligament of the midcarpal joint.
Abbreviations: DIC, dorsal intercarpal ligament; DISI, dorsal intercalated segment instability; DRC, dorsal radiocarpal; LRL, long radiolunate ligament; RSC, radioscaphocapitate ligaments; SC, scapholunate; STT, scaphotrapeziotrapezoid ligaments; UAL, ulnar arm of the palmar arcuate ligament; UCLC, ulnocarpal ligament complex; VISI, volar intercalated segment stability.
Note: A correlation with the pathoanatomy and previous classifications of midcarpal instability is provided.

27.4.1 Physical Examination

Examination findings depend on the subtypes and severity of PRI. In V-U-PRI, pain is located on the dorsoulnar aspect of the wrist, generally at the TH joint and can be aggravated by palpation. In some forms of V-R-PRI, pain occurs over the scaphoid. Traumatic avulsion of the DRC from the triquetrum may be tender at palpation over the dorsum of the triquetrum. Patients may show an apparent prominent ulnar head, which is actually related to the volar sag of the wrist (▶ Fig. 27.5). This is related to a volar translocation of the ulnar column of the wrist, producing also carpal supination, and is confirmed by an increased pisostyloid distance, compared to the contralateral wrist[50] (▶ Fig. 27.6). A dorsally directed force applied on the pisiform, correcting the volar sag, may alleviate the pain by supporting the volar ulnar side of the wrist and also reducing carpal supination[50] (▶ Fig. 27.7). When the force is discontinued, the wrist moves back into carpal supination, with or without a clunk.[52] Beighton's hypermobility test may be used to assess generalized ligamental laxity.[50,54] Radioulnar ballottement test may be performed and compared on contralateral side to exclude distal radioulnar joint instability.[56] Wrist range of motion is usually normal. Patients may spontaneously reproduce the catch-up clunk on wrist ulnar deviation, which is often audible to the examiner. The midcarpal shift test (MCST), described

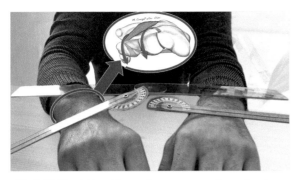

Fig. 27.5 The right wrist may show an apparent prominent ulnar head, which is actually related to carpal supination and the volar sag, as depicted in the artist's drawing.

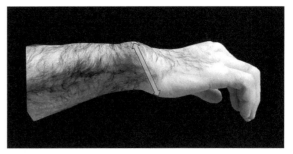

Fig. 27.6 Measurement of pisostyloid distance, according to Ho et al.[50]

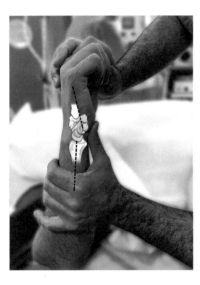

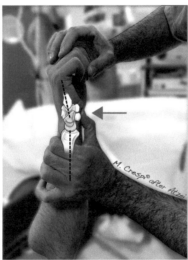

Fig. 27.7 The volar sag is corrected by applying a dorsally directed force on the pisiform, supporting the volar ulnar side of the wrist and also reducing flexion of the proximal carpal row and carpal supination. When the force is discontinued, the wrist moves back into carpal supination, with or without a clunk.

by Lichtman and Wroten,[5] is the specific provocative maneuver to elicit findings of V-PRI.

To perform the MCST on a right wrist, the examiner uses the left hand to stabilize the subject's forearm in a pronated position. The examiner then takes the subject's right hand with his right hand and positions his thumb over the dorsal distal capitate region of the patient's wrist. He then exerts a palmarly directed force onto the subject's wrist, allowing the carpus to translate palmarly. The wrist is then ulnarly deviated while maintaining palmarly directed pressure. As the wrist is ulnarly deviated, there is a clunking as the wrist approaches full ulnar deviation. Hand positions are switched when the contralateral hand is examined. The test is positive if it recreates the catch-up clunk and patient's symptoms. The test is also confirmed if the clunk is eliminated when the test is repeated while pressing the pisiform in a dorsal direction.[2,52] Symptoms can also be elicited with simple axial wrist loading during radial to ulnar deviation. In this test, the patient's forearm is pronated and the examiner applies an axial load on the patient's wrist, while moving it

from radial to ulnar deviation. The test is positive if clunk is felt when the wrist is ulnarly deviated.[57] The MCST and the carpal loading test may be positive also in normal patients with no wrist problems; however, in the absence of pain, these tests should not be considered pathologic. Grading the severity of the clinical presentation of PRI remains a challenging task. Lichtman et al[58] proposed a score system based on the findings of the MCST (▶ Table 27.2). The score ranges from Grade I to V, indicating greater laxity around the PCR. The higher grade corresponds to the greater amount of palmar translation of the PCR produced by the examiner's thumb pressure over the dorsal capitate as well as to the greater amount of ulnar deviation required to reproduce the catch-up clunk. Grade V is assigned to individuals who can spontaneously reproduce the painful clunk without assistance from the examiner. This self-induced clunking differentiates Grade V from Grade IV. Quantitative assessment of the MCST showed that ulnar deviation required to reproduce the clunk ranges from about 35 degrees to 40 degrees from Grade I to III, with some overlapping for

27

Grade III and IV. Due to these small differences, fine assessment using the MCST is rather subjective and highly dependent on the skills of the examiner.[52,58] Based on the combination of clinical presentation and the radiographic assessment of VISI deformity on lateral views at rest, Hargreaves[51] introduced a classification system of V-PRI including presymptomatic, dynamic, and static grades and relative subtypes (► Table 27.3) and proposing options of management for each grade. However, this system does not take into account the amount of pain and functional loss. Therefore, subjective functional questionnaires, such as the Disabilities of the Arm, Shoulder, and Hand (DASH) and Patient-Rated Wrist Evaluation (PRWE), may also be used in conjunction. Mason and Hargreaves[59] also proposed to infer a subjective measure of instability from the ability to pour a kettle, or pour water from a jar. They categorized patients into five groups (never; rarely; sometimes; often; always), according to the frequency of symptoms occurring while pouring. The provocative test to assess D-PRI are performed under fluoroscopy. According to the original description of the capitolunate (CL) instability pattern, the most common form of D-PRI,[17] the wrist is placed under fluoroscopy in a slightly flexed position and a dorsally directed pressure is put on the scaphoid tubercle while using longitudinal traction. Fluoroscopy permits to identify the dorsal subluxation of the capitate from the lunate, as well as the DISI malalignment of the PCR. Similar radiographic findings were described by Johnson and Carrera[19] related to what they called the CCI. Clinical assessment should always include provocative maneuvers to exclude lunotriquetral (LT) dissociation, which is the more common pathology to mimic PRI symptoms and dysfunction. Kleinman's "LT shear test"[60] is the easier way to assess instability of the LT joint. The test is said to be positive when dorsal loading of the pisiform with the thumb, while the dorsal aspect of the lunate is stabilized with one finger, reproduces patient's pain or discomfort and causes joint hypermobility.

27.4.2 Advanced Investigations

Clinical history and examination remain the gold standard[61]; however, advanced investigations, such as imaging and arthroscopy, are recommended to implement the diagnostic work-up of PRI. Imaging is not usually helpful in confirming a diagnosis of PRI.[51,62] Plain X-rays are generally normal. A static VISI deformity is indicative of V-PRI (► Fig. 27.8). DISI deformity can be demonstrated in D-PRI (► Fig. 27.9).[52,54,63] In posttraumatic cases a chip fracture of the dorsum of the triquetrum may be evident, suggesting a fracture avulsion of the DRC from the triquetrum.

Table 27.2 Lichtman's grading for midcarpal laxity (modified)

Grade	Palmar midcarpal translation	Amount of ulnar deviation required to reproduce the clunk
I	None	None; no true clunk
II	Minimal	Minimal
III	Moderate	Moderate
IV	Maximal	Significant
V	Self-induced	Self-induced

Note: For clarity, rightmost column description was changed from just "clunk" to specify that it refers to the amount of ulnar deviation required to reproduce the clunk.

Table 27.3 Hargreaves' grading system for palmar midcarpal instability, i.e., V-PRI

Grade	Definition	Description
0	Presymptomatic	No symptoms of instability but able to perform voluntary catch-up clunk Patient at risk of symptoms
1	Dynamic	Symptoms of giving way Symptoms reproduced with a positive MCST No voluntary clunk or sag
2	Voluntary dynamic	Symptomatic giving way with voluntary subluxation (ulnar sag sign or voluntarily performed catch-up clunk)
3	Static reducible	VISI deformity on lateral X-ray at rest Deformity easily reducible on manipulation
4	Static irreducible	Fixed VISI deformity on lateral X-ray Not easily reducible Locked

Abbreviations: DASH, disabilities of the arm, shoulder, and hand; MCST, midcarpal shift test; VISI, volar intercalated segment instability; V-PRI, volar proximal row instability.
Note: Separate assessment of pain and functional loss using the DASH questionnaire is recommended.

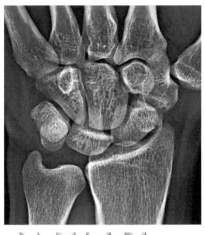
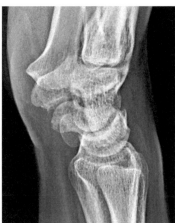

Fig. 27.8 A static volar intercalated segment instability (VISI) deformity is indicative of volar proximal row instability (V-PRI). On plain X-rays and artist's rendering, the posteroanterior (PA) view shows intact Gilula's arcs. The lateral view shows lunate and scaphoid flexion with preserved scapholunate angle.

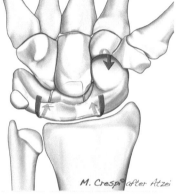
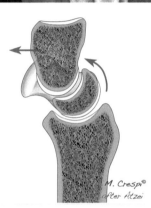

As plain X-rays portray a static view of the carpal bones at rest, radiographic findings, such as the values of CL, RL, and LT angles, should be expected normal in true PRI. In these cases, only stress view radiographs (possibly performed with patient's muscular relaxation) may show pathological values of various carpal angles, which infer some carpal "malalignment" (a more appropriate definition to be used instead of "instability"). Subsequently, when pathological values of these angles are measured on plain X-rays, as it occurs in most severe cases of PRI, they actually suggest the degree of PCR "subluxation/dislocation," other than "instability" proper. The "open mouth sign," described by Garcia-Elias,[6] consists in a subtle opening of the STT joint (▶ Fig. 27.10), which can be seen on radially deviated posteroanterior (PA) view, is helpful to rule out V-R-PRI caused by insufficiency of the ST ligaments. Video fluoroscopy in different planes enables dynamic assessment of PRI. It may illustrate the pathognomonic catch-up clunk and volar carpal sag.[9] Newer imaging techniques, including four-dimensional CT-scans or 3 T magnetic resonance imaging (MRI), have been introduced as promising noninvasive methods to investigate carpal alignment and kinematics.[64] However, so far, their role is limited to the exclusion of other wrist pathologies, which could cause similar symptoms that can be quite difficult to differentiate from those of PRI. If a VISI deformity is noted,

it is important to exclude other more common causes, such as LT dissociation. Yet, even more advanced imaging is of limited help in differentiating between LT instability and V-PRI. Diagnostic arthroscopy is crucial as it permits direct visualization and probing of intrinsic and extrinsic ligaments and rules out other intra-articular pathologies.[65] Wrist arthroscopy is the gold standard for the assessment of intra-articular disorders. In PRI, arthroscopy is recommended to exclude LT dissociation and other pathology as well as to assess the quality of the joint surfaces before reconstructive surgery. Usually joint inspection is not difficult to perform, as the joint spaces are generally quite spacious, due to the laxity of the joint. The 1–2 and 6-R portals are recommended for the inspection of the radiocarpal joint. The use of the 1–2 portal prevents additional damage of the DRC and is very helpful for the evaluation of the DRC, clearly visible along its entire length. Thorough radiocarpal exploration through the 1–2 portal is facilitated by the widened joint space. MCR and MCU portals are used for midcarpal exploration. Sometimes synovitis may make joint exploration difficult, especially on the dorsal aspect of both the radiocarpal and midcarpal joints and over the ulnocarpal ligaments in the prestyloid area of the radiocarpal joint. In long-standing cases, some degenerative changes of the cartilage of the proximal lunate or the proximal hamate may be found.

27

V

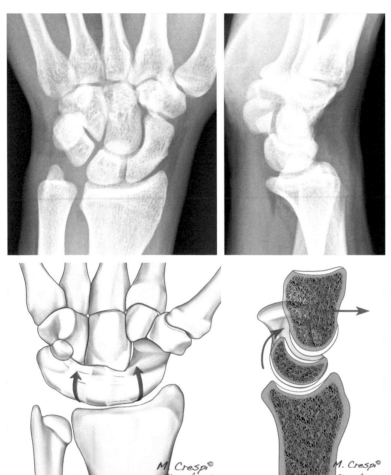

Fig. 27.9 A static dorsal intercalated segment instability (DISI) deformity is indicative of dorsal proximal row instability (D-PRI). On plain X-rays and artist's rendering, the posteroanterior (PA) view shows intact Gilula's arcs. The lateral view shows lunate and scaphoid extension with preserved scapholunate angle.

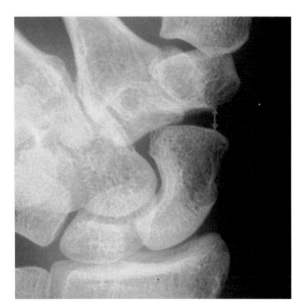

Fig. 27.10 The "open mouth sign" consists in the widening of the scaphotrapeziotrapezoid (STT) joint (arrow), when the wrist is forcedly ulnarly deviated. (Reproduced with permission from Garcia-Elias M. The non-dissociative clunking wrist: a personal view. J Hand Surg Eur Vol. 2008;33(06):698–711.[6])

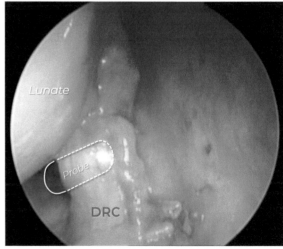

Fig. 27.11 Arthroscopy reveals a prominent and slack dorsal radiocarpal (DRC).

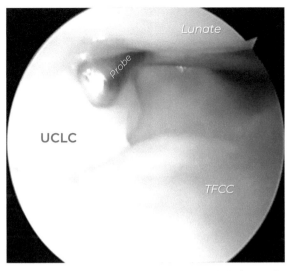

Fig. 27.12 Arthroscopy reveals a prominent and slack ulnocarpal ligament complex (UCLC).

In the radiocarpal joint, usually synovectomy reveals a prominent and slack DRC (▶ Fig. 27.11).[46] The UCLC may also appear relaxed and free-floating when probed (▶ Fig. 27.12). In the midcarpal joint, the ulnar palmar surface of the midcarpal joint, and particularly the UAL, generally shows a normal appearance. Thus, no obvious widening of the TH interval can be detected. Probing shows normal tension of the TH ligament. Widening of the STT joint space and ST ligament laxity are difficult to detect. It may be present in most severe PRI.

▶ Table 27.4 summarizes the subtypes of PRI correlating with the clinical and radiographic findings.

27.5 Options of Treatment for Proximal Row Instability

Management of PRI includes conservative methods and surgical procedures. Most cases of developmental PRI respond to conservative treatment. Indications for treatment

Table 27.4 Correlation of the different subtypes of proximal row instability (PRI) with the pathoanatomy and clinical and radiographic findings

PRI, proximal row instability					
Categories		Developmental/Posttraumatic			
Subtypes		VISI alignment V-PRI		DISI alignment D-PRI	Combined VISI/DISI alignment C-PRI
		Ulnar sided V-U-PRI	Radial sided V-R-PRI		
Ligaments involved	Dorsal ligament	*DRC		^DIC	Combination of palmar and/or dorsal radio- and/or midcarpal ligaments
	Palmar ligament	[^UAL] *UCLC	^STT ^SC *UCLC	*LRL *RSC [*UCLC]	
Pain location		Dorsal TH area	Palmar periscaphoid area	Vague Mostly dorsal-central	Vague Mostly dorsal
Clinical findings		Clunking in UD along reverse DTM Palmar sag Positive "palmar passive displacement" test Positive midcarpal shift test		Positive "dorsal passive displacement" test	Clunking in UD along reverse DTM Palmar sag Positive palmar and dorsal passive displacement test
Radiographs		VISI		DISI/Neutral	Variable VISI/DISI or even neutral
Fluoroscopy		Catch-up of the PCR in UD (from flexion to extension)		Passive dorsal displacement of capitate at CL-j	Hypermobile PCR Catch-up of the PCR Passive dorsal displacement of capitate
		[widening of TH-j in RD]	widening of STT-j in UD	Capitate relocates from extreme UD toward neutral	

*Indicates a ligament of the radioulnocarpal joint.
^Indicates a ligament of the midcarpal joint.
Abbreviations: DIC, dorsal intercarpal ligament; DISI, dorsal intercalated segment instability; DRC, dorsal radiocarpal ligament; DTM, "dart-throwing" motion; LRL, long radiolunate ligament; PCR, proximal carpal row; RD, radial deviation; RSC, radioscaphocapitate ligaments; SC, scapholunate; STT, scaphotrapeziotrapezoid ligaments; STT-j, scaphotrapeziotrapezoid joint; TH-j, triquetrohamate joint; UAL, ulnar arm of the palmar arcuate ligament; UCLC, ulnocarpal ligament complex; UD, ulnar deviation; VISI, volar intercalated segment stability.

27

are based on clinical grading. Hargreaves' grading system[51] is suitable for this purpose (▶ Table 27.3). Surgery is usually reserved for posttraumatic PRI or Stage 3 (Static Reducible) developmental PRI, refractory to conservative measures, and in Stage 4 (Static Irreducible) PRI. Aim of surgical procedures is to stabilize the PCR by means of soft tissue procedure or limited carpal fusions (LCFs). Soft tissue procedures permit to preserve a greater arc of motion than LCF, and are largely preferred by the patient. However, LCFs are generally more reliable and can be performed when soft tissue stabilization fails. Numerous techniques have been described, but long-term data are lacking. Recently, Jing and coworkers[61] published a comprehensive review of the currently available literature. Based on the authors' personal experience, the following strategy of treatment is recommended.

27.5.1 Treatment of Volar Proximal Row Instability (V-PRI)

Neuromuscular rehabilitation with proprioceptive exercises and muscular strengthening is particularly effective in V-PRI. A minimum 3-month rehabilitation program is recommended in all cases of developmental V-PRI, regardless of the clinical severity and radiographic appearance. The program includes activity modification, improvement of ergonomics at the workplace, and patient general education on how to minimize clunking. Passive reduction of the PCR may be achieved with the ulnar-boost splint, which uses a three-point dynamic design acting on the pisotriquetral unit. It pushes dorsally the pisiform and applies a volar-directed pressure on the ulnar head and the dorsum of the hand to correct VISI malalignment.[66] The ulnar-boost splint can provide prompt pain relief and improved function in V-PRI. Dynamic correction of the carpal supination can be achieved by activating the extrinsic stabilizers of the PCR. Cocontraction of the flexor and extensor carpi ulnaris and hypothenar muscles, actively pushing the pisiform dorsally, produces pronation and extension of the PCR and reduces the palmar sag.[67] For the V-PRI of radial origin (V-R-PRI) strengthening exercises should be associated to the flexor carpi radialis.[11] Neuromuscular training generates an extrinsic support to the ulnar side of the wrist which decreases instability, thus improving symptoms. Most severe cases may benefit from the use of the Dart Splint.[68] It is a hinged orthosis, which restricts wrist movement to DTM only, thus preventing the triggering of the clunking. It is very effective in educating the patient on proper wrist movement, also facilitating postoperative rehabilitation.

For those refractory cases requiring surgery, a preliminary arthroscopic assessment is recommended. The main goal is to exclude other pathology, in particular, LT dissociation and joint degeneration. Then, it is important to assess the severity and the reparability of the ligamentous damage. Arthroscopic findings vary according to the category and the subtype. In the developmental V-PRI of ulnar origin (V-U-PRI), which is the most common condition, attenuation, or even absence, of the DRC ligament is a constant finding. When suspected, this detail of the DRC ligament is better observed using a 1–2 portal.[46] Another common finding at radiocarpal exploration is the bulging of the UCLC, which have a markedly loose appearance and texture when probed.[46] Midcarpal exploration usually does not provide striking findings. The TH space may appear somehow "widened," but a distinct attenuation, or rupture, is hardly seen.[46,50,59]

Atzei et al[46] described an all-inside technique of arthroscopic plication of the loose and attenuated DRC, which is also sutured to the DIC. By narrowing the gap between the DIC and DRC ligaments, the procedure stabilizes both midcarpal joint and radiocarpal joint. Von Schroeder[54] performed the same procedure as an open technique. Both techniques reported encouraging results. When the DRC is absent, a strip of the ECU, anchored on the triquetrum tubercle and then on the dorsal rim of the radius, can be used for reconstruction of the DRC ligament. A side-to-side arthroscopic plication of the UCLC[69] is recommended as an ancillary procedure along with the DRC ligament plication, in those cases showing a marked carpal sag.[46] In order to recreate both the UAL and the DRC ligament, Garcia-Elias and Geissler[70] suggested to use a strip of the ECRB tendon, tunneled through the capitate and then through the triquetrum, to be finally secured on the dorsal rim of the radius. Although rather demanding, the technique produced excellent results.[9] As an alternative, Ho et al[50] proposed use of a distally based strip, the flexor carpi ulnaris, to reinforce the palmar TH joint and recreate the DRC ligament. The authors have no experience on capsuloligamentous thermal shrinkage using radiofrequency probes. Promising results have been reported[59]; however, questions remain as regards the potential loss of proprioception or the risk of thermal chondral lesions and injury to extensor tendons. In the posttraumatic V-U-PRI, arthroscopy may confirm either the avulsion of the DRC ligament from the triquetrum or lunate, or more uncommonly from its radial origins or midsubstance. Arthroscopic-assisted bone anchor fixation of the DRC ligament to the triquetrum or arthroscopic midsubstance repair is recommended.[71]

The V-PRI of radial origin (V-R-PRI) is a more uncommon condition as both developmental and posttraumatic. Arthroscopy may confirm the same findings regarding the DRC and UCLC, but may fail to show damage of STT ligaments. Therefore, just before surgery, a dynamic assessment under fluoroscopy with patient relaxation is recommended. Widening of the SC joint is even a more uncommon finding, usually associated to a high-energy injury. STT capsular plication is indicated along the plication/repair or reconstruction of the DRC and UCLC. In case of failure, a modified Brunelli reconstruction can be used to reinforce the palmar aspect of the STT joint.[11] LCF are indicated in revision cases of failed soft tissue procedures or as primary treatment of static irreducible deformities. Triquetrohamate,[72] four-corner arthrodesis,[73] and STT[27] fusions have been proposed. The downside of these procedures is that they block the midcarpal joint, preventing the useful DTM. A more physiological alternative is the radio(scapho)lunate fusion that preserves the DTM.[74]

27.5.2 Treatment of Dorsal Proximal Row Instability (D-PRI)

Patients presenting with a short duration of symptoms and no history of trauma tend to improve with conservative treatment. Proprioceptive re-education is based on the strengthening of the ECU, ECRL, and ECRB muscles. Developmental D-PRI, secondary to congenital hypoplasia of the DIC, may benefit from an augmentation capsulodesis of the DIC, as suggested by Szabo et al[75] for scapholunate dissociation, or a tenoplasty in order to deepen the scapholunate socket.[6]

Posttraumatic D-PRI are mostly secondary to an avulsion of the DIC from the dorsal scaphoid or lunate.[15] Midcarpal arthroscopy may reveal the rupture, provided the viewing portal, usually the MCU portal, is established at a distance from the avulsion site (i.e., more distal and ulnar than usual) to get proper view. Arthroscopic repair, or bone-anchor refixation, is usually very effective in relieving pain and restoring carpal kinematics. In the rare cases when surgery is required, especially in young hyperlax women, reefing of the space of Poirier through a volar approach[19] is recommended, although it may cause a certain loss of extension of the wrist.[76]

27.5.3 Treatment of Combined Proximal Row Instability (C-PRI)

Patients with combined dorsal and palmar MCI usually have marked laxity of the wrists, and they should be treated nonoperatively as far as possible.[11] The reported results of soft tissue procedures in multidirectional instabilities are unsatisfactory. If conservative management fails and the patient is very symptomatic, the best option is a radio(scapho)lunate fusion, or a midcarpal fusion in some cases.[74] This procedure restores appropriate lunate posture, especially when there is a gross radiocarpal hypermobility, and provides a satisfactory physiological range of movement in DTM.

27.6 Conclusions

Nondissociative carpal instabilities are a broad spectrum of poorly understood disorders. Proper understanding is complicated by confusing nomenclature and poor evidence due to paucity of cases. This review summarizes the diagnostic and therapeutic conceptions of the authors according to the current acquisitions. Introducing the definition of PRI, and its subtypes, to address the kinematic dysfunctions of the PCR may help to unify the preexisting different pathomechanic and clinical approaches and facilitate the choice of appropriate treatment.

References

[1] Dobyns JH, Linscheid RL, Macksoud WS. Proximal carpal row instability non-dissociative. Orthop Trans. 1985; 9:574

[2] Wright TW, Dobyns JH, Linscheid RL, Macksoud W, Siegert J. Carpal instability non-dissociative. J Hand Surg [Br]. 1994; 19(6):763–773

[3] Rayhack JM, Linscheid RL, Dobyns JH, Smith JH. Posttraumatic ulnar translation of the carpus. J Hand Surg Am. 1987; 12(2):180–189

[4] Lichtman DM, Schneider JR, Swafford AR, Mack GR. Ulnar midcarpal instability-clinical and laboratory analysis. J Hand Surg Am. 1981; 6 (5):515–523

[5] Lichtman DM, Wroten ES. Understanding midcarpal instability. J Hand Surg Am. 2006; 31(3):491–498

[6] Garcia-Elias M. The non-dissociative clunking wrist: a personal view. J Hand Surg Eur Vol. 2008; 33(6):698–711

[7] Viegas SF, Patterson RM, Peterson PD, et al. Ulnar-sided perilunate instability: an anatomic and biomechanic study. J Hand Surg Am. 1990; 15(2):268–278

[8] Kuhlmann JN, Boabighi A, Fahed I, Baux S. [Severe and chronic lateral sprains of the wrist with axial deviation, and their treatment]. Acta Orthop Belg. 1993; 59(1):1–9French.

[9] Heras-Palou C, Lindau T. Midcarpal instability. In: Trumble TE, Budoff JE, eds. Wrist and elbow reconstruction and arthroscopy. Rosemont: American Society for Surgery of the Hand; 2006:141–150

[10] Shiga SA, Werner FW, Garcia-Elias M, Harley BJ. Biomechanical analysis of palmar midcarpal instability and treatment by partial wrist arthrodesis. J Hand Surg Am. 2018; 43(4):331–338.e2

[11] Heras-Palou C. Midcarpal instability. In: Slutsky DJ, Osterman AL, eds. Fractures and injuries of the distal radius and carpus: the cutting edge. Philadelphia, PA: Saunders Elsevier; 2008:417–423

[12] Wolfe SW, Garcia-Elias M, Kitay A. Carpal instability nondissociative. J Am Acad Orthop Surg. 2012; 20(9):575–585

[13] Atzei A, Luchetti R, Braidotti F, Hagert E. [Options of arthroscopic treatment of palmar midcarpal instability]. Riv Chir Mano. 2013; 50 (2):205–207

[14] Fok MWM, Fernandez DL, Maniglio M. Carpal instability nondissociative following acute wrist fractures. J Hand Surg Am. 2020; 45(7):662.e1–662.e10

[15] Loisel F, Orr S, Ross M, Couzens G, Leo AJ, Wolfe S. Traumatic nondissociative carpal instability: a case series. J Hand Surg Am. 2022; 47(3):285.e1–285.e11

[16] Mouchet A, Belot J. Poignet en ressaut: subluxation mediocarpienne en avant. Bull Mem Soc Chir. 1934; 60:1243–1244

[17] Louis DS, Hankin FM, Greene TL, Braunstein EM, White SJ. Central carpal instability-capitate lunate instability pattern: diagnosis by dynamic displacement. Orthopedics. 1984; 7(11):1693–1696

[18] Schernberg F. [Mediocarpal instability]. Ann Chir Main. 1984; 3(4):344–348

[19] Johnson RP, Carrera GF. Chronic capitolunate instability. J Bone Joint Surg Am. 1986; 68(8):1164–1176

[20] Zancolli ER, III. Localized medial triquetral-hamate instability: anatomy and operative reconstruction-augmentation. Hand Clin. 2001; 17(1):83–96, vii

[21] Lichtman DM, Pientka WF, II. Midcarpal instability: a historical and etymological review. J Hand Surg Am. 2023; 48(2):188–192

[22] Wolfe SW, Crisco JJ, Orr CM, Marzke MW. The dart-throwing motion of the wrist: is it unique to humans? J Hand Surg Am. 2006; 31(9):1429–1437

27

[23] Crisco JJ, Coburn JC, Moore DC, Akelman E, Weiss AC, Wolfe SW. In vivo radiocarpal kinematics and the dart thrower's motion. J Bone Joint Surg Am. 2005; 87(12):2729–2740

[24] Ishikawa J, Cooney WP, III, Niebur G, An KN, Minami A, Kaneda K. The effects of wrist distraction on carpal kinematics. J Hand Surg Am. 1999; 24(1):113–120

[25] Moritomo H, Murase T, Goto A, Oka K, Sugamoto K, Yoshikawa H. Capitate-based kinematics of the midcarpal joint during wrist radioulnar deviation: an in vivo three-dimensional motion analysis. J Hand Surg Am. 2004; 29(4):668–675

[26] Weber ER. Concepts governing the rotational shift of the intercalated segment of the carpus. Orthop Clin North Am. 1984; 15(2):193–207

[27] Caputo AE, Watson HK, Weinzweig J. Midcarpal instability. In: Watson HK, Weinzweig J, eds. The wrist. Philadelphia, PA: Lippincott, Williams and Wilkins, 2001: 511–520

[28] Gilula LA, Mann FA, Dobyns JH, Yin Y. Wrist terminology as defined by the International Wrist Investigators' Workshop (IWIW). J Bone Joint Surg. 2002; 84 Suppl 1:1–66

[29] Lichtman DM, Bruckner JD, Culp RW, Alexander CE. Palmar midcarpal instability: results of surgical reconstruction. J Hand Surg Am. 1993; 18(2):307–315

[30] Wright TW, Dobyns JH. Carpal instability non-dissociative. In: Cooney WP, Linscheid RL, Dobyns JH, eds. The wrist. Diagnosis and operative treatment. Vol. 1. St. Louis, MO: Mosby; 1998:550–568

[31] Fernandez DL, Capo JT, Gonzalez E. Corrective osteotomy for symptomatic increased ulnar tilt of the distal end of the radius. J Hand Surg Am. 2001; 26(4):722–732

[32] Berger RA, Garcia-Elias M. General anatomy of the wrist. In: An KN, Berger RA, Cooney WP, eds. Biomechanics of the wrist joint. New York: Springer; 1991:1–22

[33] Trumble TE, Bour CJ, Smith RJ, Glisson RR. Kinematics of the ulnar carpus related to the volar intercalated segment instability pattern. J Hand Surg Am. 1990; 15(3):384–392

[34] Viegas SF, Patterson RM, Peterson PD, et al. Ulnar-sided perilunate instability: an anatomic and biomechanic study. J Hand Surg Am. 1990; 15(2):268–278

[35] Sandow MJ. Computer modelling of wrist biomechanics: translation into specific tasks and injuries. Curr Rheumatol Rev. 2020; 16(3):178–183

[36] Sandow M, Fisher T. Anatomical anterior and posterior reconstruction for scapholunate dissociation: preliminary outcome in ten patients. J Hand Surg Eur Vol. 2020; 45(4):389–395

[37] Moritomo H, Murase T, Goto A, Oka K, Sugamoto K, Yoshikawa H. Capitate-based kinematics of the midcarpal joint during wrist radioulnar deviation: an in vivo three-dimensional motion analysis. J Hand Surg Am. 2004; 29(4):668–675

[38] Moritomo H, Murase T, Goto A, Oka K, Sugamoto K, Yoshikawa H. In vivo three-dimensional kinematics of the midcarpal joint of the wrist. J Bone Joint Surg Am. 2006; 88(3):611–621

[39] Drewniany JJ, Palmer AK, Flatt AE. The scaphotrapezial ligament complex: an anatomic and biomechanical study. J Hand Surg Am. 1985; 10(4):492–498

[40] Pérez AJ, Jethanandani RG, Vutescu ES, Meyers KN, Lee SK, Wolfe SW. Role of ligament stabilizers of the proximal carpal row in preventing dorsal intercalated segment instability: a cadaveric study. J Bone Joint Surg Am. 2019; 101(15):1388–1396

[41] Craigen MA. Recurrent locking of the wrist due to dorsal midcarpal subluxation. J Bone Joint Surg Br. 1996; 78(4):664–666

[42] Yasuda M, Kusunoki M, Kazuki K, Yamano Y. Correction of dorsiflexed intercalated segment instability after restoration of scaphoid height in a cadaver model of scaphoid non-union. J Hand Surg [Br]. 1995; 20(5):596–602

[43] Moritomo H, Murase T, Arimitsu S, Oka K, Yoshikawa H, Sugamoto K. Change in the length of the ulnocarpal ligaments during radiocarpal motion: possible impact on triangular fibrocartilage complex foveal tears. J Hand Surg Am. 2008; 33(8):1278–1286

[44] Wiesner L, Rumelhart C, Pham E, Comtet JJ. Experimentally induced ulnocarpal instability: a study on 13 cadaver wrists. J Hand Surg Am. 1996; 21B:24–29

[45] Margulies IG, Xu H, Gopman JM, et al. Narrative review of ligamentous wrist injuries. J Hand Microsurg. 2021; 13(2):55–64

[46] Atzei A, Hagert E, Braidotti F, Luchetti R. Arthroscopic ligament plication for palmar midcarpal instability. 30th IWIW Meeting, September 17, 2014, Boston, USA

[47] Sandow MJ, Fisher TJ, Howard CQ, Papas S. Unifying model of carpal mechanics based on computationally derived isometric constraints and rules-based motion: the stable central column theory. J Hand Surg Eur Vol. 2014; 39(4):353–363

[48] Wolfe SW. A ligament-based classification and treatment algorithm. 74th ASSH Annual Meeting. IC11: The 2019 Linscheid-Dobyns Instructional Course Lecture: The Critical Stabilizers of the Intercalated Segment, September 5, 2019, Las Vegas, USA

[49] Larsen CF, Amadio PC, Gilula LA, Hodge JC. Analysis of carpal instability: I. Description of the scheme. J Hand Surg Am. 1995; 20(5):757–764

[50] Ho PC, Tse WL, Wong CW. Palmer midcarpal instability: an algorithm of diagnosis and surgical management. J Wrist Surg. 2017; 6(4):262–275

[51] Hargreaves DG. Midcarpal instability. J Hand Surg Eur Vol. 2016; 41(1):86–93

[52] Feinstein WK, Lichtman DM. Recognizing and treating midcarpal instability. Sports Med Arthrosc Rev. 1998; 6:270–277

[53] Linscheid RL, Dobyns JH, Beabout JW, Bryan RS. Traumatic instability of the wrist. Diagnosis, classification, and pathomechanics. J Bone Joint Surg Am. 1972; 54(8):1612–1632

[54] von Schroeder HP. Dorsal wrist plication for midcarpal instability. J Hand Surg Am. 2018; 43(4):354–359

[55] Urbanschitz L, Pastor T, Fritz B, Schweizer A, Reissner L. Posttraumatic carpal instability nondissociative. J Wrist Surg. 2021; 10(4):290–295

[56] Raskin KB, Beldner S. Clinical examination of the distal ulna and surrounding structures. Hand Clin. 1998; 14(2):177–190

[57] Zelenski NA, Shin AY. Management of nondissociative instability of the wrist. J Hand Surg Am. 2020; 45(2):131–139

[58] Lichtman DM, Gaenslen ES, Pollock GR. Midcarpal and proximal carpal instabilities. In: Lichtman DM, Alexander AH, eds. The wrist and its disorders. 2nd ed. Philadelphia, PA: WB Saunders, 1997:316–328

[59] Mason WT, Hargreaves DG. Arthroscopic thermal capsulorrhaphy for palmar midcarpal instability. J Hand Surg Eur Vol. 2007; 32(4):411–416

[60] Kleinman WB. Stability of the distal radioulna joint: biomechanics, pathophysiology, physical diagnosis, and restoration of function what we have learned in 25 years. J Hand Surg Am. 2007; 32(7):1086–1106

[61] Jing SS, Smith G, Deshmukh S. Demystifying palmar midcarpal instability. J Wrist Surg. 2021; 10(2):94–101

[62] Lindau TR. The role of arthroscopy in carpal instability. J Hand Surg Eur Vol. 2016; 41(1):35–47

[63] Toms AP, Chojnowski A, Cahir JG. Midcarpal instability: a radiological perspective. Skeletal Radiol. 2011; 40(5):533–541

[64] McLean JM, Bain GI, Watts AC, Mooney LT, Turner PC, Moss M. Imaging recognition of morphological variants at the midcarpal joint. J Hand Surg Am. 2009; 34(6):1044–1055

[65] Van Overstraeten L, Camus EJ. A systematic method of arthroscopic testing of extrinsic carpal ligaments: implication in carpal stability. Tech Hand Up Extrem Surg. 2013; 17(4):202–206

[66] O'Brien MT. An innovative orthotic design for midcarpal instability, non-dissociative: mobility with stability. J Hand Ther. 2013; 26(4):363–364

[67] Esplugas M, Garcia-Elias M, Lluch A, Llusá Pérez M. Role of muscles in the stabilization of ligament-deficient wrists. J Hand Ther. 2016; 29(2):166–174

[68] Braidotti F, Atzei A, Fairplay T. Dart-Splint: an innovative orthosis that can be integrated into a scapho-lunate and palmar midcarpal instability re-education protocol. J Hand Ther. 2015; 28(3):329–334, quiz 335

[69] Moskal MJ, Savoie FH, III, Field LD. Arthroscopic capsulodesis of the lunotriquetral joint. Clin Sports Med. 2001; 20(1):141–153, ix–x

V

[70] Garcia-Elias M, Geissler WB. Carpal instability. In: Green DP, Hotchkiss RN, Pederson WC, et al ed. Green's operative hand surgery. 5th ed. Churchill Livingstone; 2005:535–604

[71] Slutsky DJ. Arthroscopic dorsal radiocarpal ligament repair. Arthroscopy. 2005; 21(12):1486

[72] Rao SB, Culver JE. Triquetrohamate arthrodesis for midcarpal instability. J Hand Surg Am. 1995; 20(4):583–589

[73] Goldfarb CA, Stern PJ, Kiefhaber TR. Palmar midcarpal instability: the results of treatment with 4-corner arthrodesis. J Hand Surg Am. 2004; 29(2):258–263

[74] Garcia-Elias M, Lluch A, Ferreres A, Papini-Zorli I, Rahimtoola ZO. Treatment of radiocarpal degenerative osteoarthritis by radioscapholunate arthrodesis and distal scaphoidectomy. J Hand Surg Am. 2005; 30(1):8–15

[75] Szabo RM, Slater RR, Jr, Palumbo CF, Gerlach T. Dorsal intercarpal ligament capsulodesis for chronic, static scapholunate dissociation: clinical results. J Hand Surg Am. 2002; 27(6):978–984

[76] Apergis EP. The unstable capitolunate and radiolunate joints as a source of wrist pain in young women. J Hand Surg [Br]. 1996; 21(4):501–506

27

Section VI

Other Injuries

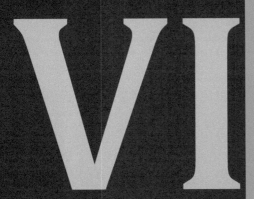

28 Ligament Injuries Associated to Distal Radius Fractures

Tommy R. Lindau

Abstract

Intra-articular congruity is essential to improve outcome in distal radius fractures. A part of this is achieved with improved fixation, such as the volar-locking plates, and another part of this can only be achieved by using arthroscopy. In addition to improving the intra-articular congruity, associated ligament injuries can be detected and treated.

The aim of this chapter is to outline various types of associated injuries with suggested management in a stepwise fashion whereas other chapters present more details regarding operative options in cases where there is no associated radius fracture. Hence, once patient- and treatment-related factors are managed, focus should be on identifying and managing associated ligament injuries.

Keywords: arthroscopy, chondral, distal radius fracture, DRU joint, intra-articular, lunotriquetral ligament, scapholunate advanced collapse, scapholunate ligament, TFCC

28.1 Introduction

The outcome of distal radius fracture treatment can still not be fully predicted today. In fact, there is little scientific evidence for most things that are done in the management of distal radius fractures.[1] In addition to the fact that arthroscopic evaluation is superior in assessing the articular step-off and the rotation of fractured fragments, it is also possible to recognize ligament injuries (▶ Table 28.1).[2,4] There is a high incidence of soft tissue injuries associated with distal radius fractures, which are frequently missed when the fracture is managed by conventional methods of treatment (▶ Table 28.1).[2,3]

These associated injuries should not be surprising as the radius is involved in the greater arch mechanism in perilunate dislocations described by Mayfield et al.[5] This is particularly noted in nonosteoporotic patients who more often present with intra-articular fractures caused by a severe, high-energy trauma, whereas, in contrast, such associated injuries are uncommon in osteoporotic patients where most fractures are extra-articular due to low-energy trauma. Arthroscopy should therefore be considered predominately in younger patients with a more high-energy trauma, in particular radial styloid fractures, in order to detect ligament injuries in addition to improving intra-articular congruency.

28.2 Indications for Arthroscopy

The primary indication for arthroscopy in the management of distal radius fractures is an intra-articular step-off more than 1 mm after an attempted closed reduction or an initial fixation with a volar plate. Second, radius fractures with associated scaphoid fractures and/or obvious ligament injuries will benefit from arthroscopic management (▶ Fig. 28.1). Radiological signs may suggest associated soft tissue injuries, such as widening of intercarpal joint spaces and/or radiographic disruption of the carpal arches of the so-called Gilula lines, i.e., the three arches that can be drawn along the proximal and distal carpal rows (▶ Fig. 28.1). Third, a radiological widening of the distal radioulnar joint (DRUJ) may be another sign of a ligament injury to the triangular fibrocartilage complex (TFCC) that may need arthroscopic assessment and treatment.

Simple radial styloid fractures are most often two-part fractures and may be part of an incomplete greater arch

Table 28.1 Ligament injuries associated to distal radius fractures

Study (y)	Number and type of injury	TFCC injury (%)	SL injury (%)	LT injury (%)
Fontes (1995)	30, intra- and extra-articular	70	40	17
Geissler (1996)	60, intra-articular	49	32	15
Lindau (1997)	50, intra- and extra-articular	78	54	16
Richards (1997)	118, intra- and extra-articular	35 (intra) 53 (extra)	21 (intra) 7 (extra)	7 (intra) 13 (extra)
Mehta (2000)	3, intra-articular	58	85	61
Hanker (2001)	173, intra-articular	61	8	12

Abbreviations: LT, lunotriquetral; SL, scapholunate; TFCC, triangular fibrocartilage complex.

28

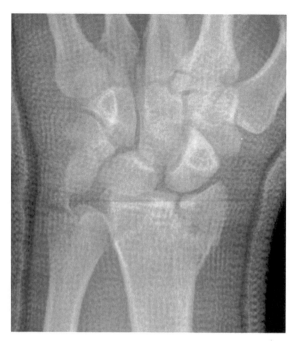

Fig. 28.1 Radius fracture with associated scapholunate (SL) ligament injury diagnosed with the "ring sign" of the scaphoid.

injury according to the Mayfield mechanism,[5] but without a dislocation of the lunate.

Complex, impacted fractures such as the "die-punch" fractures warrant arthroscopic assessment, reduction, and fixation. Three- or four-part fractures or even more complex injuries with high-grade intra-articular comminution ("explosion fractures") are challenging but will benefit from arthroscopic management in expert hands.

28.2.1 The Arthroscopic Procedure—"Dry" or Wet?

The "dry" arthroscopic technique will minimize the risk of further soft-tissue swelling and subsequent risk of secondary compartment syndrome, compared to the wet technique with continuous saline irrigation, but it may make the procedure slightly more difficult.[6] "Dry" should not be taken literally, as there might be intra-articular debris and hemarthrosis, which will have to be cleared by irrigating the joint, before continuing with a "dry" arthroscopy technique.[6] If a "dry" arthroscopy technique is preferred, the air valve should be kept open to permit free circulation of air through the joint.

28.2.2 The Arthroscopic Procedure—Arthroscopic Assessment

The examination starts by assessing the radiocarpal joint surface regarding intra-articular congruency and possible

need for optimizing the provisionally closed or open reduction. A 2-mm probe is helpful, inserted through the 4–5 or the 6-R portal, to accurately evaluate the gap, separation, and step-off of fragments. Once articular congruity is achieved, associated ligament or cartilage injuries are assessed: integrity of the scapholunate (SL) ligament, the lunotriquetral (LT) ligament, and the TFCC or any other intra-articular pathology is visualized and the sequence of surgery can be planned.

TFCC injuries appear to be the most common associated ligament injury. They are found in around three-fourth of the fractures (▶ Table 28.1).[2,3] SL ligament injuries are the second most frequent injuries. They are found in one-third to one-half of cases (▶ Table 28.1).[2,3] LT ligament tears (▶ Table 28.1) are less common and are seen in about one-sixth of the fractures.[2,3] Chondral lesions have been found[2] with a possible long-term development of secondary osteoarthritis (OA).[7]

28.2.3 Triangular Fibrocartilage Complex (TFCC) Injuries

TFCC injuries are the most common associated intra-articular injuries in distal radius fractures in nonosteoporotic patients (▶ Table 28.2; ▶ Fig. 28.2a, b; ▶ Fig. 28.3).[2,3] Cadaveric studies suggest that a displacement of the distal radius has to be more than 4 mm of radial shortening, down to 0 degree of radial inclination, and a dorsal tilt of minimum 10 degrees in order for an ulnar attachment of TFCC to be compromised. In a 1-year outcome study they found that peripheral tears to the TFCC (▶ Fig. 28.2b) will cause instability and subsequent worse outcome.[8] However, in a 15-year prospective longitudinal outcome study of untreated TFCC tears this seems to be less of a problem than anticipated, as only one patient needed a stabilizing procedure due to painful instability.[9] In the absence of scientific evidence, clinical experience supports TFCC treatment in association with distal radius fractures as described in ▶ Table 28.2.

28.2.4 Intercarpal Ligament Injuries

Intercarpal ligament injuries to the SL and the LT ligaments associated with distal radius fractures can be looked upon as incomplete greater arch injuries described by Mayfield et al.[5] It is important to assess and diagnose these ligament injuries.

In the absence of arthroscopy, fluoroscopic assessment in ulnar and radial deviation will diagnose severe intercarpal ligament injuries.

Arthroscopic assessment will not only diagnose them, but also allow grading based on a combined radiocarpal and midcarpal assessment[2,3] (▶ Table 28.3, Box 28.1). Depending on the grading, severity is controlled and further management is decided. The ligament injuries are visualized at radiocarpal arthroscopy and are classified

Table 28.2 TFCC classification according to Palmer[10]

Central perforation tears (Palmer,[10] ► Fig. 28.2a)	... are stable and can be debrided to leave smooth edges with a suction punch, a shaver, or a radiofrequency probe. Care should be taken to avoid jeopardizing the stability provided by the important palmar and dorsal ulnoradial ligaments. This treatment does not change the overall rehabilitation plan for the radius fracture.
Peripheral tears (Palmer,[10] ► Fig. 28.2b)	... may come with or without associated DRUJ instability. The distal tears may be debrided and possibly sutured back to the capsule and ECU subsheath. The proximal tears cannot be seen at radiocarpal arthroscopy alone, but need reattachment to the fovea of the ulna. The combined tears are diagnosed due to the distal component and should also be reattached. Reattachment can be done with arthroscopy assistance or with an open technique with similar good outcome. Arthroscopically assisted reattachment is done with two or three 2-0 absorbable (PDS) sutures that are passed through the periphery of the TFCC and fixed to the distal ulna, either through drill holes or with any one of the many varieties of TFCC techniques. The repair Is protected from supination and pronation for 4 wk, followed by 2–4 wk in a short-arm cast.
Ulnocarpal ligament tears (Palmar[10] ► Fig. 28.2c)	... are very rare. A reinsertion technique directly through the palmar approach in line with the exposure of the critical corner in the intermediate column is the simplest option. This repair should be protected for 4 wk in relation to the rehabilitation for the radius fracture.
Radial avulsion tears (Palmar[10] ► Fig. 28.2d)	... are uncommon, but may often be associated with a dorsoulnar fracture fragment. If found in isolation, i.e., true avulsions from the radial insertion site of the ulnoradial ligament, they most likely ought to be reattached. Due to the need for internal fixation of the distal radius fracture, the techniques based on drill holes through the radius are not suitable, but rather with suture anchors with a mini–open approach.

Abbreviations: DRUJ, distal radioulnar joint; ECU, extensor carpi ulnaris; PDS, polydioxanone suture; TFCC, triangular fibrocartilage complex.

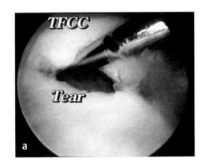
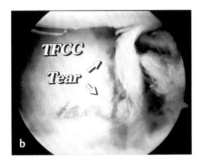

Fig. 28.2 (a) Central perforation tear of the triangular fibrocartilage complex (TFCC) ligament. This may be painful and debridement should be considered, but it never leads to instability of the distal radioulnar joint (DRUJ). **(b)** Peripheral TFCC tear with detachment from the fovea of the ulnar head.

as partial or complete (► Table 28.3, Box 28.1; ► Fig. 28.4a). The ligaments are examined along their different portions: dorsal, membranous, and palmar.

From the midcarpal joint, the joint space, not the ligament, is assessed for widening and step-off (► Fig. 28.4b). A probe with known size (e.g., 1 mm thickness and 2 mm tip length) is useful as a gauge for measurement (► Table 28.3, Box 28.1). The widening and the step-off reflect the degree of mobility of the affected intercarpal joint as a consequence of the ligament injury. This mobility is not necessarily a pathological laxity. Once the traction is released, the assessed joint can be tested, by checking signs of pathological excessive mobility with the arthroscope in the midcarpal joint. Thus, the intercarpal ligament injury can be fully classified and graded (► Table 28.3, Box 28.1).

28.2.5 Scapholunate (SL) Ligament Injuries

SL ligament injuries occur in half of the displaced distal radius fractures, at least in younger patients.[2] If left untreated, high-grade SL tears are likely to progress first to SL dissociation and symptomatic wrist instability.[11] This will, in the long term, further lead to posttraumatic scapholunate advanced collapse (SLAC) OA. Being aware of the long-term consequences of untreated SL tears, it is important to detect SL tears early and to consider treatment. If found and treated early, arthroscopic reduction and percutaneous pinning is the simplest option and has a good outcome in 85% of the patients. It is noteworthy that there is no strong evidence (level 1 or 2) for management of these injuries and recommendations published are mainly experience-based.[12]

28

Grade I-II SL Injuries

Low-grade injuries are best managed with immobilization, as most patients are asymptomatic at 1 year.[11] Therefore, the protocol for mobilization of the distal radius

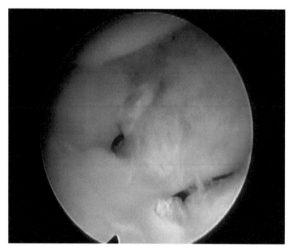

Fig. 28.3 Repair of peripheral tears has to be through the fovea of the ulnar head to regain stability. Suture anchors, drill holes, and other techniques are available (▶ Table 28.2).

fracture after volar-locking plate fixation may have to be adjusted.[12]

Grade III-IV SL Injuries

Radiographic SL dissociation and long-term SLAC wrist is more likely with Grade III-IV injuries (▶ Fig. 28.4a, b) if untreated, and consequently early treatment is important.[11] Grade III can be treated with arthroscopic reduction and Kirschner-wire (K-wire) pinning (▶ Fig. 28.5a-c). While protecting the sensory branches of the radial nerve, a skin incision is made slightly palmar to the anatomical snuffbox. K-wires into the scaphoid are used as a joystick to achieve arthroscopic reduction, which can be assessed from the midcarpal joint (▶ Fig. 28.5a). Once reduction is achieved, the K-wire is advanced into the lunate (▶ Fig. 28.5b). An additional K-wire should be inserted into the scaphocapitate (SC) joint (▶ Fig. 28.5c). Pins can be removed at 6 weeks.[12]

Grade IV injuries, especially if found with radiologically visible dissociation already on the trauma films, can be difficult to reduce arthroscopically and should most likely be treated with an open repair.[12] Open direct repair is followed by protective K-wires as described above. During closure, dorsal capsulodesis can be added to augment the repair.

Table 28.3 Arthroscopic classification of scapholunate ligament tears according to Geissler

Grade	Radiocarpal joint	Midcarpal instability	Step-off
1	Hemorrhage of interosseous ligament (IOL), no attenuation	None	None
2	Incomplete, partial, or full-substance tear, no attenuation	Slight gap (<3 mm)	Midcarpal only
3	Ligament attenuation incomplete, partial, or small full-substance tear	Probe can be passed between carpal bones	Midcarpal and radiocarpal
4	Complete tear	Gross instability; 2.7-mm scope can be passed thru (drive thru sign)	Midcarpal and radiocarpal

Reproduced with permission from Geissler WB, Freeland AE, Savoie FH, McIntyre LW, Whipple TL. Intracarpal soft-tissue lesions associated with an intra-articular fracture of the distal end of the radius. J Bone Joint Surg Am. 1996; 78(3):357–365.[3]

Box 28.1 Lindau classification system for intercarpal SL and LT ligament injuries and mobility of the joints

Grade 1: Hematoma or distension; diastasis nil; step-off nil
Grade 2: As above and/or partial tear; diastasis 0–1 mm; step-off < 2 mm
Grade 3: Partial or total tear; diastasis 1–2 mm; step-off < 2 mm
Grade 4: Total tear; diastasis > 2 mm; step-off > 2 mm

Based on Lindau T, Arner M, Hagberg L. Intraarticular lesions in distal fractures of the radius in young adults. A descriptive arthroscopic study in 50 patients. J Hand Surg [Br]. 1997; 22(5):638–643.

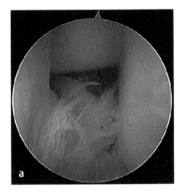
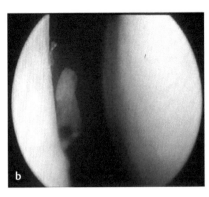

Fig. 28.4 **(a)** Arthroscopic view from the radiocarpal portal with a so-called "drive through sign"; i.e., the head of the capitate can be seen and the scope can be passed through the scapholunate (SL) joint, a Grade IV SL tear (▶ Table 28.3). **(b)** Midcarpal arthroscopy shows a step and a gap that can be measured for grading, in this case a Grade III (Box 28.1).

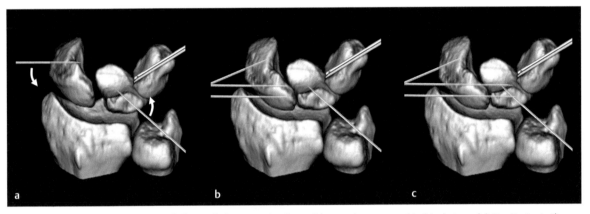

Fig. 28.5 Repair of a Grade III-IV scapholunate (SL) tear can be done with an arthroscopy-assisted technique. **(a)** One K-wire in the scaphoid and lunate, respectively, is used and a joystick maneuver used with the scope in the midcarpal joint to secure adequate reduction of the joint **(b)**. **(b,c)** K-wires are inserted into the scaphoid and once reduction has been achieved the wires are advanced over the SL joint and a final one into the capitate to protect the torn ligament and allow healing.

28.2.6 Lunotriquetral (LT) Ligament Injuries

The incidence of LT ligament injuries is about one-sixth (▶ Table 28.1). So far, there is no evidence that LT tears lead to long-term problems when associated with distal radius fractures.[11] Stable LT injuries (Grade I-III) may benefit from immobilization, where the distal radius fracture mobilization protocol needs to be reconsidered. Grade IV injuries may need arthroscopic debridement of the tear and pinning of the joint. K-wires are introduced from a dorsoulnar approach. The LT dissociation is reduced with a joystick maneuver and two to three wires are advanced across the joint. Wires are kept for 6 weeks.

28.2.7 Chondral Lesions

Acute chondral lesions can be seen as subchondral hematomas (with or without cartilage cracks), avulsed cartilage flakes, or complete avulsions of the cartilage with visible bare bone.[2] There is weak evidence that subchondral hematoma can lead to the development of early onset of mild, radiographic OA.[7] Currently, no other treatment option is

available other than debridement for these injuries. A tempting, but unproven, option is the microfracture treatment as familiar from the knee joint. Chondral lesions may lead to treatment changes, as a comminuted intra-articular fracture might be treated with a primary partial wrist fusion or even a hemiarthroplasty instead of a lengthy attempt of reducing a multifragmentary joint surface with loss of cartilage, as there is increased awareness of an expected bad outcome with these associated lesions. Together with the associated ligament injuries, chondral lesions reflect the complexity of distal radial fractures, especially in younger patients.[6]

28.3 Outcomes

Currently, there is no scientific evidence that arthroscopy is necessary in the management of distal radius fractures. In spite of that, there seems to be increasing support regarding the benefit of arthroscopy in the management of distal radius fractures.[9,13,14] Further, there is limited experience in arthroscopically assisted treatment of associated injuries. However, TFCC repairs in conjunction with distal

28

Table 28.4 Pearls, pitfalls, and tips in understanding the usefulness of wrist arthroscopy as an adjuvant investigation in the treatment of distal radius fractures

1	There is a wide spectrum of injury pattern after a fall onto the outstretched hand such as sprain, radial styloid fracture in isolation, and radial styloid fracture as part of the greater arch injury, thereby as part of a complete or incomplete perilunate dislocation mechanism.[6]
2	Arthroscopy as an adjunct in the management of distal radius fractures has been available for over 20 years, yet still requires experience and management in expert centers. Successful management of this complex fracture requires thorough understanding of the anatomy, understanding the relevance of individual fracture fragments, and awareness of associated soft tissue injuries.
3	Displaced fractures in nonosteoporotic patients have a high incidence of associated soft tissue injuries. Associated injuries will affect the long-term outcome. Arthroscopy plays its role to establish the complete diagnosis and facilitate early treatment to optimize the overall outcome of these complex injuries.
4	Arthroscopy will in descending frequency diagnose TFCC injuries, intracarpal SL and LT ligament tears, and chondral lesions. Once diagnosed and graded, the appropriate surgical treatment of these lesions can be added to the fracture fixation with further modification of the postoperative rehabilitation protocol.
5	Undetected associated injuries may explain the absence of improved outcome in studies comparing volar-locking plate fixation and early mobilization to external fixation or pinning.

Abbreviations: LT, lunotriquetral; SL, scapholunate; TFCC, triangular fibrocartilage complex.

VI

radius fixation resulted in a high degree of patient satisfaction and good to excellent clinical outcomes.[15]

28.4 Conclusion

There is an increasing awareness in the complexity of distal radius fractures as it should not only be seen as a bony injury, but rather as a bony consequence of the energy passing the wrist while fracturing the radius (▶ Table 28.4). The main advantage of arthroscopically assisted management of distal radius fractures is to improve intra-articular accuracy to less than 1 mm of incongruency. Second, to combine this with complete assessment, management, and treatment of TFCC, intercarpal ligament, and cartilage injuries. Third, the surgeon has complete control of all fracture- and treatment-related factors in distal radius fractures. The author hopes that this concept will continue to evolve in the future for the benefit of the patients.

References

[1] Cochrane library; Handoll H, Elstub L, Elliott J, et al. Cochrane Bone, Joint and Muscle Trauma Group. About The Cochrane Collaboration (Cochrane Review Groups (CRGs)) 2008, Issue 4

[2] Lindau T, Arner M, Hagberg L. Intraarticular lesions in distal fractures of the radius in young adults. A descriptive arthroscopic study in 50 patients. J Hand Surg [Br]. 1997; 22(5):638–643

[3] Geissler WB, Freeland AE, Savoie FH, McIntyre LW, Whipple TL. Intracarpal soft-tissue lesions associated with an intra-articular fracture of the distal end of the radius. J Bone Joint Surg Am. 1996; 78(3):357–365

[4] Cognet JM, Martinache X, Mathoulin C. [Arthroscopic management of intra-articular fractures of the distal radius]. Chir Main. 2008; 27(4): 171–179

[5] Mayfield JK, Johnson RP, Kilcoyne RF. The ligaments of the human wrist and their functional significance. Anat Rec. 1976; 186(3): 417–428

[6] Del Piñal F. Technical tips for (dry) arthroscopic reduction and internal fixation of distal radius fractures. J Hand Surg Am. 2011; 36 (10):1694–1705

[7] Lindau T, Adlercreutz C, Aspenberg P. Cartilage injuries in distal radial fractures. Acta Orthop Scand. 2003; 74(3):327–331

[8] Lindau T. Treatment of injuries to the ulnar side of the wrist occurring with distal radial fractures. Hand Clin. 2005; 21(3):417–425

[9] Mrkonjic A, Geijer M, Lindau T, Tägil M. The natural course of traumatic triangular fibrocartilage complex tears in distal radial fractures: a 13–15 year follow-up of arthroscopically diagnosed but untreated injuries. J Hand Surg Am. 2012; 37(8):1555–1560

[10] Palmer AK. Triangular fibrocartilage complex lesions: a classification. J Hand Surg Am. 1989; 14(4):594–606

[11] Forward DP, Lindau TR, Melsom DS. Intercarpal ligament injuries associated with fractures of the distal part of the radius. J Bone Joint Surg Am. 2007; 89(11):2334–2340

[12] Chennagiri RJR, Lindau TR. Assessment of scapholunate instability and review of evidence for management in the absence of arthritis. J Hand Surg Eur Vol. 2013; 38(7):727–738

[13] Ono H, Katayama T, Furuta K, Suzuki D, Fujitani R, Akahane M. Distal radial fracture arthroscopic intraarticular gap and step-off measurement after open reduction and internal fixation with a volar locked plate. J Orthop Sci. 2012; 17(4):443–449

[14] Scheer JH, Adolfsson LE. Patterns of triangular fibrocartilage complex (TFCC) injury associated with severely dorsally displaced extra-articular distal radius fractures. Injury. 2012; 43(6):926–932

[15] Ruch DS, Yang CC, Smith BP. Results of acute arthroscopically repaired triangular fibrocartilage complex injuries associated with intra-articular distal radius fractures. Arthroscopy. 2003; 19(5): 511–516

29 Pisotriquetral Instability

Eduardo R. Zancolli III

Abstract

Current literature only describes severe instabilities (usually dislocations) of the pisotriquetral (PT) joint. We should ask ourselves why this joint cannot present, as in the grading of instabilities of any other joint, mild and moderate instabilities.

The elongation or lesion of the medial PT ligament (with indemnity of the pisohamate and pisometacarpal ligaments) causes these mild and moderate instabilities of the PT joint which should be diagnosed and treated when treating other associated pathologies (i.e., triangular ligament) in order to reduce residual pain after surgery.

Plicature and augmentation (with the dorsal retinaculum) of the medial PT ligament (plus local synovectomy) leads to better results and reduces the number of cases with residual pain (avoiding pisiformectomy).

Keywords: pisotriquetral mild and moderate instabilities, medial pisotriquetral ligament, peritriquetral lesional ring, inverted dart throwing motion, swing arc motion

29.1 Introduction

During the past few decades, hand surgeons have had huge interest in pathologies of the ulnar side of the wrist. Many biomechanical, diagnostic, arthroscopic, and surgical advances, reflected in an enormous number of papers, have been achieved particularly in the assessment and treatment of the distal radioulnar joint (DRUJ) and the lunotriquetral joint (LTJ).

Despite such advances, a critical analysis of the results show that a significant percentage of patients did not finish with complete pain-free wrists and full return to previous activities, especially sports.[1,2] Upon repairing the triangular ligament, between 36[1] and 62.5%[2] of the patients reported residual pain. The same occurs with operations for the LT lesions (reparations and mini-arthrodesis): between 52 and 64%[3] of the cases reported residual pain. Hence it can be said that pain is usually the main or only presenting symptom on the ulnar side of the wrist in the great majority of patients.

One possibility for residual pain is not diagnosing other associated pathologies, near in localization. Can this be happening? Why? Not all the ulnar-side regions have been studied with the same detail and intensity. The pisotriquetral (PT) joint still remains not well understood by many hand surgeons, resulting in lack of diagnosis and correct treatment for PT joint instabilities (nearly the same, or worse, happening with the triquetral hamate [TH] joint[4]).

Therefore, there is doubt about the completeness of the actual paradigm with the understanding of the ulnar side of the wrist. A more inclusive paradigm could be developed by reconsidering differently three of the components of the paradigm: (1) the wholeness of the ulnar-side territory; (2) biomechanics; and (3) the grades of instability.

The actual paradigm only comprehends the problem with a limited view, as happens with an "iceberg view"[5] (i.e., considering only what is seen above the surface and ignoring what is not seen because it is still below water). The three "missing" components mentioned earlier would be the underwater part of the iceberg that are not visible.

29.2 The Underwater Part of the Iceberg: Three Components

29.2.1 The Whole Territory of the Ulnar Side

For not missing the forest for the trees, not only the DRUJ and LTJ but also the PT and TH joints should be considered. PT and TH joints are part of the same territory and may present associated lesions when the territory has been injured.

There is rarely any report on PT joint if osteoarthritis is excluded, but there are reports of complete dislocations of the triquetrum[6] and of the pisiform.[7,8] One paper refers to the pathology of the PT joint in racquet players[9] and a few more refer to PT joint instability.[10,12]

Same is the case with TH joint minor instabilities. Current knowledge gives credit to the TH joint for being responsible for midcarpal instability which is an extremely severe instability. No minor instabilities at this joint are considered in everyday clinical situations. These not so severe TH joint instabilities (not midcarpal instability) are already described in a couple of articles.[4,5]

When considering the ulnar-side territory it would be strange to have all degrees of pathology only in two areas (DRUJ and LTJ) and not "minor" instabilities in the other two (TH and PT joints).

29.2.2 Biomechanics: Need of New Biomechanical Considerations

Pathology is usually interpreted based on models. The only biomechanical model that is available for understanding the ulnar side is the Columnar Theory of Navarro[13]/Taleisnik.[14] Although this model is helpful, it is a basic model for the interpretation of the different possible complex lesions. For carpal fracture-dislocations the more detailed model by Mayfield[15] develops the possible

29

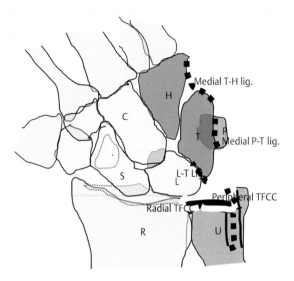

Fig. 29.1 "Peritriquetral lesional ring" and the ulnar-side possible associations according to the lesional energy: triangular fibrocartilage complex (TFCC) radial to peripheral, Bourgery's ligament (extensor carpi ulnaris [ECU] subluxation), lunotriquetral (LT) ligament, pisotriquetral (PT) ligaments, and medial triquetral hamate (TH) ligament.

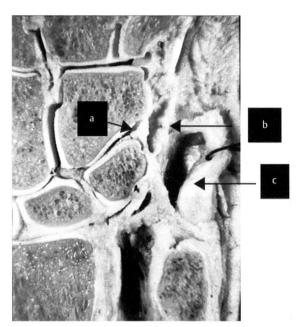

Fig. 29.2 Anatomy: (a) medial triquetral hamate (TH) Ligament; (b) reinforcement by the floor of the sixth dorsal compartment; (c) extensor carpi ulnaris (ECU) retracted with a hook. (Courtesy of Eduardo A. Zancolli, MD.)

pathological progression depending on the amount of lesional energy.

Based on this idea, considering that a similar concept could be applied to the ulnar column, in 2001 the author presented a more expanded biomechanical model: the "Peritriquetral Lesional Ring,"[4] which considers the progression of high forces over the ulnar side of the wrist.

As the triquetrum is the most fixed bone of the carpus it seems logical that with increasing energy other ulnar structures/areas around the triquetrum can be affected, i.e., the triangular ligament, the Bourgery's ligament[16] (producing extensor carpi ulnaris [ECU] subluxation), the LT ligament, the PT ligament, and the medial TH ligament (▶ Fig. 29.1).

Another concept that could be reevaluated, for a thorough understanding, is the "dart-throwing" motion.[17,18] This motion from extension-radial deviation to flexion-ulnar deviation has been demonstrated to be an important movement for daily wrist function. Here is the reevaluation. The author believes that the "dart-throwing" motion should be studied in the opposite direction also, which can be referred to as "inverse dart-throwing," or maybe, more appropriately the "swing arc." This opposite direction motion is important as it reproduces the way the midcarpal joint is used in many sports. The swings in tennis, golf, and polo need a great acceleration of the wrist utilizing this inverse dart-throwing direction, which is called the "swing arc." All these swings begin in flexion-ulnar deviation and accelerate to extension-radial deviation. It is interesting to note that this strenuous acceleration must, inevitably, have an end

point and some anatomical structure for the limit. It is mainly restrained by the medial side of the TH joint. Thus, the medial TH ligament, usually not considered in much detail in current medical literature, has an action as the final limiting structure of this motion (▶ Fig. 29.2).[4]

29.2.3 Grades of Instability

Surgeons diagnose ulnar-sided wrist "instabilities." In their diagnosis the first consideration is that patients usually suffer and complain of pain, weakness, and reduced function. Only in some of the most severe cases, specially happening in the case of midcarpal instability,[19,21] patients may manifest a sensation of instability, a symptom commonly seen in other joints (e.g., the shoulder, elbow, knee, and ankle).

Surgeons also recognize progressive degrees of instability in many joints, often graded as mild, moderate, and severe (or sometimes as subluxation and dislocation). Going against this observable and demonstrated concept, there are only reports on complete dislocations at the PT and TH joints. This begs the question as to why these joints cannot also suffer symptomatic progressive instability?

Although the precise anatomy of the ligaments of the PT joint has been described,[10,12] study is scarce on PT instability. If diagnosed, a situation that rarely occurs, the proposed treatment is pisiform bone excision.[22,24] Based on this indication another question arises. Why is

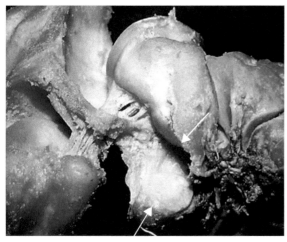

Fig. 29.3 Anatomy: the pisotriquetral (PT) joint opened by sectioning the medial PT ligament (*arrows*).

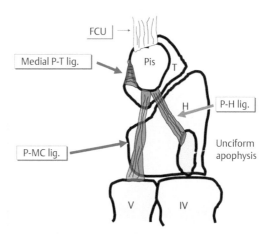

Fig. 29.4 Anatomy: ligaments of the pisotriquetral (PT) joint.

pisiform removal indicated instead of a ligament reconstruction as done in so many other joints?

In 1996, the author presented PT joint instability for the first time at the Kleinert Institute[25,26] and in 2004 presented a paper at the IFSSH Congress.[27] One year later, in 2005, Rayan presented two papers referring to PT instability.[10,11]

29.3 Anatomy

The anatomy of the PT joint has been described by several authors.[10,12,25,30] The pisiform is stabilized longitudinally by two ligaments: the pisohamate ligament (PHL), from the pisiform to the unciform apophysis, and the pisometacarpal ligament (PML), from the pisiform to the base of the little finger metacarpal (volarly). They prevent proximal dislocation of the pisiform with the vigorous contraction of the flexor carpi ulnaris (FCU).

The author described a third ligament: the medial pisotriquetral ligament[25,26] (MPTL) and, as already mentioned, it was also reported in the paper of 2004.[27] This ligament prevents excessive opening between the pisiform and the triquetrum in an anteroposterior plane. One year after this presentation Rayan[10,11] presented papers studying the ligaments but calling the medial ligament the "ulnar" PT ligament (▶ Fig. 29.3, ▶ Fig. 29.4, ▶ Fig. 29.5, ▶ Fig. 29.6, ▶ Fig. 29.7).

29.4 Symptoms

Patients can present with pain isolated at the PT joint or associated with other ulnar-sided pathology, e.g., the DRUJ. They usually complain of pain with demanding activities, but sometimes also with daily life activities which demand active contraction of the FCU. The symptoms are usually in their dominant hand.

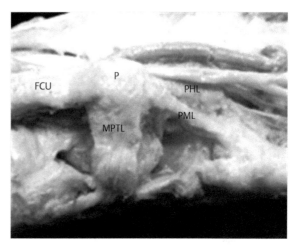

Fig. 29.5 Anatomical dissection of the pisotriquetral (PT) joint ligaments. (Courtesy of Carlos Zaidenberg.) FCU, flexor carpi ulnaris; P, pisiform; MPTL, medial pisotriquetral ligament; PML, pisometacarpal ligament; PHL, pisohamate ligament.

29.5 Physical Examination

Meticulous physical examination reveals localized pain at the medial side of the PT joint when palpating with the examiner's thumb. When pain is elicited with this maneuver the patient should be asked if that pain is same as the pain they are complaining of (▶ Fig. 29.8).

29.6 Imaging Studies

The key tests for diagnosis are radiographs and a magnetic resonance imaging (MRI) scan.

Radiographs are performed with a lateral view, 20-degree supinated. This view allows to measure the opening of the PT joint. It can also be done tangential to Lister's tubercle.[31]

29

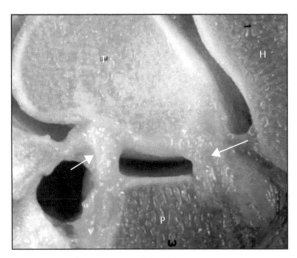

Fig. 29.6 Medial pisotriquetral (PT) ligament insertions (*arrows*). (Courtesy of Marc Garcia-Elias, MD.)

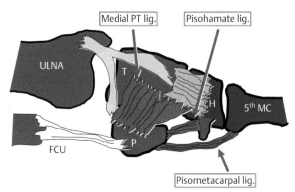

Fig. 29.7 Pisotriquetral (PT) ligamentary complex.

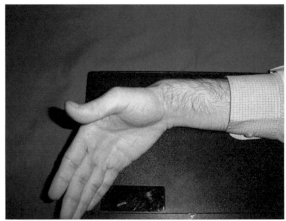

Fig. 29.9 Incidence for the pisotriquetral (PT) joint: lateral 20-degree supinated with 20-degree wrist flexion.

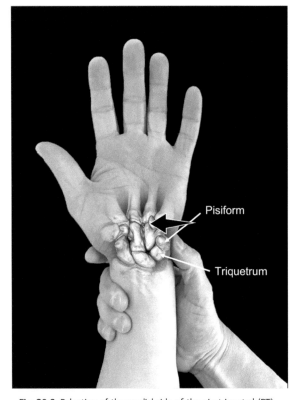

Fig. 29.8 Palpation of the medial side of the pisotriquetral (PT) joint.

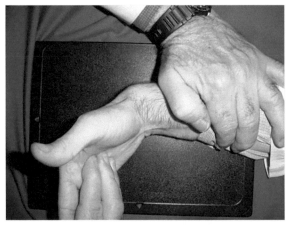

Fig. 29.10 Same incidence but with resisted wrist flexion.

In this resting position, Jameson et al[32] established that the mean opening is 1.5 mm. They also studied that same view but with active 20 degrees of wrist flexion where the mean opening is 3.5 mm. An extra study has been added with this last view: with resisted wrist flexion. In author's experience a gap of more than 3.5 mm may be pathological. It is important to note that patients with increased ligamentous laxity may have an opening of more than 3.5 mm; therefore, comparative radiographs of the opposite side should be performed (▶ Fig. 29.9, ▶ Fig. 29.10, ▶ Fig. 29.11).

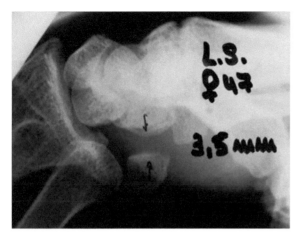

Fig. 29.11 The X-ray incidence showing opening of the pisotriquetral (PT) joint.

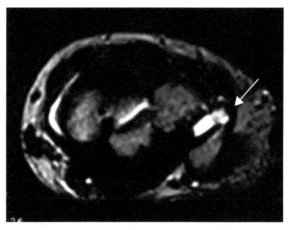

Fig. 29.12 Pisotriquetral (PT) joint synovitis and lesion of the medial PT ligament.

The T2-axial MRI scan views with fat suppression can show elongation or disruption of the medial PT ligament and increased fluid in the joint (▷ Fig. 29.12, ▷ Fig. 29.13).

29.7 Pathology and Classification

In 2005, Rayan and colleagues[10] defined the "pisiform ligament complex syndrome" as ulnar pain on the vicinity of the pisiform caused by lesion of one or more of the components of the ligamentary complex of the pisiform which unleash instability of the PT joint.

In minor or moderate instabilities, the only affected structure is the medial PT ligament. In a severe instability not only the medial ligament is compromised but also the PH and PM ligaments are affected. In this latter situation, proximal dislocation of the pisiform can manifest on unloaded radiographs.

Based on all these factors, the following classification is proposed:
- *Type I*: pathologic medial opening (medial PT ligament injury or elongation).
- *Type II*: pathologic medial opening with proximal translation of the pisiform (subluxation or dislocation) (medial PT + PH + PMC ligament injuries).

29.8 Treatment

Patients with symptoms only at the PT joint (Type I instability) are initially treated with conservative treatment: ice, nonsteroidal anti-inflammatory drugs (NSAIDs), splinting, and physiotherapy. If at 3 to 4 weeks they do not improve, then a steroid injection is given into the TH joint. If symptoms persist thereafter, surgical treatment is recommended.

If symptoms at the PT joint are associated with other pathology (e.g., triangular fibrocartilage complex [TFCC]

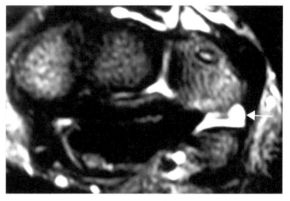

Fig. 29.13 Pisotriquetral (PT) joint synovitis and elongation of the medial PT ligament.

lesion) the initial indication can be conservative or surgical depending on the whole clinical picture and the indication for the associated pathology.

29.9 Surgical Technique

All the affected ligaments (all associations) should be repaired at the same surgical stage.

For *Type 1 instability* without associations, the skin incision is made following the trajectory of the dorsal cutaneous branch of the ulnar nerve. In the cases associated with DRUJ instability, the incision begins dorsally, i.e., radial to the ECU and is directed in a smooth "S" shape distal to the medial side of the V carpometacarpal joint. The dorsal cutaneous branch is found and protected. The dorsal retinaculum is transversally cut volar to the PT joint and carefully elevated from volar to dorsal. The PT joint is identified, using a needle or palpation, and a transverse incision is made over the medial PT ligament.

29

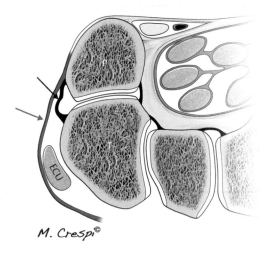

Fig. 29.14 Elongated medial pisotriquetral (PT) ligament (*black arrow*); extensor retinaculum (*red arrow*).

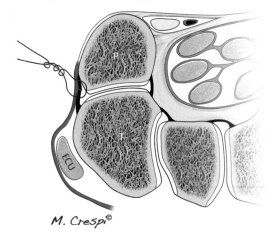

Fig. 29.15 Plicature of the medial pisotriquetral (PT) ligament (*black arrow*); augmentation with the extensor retinaculum (*red arrow*).

Once the joint is opened, synovectomy is usually required. Following this, a repair or retensioning of the ligament is performed with 3–0 or 4–0 absorbable sutures (usually three) at maximum tension. Subsequently, augmentation with the dorsal retinaculum is performed to reinforce the medial ligament (sutured with the previous stitches) (▶ Fig. 29.14, ▶ Fig. 29.15, ▶ Fig. 29.16).

In *Type 2 injuries* the medial ligament and the PH ligament are reconstructed. For the latter reconstruction a volar incision is added and the PH ligament is reconstructed with one-third of the FCU cut proximally and taken and sutured to the unciform apophysis (▶ Fig. 29.17).

29.10 Postoperative

The wrist is immobilized for 4 weeks in a short-arm plaster cast and then supported in a removable wrist splint for another 4 weeks (with intermittent active and passive exercises). At 8 weeks, strengthening exercises are started and at 3 months postoperatively patients are allowed to return to sports.

In cases where the TFCC is also repaired, an above-elbow plaster cast is applied for the first 4 weeks.

29.11 Discussion

PT instability was diagnosed in 35 wrists. Only 40% of the symptomatic PT joints required surgery, the rest did well with conservative treatment.

The results were assessed of the 14 wrists with Type I instabilities operated on the PT joint with a mean follow-up of 2 years and 8 months. Nearly all were young patients with a mean age of 26 years. It is interesting to highlight that all the PT joints that needed surgery occurred in the dominant wrists of the patients and most

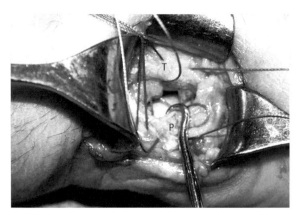

Fig. 29.16 Plicature of the medial pisotriquetral (PT) ligament after local synovectomy.

of them practiced demanding sports or were professional musicians (79%).

The mean time from onset of symptoms to surgery was 10 months. As indicated, all ulnar-side pathologies were treated with the same surgical procedure. Type I instabilities at the PT joint that required surgery were associated to other ulnar-side pathologies in 79% of the cases with a mean of 1.7 (range 1–4) associations per wrist. The second most common association was TH instability in 76% of the cases. Other associations were TFCC lesions (in 36% with PT joint instability and 48% with all ulnar-side cases) and ECU tendon subluxation. The less frequent association of PT instability was LT instability.

It is interesting to note that the percentage of associations is similar to the percentages of reported residual pain after surgery treated as monopathology (▶ Fig. 29.18, ▶ Fig. 29.19).

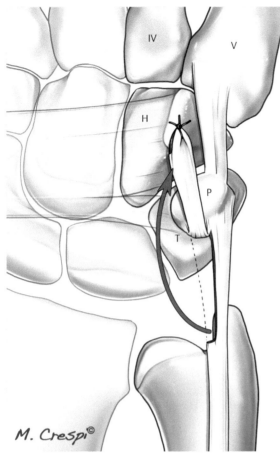

Fig. 29.17 Reconstruction of the pisohamate (PH) ligament with one-third of the flexor carpi ulnaris (FCU).

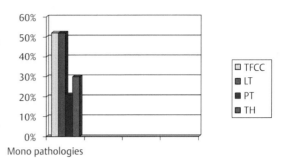

Mono pathologies

Fig. 29.18 Ulnar-side pathologies presented with a diagnosis of unique problem on the ulnar side.

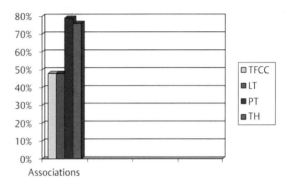

Associations

Fig. 29.19 Ulnar-side pathologies associated with other ulnar-side problems. Pisotriquetral (PT) instability resulted in the most associated pathology on the ulnar side (in 79% of the cases).

With this approach to ulnar-side pathologies, better numbers of pain-free wrists and higher percentages of full return to demanding sports (tennis, golf, polo) and professional music (guitar, violin) were achieved. At a mean follow-up of 2 years and 8 months (range 1–6 y) 86% of patients treated for PT joint instability were completely pain-free, with the remaining having mild pain and mild limitations.

29.12 Conclusion

When not diagnosed and treated, PT instability can be a cause of residual pain in cases operated for other reasons (e.g., triangular ligament). In most of the cases Type I PT instability that requires surgery presents associated to other ulnar-side pathologies (79%). All painful ulnar-side pathologies should be treated with the same surgical procedure in order to reduce residual ulnar pain. This approach results in a higher number of patients returning to demanding sports and professional musical performance.

In order to achieve completeness of the current paradigm on the ulnar side of the wrist, the author believes that the following three aspects should be considered differently: (1) the territory of the ulnar side; (2) biomechanics; and (3) the concept of grades of instability at the PT and the TH joints.

References

[1] Corso SJ, Savoie FH, Geissler WB, Whipple TL, Jiminez W, Jenkins N. Arthroscopic repair of peripheral avulsions of the triangular fibrocartilage complex of the wrist: a multicenter study. Arthroscopy. 1997; 13(1):78–84

[2] Chou KH, Sarris IK, Sotereanos DG. Suture anchor repair of ulnar-sided triangular fibrocartilage complex tears. J Hand Surg [Br]. 2003; 28(6):546–550

[3] García-Elías M. Analysis on lunotriquetral tears. Personal communication.

[4] Zancolli ER, III. Localized medial triquetral-hamate instability: anatomy and operative reconstruction-augmentation. Hand Clin. 2001; 17(1):83–96, vii

[5] Zancolli ER III. The "Iceberg View" on the ulnar side of the wrist: our disagreement and implications. Hand clinics: challenging current

29

wisdom in hand surgery. Philadelphia, PA; London; Toronto: WB Saunders Company; 2022 (in edition)

[6] Braig D, Koulaxouzidis G, Kalash Z, Bürk J, Stark B. Volar dislocation of the triquetrum: case report and review of literature. J Hand Microsurg. 2014; 6(2):87–91

[7] Cohen I. Dislocation of the pisiform. Ann Surg. 1922; 75(2):238–239

[8] Immermann EW. Dislocation of the pisiform. J Bone Joint Surg Am. 1948; 30A(2):489–22

[9] Helal B. Chronic overuse injuries of the piso-triquetral joint in racquet game players. Br J Sports Med. 1978; 12(4):195–198

[10] Rayan GM. Pisiform ligament complex syndrome and pisotriquetral arthrosis. Hand Clin. 2005; 21(4):507–517

[11] Rayan GM, Jameson BH, Chung KW. The pisotriquetral joint: anatomic, biomechanical, and radiographic analysis. J Hand Surg Am. 2005; 30(3):596–602

[12] Orozco J; Rayan G: Pisohamate ligament instability/tear. In: Slutsky DJ, ed. Principles and practice of wrist surgery. Philadelphia, PA: Saunders Elsevier; 2010:Chap. 51:528–537

[13] Navarro A: Luxaciones del Carpo. Anales de Fac de Med Montevideo. Orthop Trans. 1921:113–141

[14] Taleisnik J. The ligaments of the wrist. J Hand Surg Am. 1976; 1(2):110–118

[15] Mayfield JK. Pathogenesis of wrist ligament instability. In: Lichtman DM, ed. The wrist and its disorders. Philadelphia, PA: WB Saunders; 1988:53–73

[16] Bourgery JM, Jacob NA. Traité complet d'anatomie de l'homme. Anatomie descriptive ou phisiologique. H, CA Delanney, Paris. Vol 1. Osteologie et syndesmologie; 1832 Vol 2. Miologie, aponeurologie; 1852

[17] Kane P, VopatBGMansuripurPK, et al. Relative contributions of midcarpal and radiocarpal joints to Dart-Thrower's motion at the wrist. J Hand Surg A. 2018; 43(3):234–240

[18] Kamal RN, Rainbow M, Akelman E, Crisco JJ. In vivo triquetrum-hamate kinematics through a simulated hammering task wrist motion. J Bone Joint Surg. 2012; 94(14):e85

[19] Mouchet A, Belot J. Poignet a'ressaut: Subluxation Mediocarpienne en avant. Bulletin et Memories de la Societé Nationale de Chirurgie. 1934; 60:1243–1244

[20] Lichtman DM, Schneider JR, Swafford AR, Mack GR. Ulnar midcarpal instability-clinical and laboratory analysis. J Hand Surg Am. 1981; 6 (5):515–523

[21] García-Elías M. The non-dissociative clunking wrist: a personal view. J Hand Surg Eur Vol. 2008; 33(6):698–711

[22] Minami M, Yamazaki J, Ishii S. Isolated dislocation of the pisiform: a case report and review of the literature. J Hand Surg Am. 1984; 9A (1):125–127

[23] Carroll RE, Coyle MP, Jr. Dysfunction of the pisotriquetral joint: treatment by excision of the pisiform. J Hand Surg Am. 1985; 10(5):703–707

[24] Rietberg NT, Brown MS, Haase SC. Pisotriquetral pain treated with bilateral pisiform excision in a collegiate diver. J Wrist Surg. 2018; 7 (5):415–418

[25] Zancolli EA. Medial piso-triquetral instability. Kleinert Institute. August 1996:XXV

[26] Zancolli EA. Annual Meeting Argentine Association for Surgery of the Hand. December 1996

[27] Zancolli ER III. Medial piso-triquetral instability. Congress Abstracts 9th Congress IFSSH. Budapest, Hungary. June 2004

[28] Yamaguchi S, Nagao T, Beppu M, Tuda A, Miyoshi K. Pisotriquetral joint—anatomy and movement. J Jpn Soc Surg Hand. 1992; 9:25–28

[29] Pevny T, Rayan GM, Egle D. Ligamentous and tendinous support of the pisiform, anatomic and biomechanical study. J Hand Surg Am. 1995; 20(2):299–304

[30] Zancolli EA. Anatomía Quirúrgica de la Mano. Atlas Ilustrado. Editorial Médica Panamericana. Buenos Aires, Argentina. 2015

[31] Gardner-Thorpe D, Giddins GEB. A reliable technique for radiographic imaging of the pisotriquetral joint. J Hand Surg [Br]. 1999; 24(2):252

[32] Jameson BH, Rayan GM, Acker RE. Radiographic analysis of pisotriquetral joint and pisiform motion. J Hand Surg Am. 2002; 27 (5):863–869

VI

Index

Note: Page numbers set **bold** or *italic* indicate headings or figures, respectively.